INTEGRATED COMMUNITY HEALTHCARE

Next Generation Strategies for
Developing Provider Networks

CHRISTOPHER J. EVANS, CHE
ROBERT L. WILSON, JR.
F. GENE DePORTER, CHE

McGraw-Hill

A Division of The McGraw·Hill Companies

*New York   San Francisco   Washington, D.C.   Auckland   Bogotá
Caracas   Lisbon   London   Madrid   Mexico City   Milan
Montreal   New Delhi   San Juan   Singapore
Sydney   Tokyo   Toronto*

Library of Congress Cataloging-in-Publication Data

Evans, Christopher J.
   Integrated community healthcare : next generation strategies for
developing provider networks / Christopher J. Evans, Robert L.
Wilson, Jr., F. Gene DePorter.
      p. cm.
   Includes bibliographical references and index.
   ISBN 0-7863-1101-0
   1. Hospital-physician joint ventures—United States—
Administration.   2. Integrated delivery of healthcare—United
States.   I. Wilson, Robert L., Jr.   II. DePorter, F. Gene.
III. Title.
   RA410.58.E93   1997
   362.1'068—dc21   97-1484

McGraw-Hill
A Division of The McGraw·Hill Companies

1 2 3 4 5 6 7 8 9 0 DOC / DOC 9 0 9 8 7

ISBN 0–7863–1101–0

This publication is designed to provide accurate and
authoritative information in regard to the subject matter
covered. It is sold with the understanding that neither the
author nor the publisher is engaged in rendering legal, accounting,
or other professional service. If legal advice or other expert
assistance is required, the services of a competent professional
person should be sought.

From a Declaration of Principles jointly adopted by a Committee
of the American Bar Association and a Committee of Publishers.

McGraw-Hill books are available at special quantity discounts to use
as premiums and sales promotions, or for use in corporate training
programs. For more information, please write to the Director of Special
Sales, McGraw-Hill, 11 West 19th Street, New York, NY 10011. Or
contact your local bookstore.

PREFACE

THE BOOK FORMAT

This book is first a reference tool for practicing executives, managers, and counselors as well as a point of departure for contemporary thinking. While providing a brief overview of the IDS issues and historical attempts to deal with building provider networks, we hope to spur readers to think creatively about their current circumstances and future alternatives for positioning their organization. Discussion of provider networks, mostly of physician and hospital networking, is the predominant topic, although we discuss pure physician and pure hospital issues in some cases, most notably in Chapter 6, *Legal Issues in the Formation and Operation of IDS Organizations*. Secondly, the authors present a framework that will support discussion among baccalaureate and masters level students focused on the healthcare industry of the future. This book should become a reference shelf item for experienced administrators and students, guiding them to a deeper understanding of the why and wherefore of organizational initiatives and development, framed by historic activity and legal context.

The text moves quickly from a Chapter 1 focus on some historical perspectives on the growth of managed care to Chapter 2, which profiles some background on IDS development and provider network initiatives researched by Shortell, the authors of this book, and others pertaining to community care development activities. This section provides a more in-depth look at nonhospital/physician community care providers and the role that they can and should play in an IDS. We discuss what may be considered the process for community care network (CCN) development. We also discuss the components of high-quality integrated systems, including issues of vertical and horizontal integration and means for effecting this alignment.

In Chapter 3, *Establishing and Building Value*, we present a detailed look at the premises of value in healthcare organizations as economic entities and as structural subsystems within the industry. We discuss the attributes of economic value in healthcare and examine a considerable amount of traditional business appraisal concepts, as applied to the healthcare industry. Readers should beware this caveat: Do not expect or anticipate that this book will teach you how to appraise healthcare businesses. Business appraisal is a detailed and complicated activity that should be conducted only by trained professionals. Much like one statistics course does not qualify a student as a statistician, this text should give the reader an appreciation of concepts involved in the value estimation process. We also present a model for organizations to think of the strategic value of initiatives. Again, a conceptual approach combining subjective and objective elements that should be formulated in consultation with an experienced healthcare consultant and appraiser. The discussion leaves the reader with the conceptual framework for creating a value system for decision making.

Chapter 4, *Business Acquisitions and Financial Planning,* discusses business acquisitions and transactions including decision concepts for acquisition and partnering, transactional issues such as administrative, management and purchase agreements, and *pro forma* financial planning.

Chapter 5, *Merging Practices, Businesses, and Strategic Business Units,* discusses some of the reasons organizations and groups come together and how expectations affect the decision to pursue a business merger instead of the traditional keep, make, or buy decision. We discuss the philosophical basis for partnering and present the issues for analyzing the need to partner successfully. We believe that successful mergers are best initiated by careful planning and analysis of options for each partner and that mutual dependence be established. The section leads the reader through the do's and don'ts of relationship building and cultural integration as well as describing the operational and functional parameters for completing a successful business merger.

Chapter 6, *Legal Issues in the Formation and Operation of IDS Organizations,* provides a detailed review of the legal and regulatory issues in the formation and operation of the IDS organizations. The focus is on total system needs as they relate to provider network activity. The chapter contents describes current thinking and cases that have challenged and affected regulatory guidance in IDS development. Issues regarding physician activity and hospital activity are presented, recognizing that in many cases they are inextricably intertwined (as in the case of physician-owned hospitals or networks). Discussion of fraud and abuse, antitrust, corporate practice of medicine, tax exemption, physician organization, and special liability issues are presented.

Chapter 7, *The New Frontier*, summarizes the need for building community healthcare provider systems as learning entities and our prescriptions for system organization. We present our beliefs on why successful businesses thrive in the face of rapid change and how healthcare organizations of all sizes can assess their role and relationship in the changing market environment.

SUPPLEMENTARY MATERIAL

This book is more than a how-to book; a number of charts, tables, key step checklists, and spreadsheets are ready to work for many organizations. Many of the materials presented in the text and appendix are included on the accompanying diskette, along with several surprise files. Included in Microsoft Word® 7.0 and Excel® 7.0 for Windows® 95 formats, the items can be imported into many other software packages while retaining all formatting and imbedded commands and formulas.[1] Additional file formats may be available from The Health Service Group Corporate Services Center at (919) 460-7155.

HOW INFORMATION WAS COMPILED

The information in this book was compiled through a variety of means including extensive interviews with healthcare executives, physicians, and managers; literature review; case studies and examples from legal and consulting experience; small discussion groups; and proprietary analysis and assessment of business operations. In rare cases, we have chosen not to attribute a quote or example to an individual to maintain the confidentiality in which the comment was shared.

BRIEF CONTENTS

CONTENTS

Chapter 4

Business Acquisitions and Financial Planning   123

ACKNOWLEDGMENTS

We are deeply indebted to the contributions of many others that led, ultimately, to the production of this text. There are many people whose ideas have shaped our understanding and approach to healthcare organization, policy, delivery, and financing as it will be occurring in the new millennium. To all our colleagues with whom we have had the pleasure of working, this book would not be possible, in part, without you. We would also like to thank a variety of contributors too numerous to list, but who are referenced throughout the text in the reproductions, adaptations of their work, and the literature citations. It is through these individuals, and others, that the field of understanding grows and becomes more than what is; it becomes what is possible. Thanks to our prepublication reviewers for their comments on our text, Thomas C. Ricketts, III (author of *Partners for the Dance: Forming Strategic Alliances in Health Care*), and Ray Miles, CBA, ASA of The Institute of Business Appraisers.

CJE: I would like to thank my wife, Lynne, for her continual support of my work in general, and this project, specifically. Her outlook and uncanny way of maintaining focus never cease to amaze or challenge me. I love you very much. Many thanks to my colleagues Gene DePorter and Tom Stukes of Smith Helms Mulliss & Moore, without whom this project would never have been attempted, and to Bob Wilson without whom it never would have been realized. To Richard Janeway, M.D., Executive Vice President for Health Affairs at Wake Forest University and formerly, Dean of The Bowman Gray School of Medicine, my gratitude for sharing his wisdom on the changing face of healthcare and academic medicine, and for giving his incisive view of long-term forces in healthcare delivery, integration, and financing. To Douglas Cueny, CEO of QualChoice of North Carolina, my thanks for sharing the HMO industry story and solidifying my opinion of the optimum role of health plans in the integrated provider environment. Thanks also to James Roskelly of The Moses Cone Health System for his real world examples and encouragement. Lastly, though most importantly, I recognize the single most overriding influence and strength in my life from which all good things come, Jesus Christ, my Savior. It is only through His guidance, steadfast companionship, and love that I am able to achieve anything in this world.

RLW: I wish to acknowledge the excellent assistance of Jeri L. Kumar, my research assistant and collaborator on this project. Without Jeri's help and long hours, I would not have been able to complete the initial drafts of my portion of this work and practice law for my clients at the same time. I have found that deadlines of whatever nature wait for no one. I also wish to acknowledge my law firm, Maupin Taylor Ellis & Adams, P.A., for providing me with incomparable support during this process. Without the firm's understanding of my commitments, this work could not have been completed. I wish to acknowledge the patience and love that my family have provided over the years of my building my law practice. Alice, Rob, and Katherine have had to put up with more than anyone as I have tried to treat every client and every project as if that client or that project were my first priority. Unfortunately, the practice of law and extracurricular speaking and writing, such as this work, have intruded on what I am sure they expected to be a "normal" family life. I am truly grateful and appreciative beyond words for their steadfast support in everything I have attempted in my professional career. Finally, I wish to acknowledge with grateful appreciation my co-authors, Christopher Evans and Gene DePorter, who recruited me to this effort. Chris and Gene are consummate professionals whose attention to detail and knowledge in their areas of expertise is unsurpassed. My collaboration with them in this work has only enhanced my personal and professional respect for them and their knowledge in this area.

FGD: My thanks go out to all our spouses, Georgette, Alice and Lynne, who have supported us in this project amid the rest of our personal and working lives. I would like to thank my friend and colleague Alex McMahon for his time in review of the manuscript and advice on its completion. Thanks also to Doug Cueny at QualChoice of North Carolina and Dr. Richard Janeway at Bowman Gray/Baptist Hospital Medical Center for their input and review of our work. Finally, I would like to thank my co-authors for their patience and understanding in working on this project. I look forward to the next one with great anticipation.

INTRODUCTION

The healthcare provider industry is trying to maintain and, in some instances regain, control of its own destiny. As an industry, we have not been our own best advocates for a number of years. There have been those on the consumer and payor side of healthcare who have verbalized their concerns about cost, access, quality, and outcome strongly enough to stimulate a trilogy of government responses, namely: Regional Medical Programs, Comprehensive Health Planning, and Health Systems Agencies. The intent of these efforts has been to rationalize healthcare delivery by organizing providers into local and regional network structures. This has been complemented by a Certificate of Need program that is intended to control the amount and location of categories of health provider resources that make their way into the marketplace.

These initiatives have had various levels of success over time but were never able to achieve a collaborative momentum that could produce desired answers. Healthcare providers were viewed as disorganized and the industry was told that it needed to become systematized, integrated, collaborative, and thus efficient, effective, and economical. Healthcare providers generally continued to function on the basis of "whatever the market will bear." For a period of time the outcomes the industry could produce seemed to warrant the increasing costs, and society expected and demanded the highest quality and constant improvement regardless of the cost. The sheer dollar magnitude of the healthcare industry grew to a point where it could no longer be left to its own evolution. The dollar size, resource consumption, and the numbers of people involved have brought control of the industry to center stage. The motivations for control whether different or the same, now have the healthcare industry fending off takeover bids from the federal government, insurance companies, and business.

As these events unfolded over the past 30 years, few stopped to ask the question, Why is 12, 14, or 16% of the GDP for healthcare too much? One line of thought seems to be challenging the appropriateness of the healthcare percentage of the gross domestic product, which questions the return on investment in light of falling morbidity standards and less acceptable outcomes for dollars spent on healthcare. Given the birth rates and life expectancies enjoyed by other developed countries, the U.S. spending levels are hardly justified (given the amounts attributed to patient care versus research and education). For the last 20 years leaders of other large sectors of the economy have suggested that healthcare needed to be treated more as a business and less as an art form. The practitioners of care and the providers of care environments initially fought the concept of healthcare as a business, as a commodity. A growing cadre of individuals, however, began to push an agenda calling for the application of business concepts and the structuring of a systematic approach to delivering healthcare that resolves the issues of access, quality, and cost.

As healthcare began to take on the mantle of "a business," it shifted into high-intensity change. The healthcare industry has for the last 10 years adopted many of the management trends being utilized in other business sectors, with greater and lesser degrees of success. Nonetheless, the healthcare environment has become one of the most dynamic industries in the world and its contemporary managers have come to be viewed at times as champions or masochists of the business world for their ability to adapt to conditions of flux. For the last 10 years there have been a number of consolidations and provider close-outs in selected regions of the country that could be traced back to the influence of factors such as growing a business attitude for healthcare, the strengthening position of managed care programs, and continued pressure from government and business to reduce costs and excess capacity. But still the pace of change was not meeting expectations until one seminal event occurred: the Clinton presidential campaign. Although definitive legislation to change the healthcare industry was defeated, the Clinton administration's concept of managed competition through increased emphasis on managed care growth, within the context of regional integrated delivery systems (IDS), was the equivalent of throwing down the gauntlet. As a result the healthcare industry began to look to the visionaries in its midst and those who had been developing integrated delivery systems, to set the pace of change seldom seen among other industries. Healthcare providers have been remaking themselves rather than have the process legislated. The industry is attempting to control its own destiny and has aggressively moved to build from their experiences in delivering healthcare. The models for integrated system development were no longer the exception to the rule. Rather, they have become the objective for virtually all providers; everyone now thinks in terms of how to be "linked up" rather than be "left out."

The combination of literature profiles and industry examples of the metamorphosis from a nonsystem to an integrated delivery approach have become prolific; the texts, position papers, and articles surround us and will continue to do so for the next 5 to 10 years. Incumbent with this explosive change are the stories of organization winners and losers. In order to continue this accelerated development pace, industry researchers and futurists such as Stephen M. Shortell, Leland Kaiser, J. Daniel Beckham, and others are evaluating why some organizations have chosen particular strategies to assure their growth and survival while others with seemingly similar circumstances have failed. The information that we have access to today reflects what might be called "first generation strategies" for IDSs. However, as this analysis continues, healthcare is beginning to acknowledge that it has only completed two-thirds of a three-phase building process. The industry is moving quickly to link major institutional providers and physicians and now most also add into the recipe a strong community flavor. If one accepts that one of the objectives of an IDS is to improve community health status, then the third leg of the stool representing all other community health and human services providers must be added to the mix.

Organization development and integration have become the *modus operandi* of our changing industry. The roles of hospitals, physicians, and community care providers have and will be affected drastically by continuing changes in public perception, the business as payor impact, and continuing market and financial changes. The industry still has its opponents who are sitting by silently while other critics from government, business, and the insurance industry are suggesting "too much too late." The authors of this book believe that the healthcare industry has made astounding strides toward building the healthcare delivery system of tomorrow. Much remains to be done to strengthen and anchor the first two phases of IDS development (Phase 1—hospital to hospital, physician to physician, and Phase 2—physician to hospital links), while now aggressively building Phase 3—the community care network/community care corporation. The past does not equal the future.

WHAT HEALTHCARE EXECUTIVES MUST DO

Recognizing the need for radical change is only a first step. The second is to take action in a concise, effective and accountable manner. The third step is to see this process of change through to an acceptable end. Healthcare now maintains that it is a market-driven industry and as such it must compete to be a player. As this belief becomes accepted industrywide, healthcare providers must search continually for ways to position themselves to creatively counter future challenges. Much like the evolution from Total Quality Management (TQM) to Continuous Quality Improvement (CQI), so must healthcare providers become learning entities prepared for constant change to improve outcomes and market position. This does not mean that they should spend all of their time in refining existing, outmoded activities; the best method to perform a useless task still makes the task useless.[2] It is the usefulness of the service or process that distinguishes the delivery system of tomorrow. Healthcare executives must accept that organizing hospitals and physicians is not the end of the transition; it is not an integrated delivery system. There is a need for additional infrastructure based upon an accepted vision of where IDSs go after they are built and what third-generation expectations will be that will drive healthcare after cost, access, and quality are non-issues. Former Sony chairman Akio Morita argued that an organization is a community bound together by a common destiny.[3] J. Philip Lathrop provides at least one perspective on the competitive strategies necessary for a viable integrated delivery system in a managed care marketplace.[4] Among his most helpful suggestions include growing markets into smaller areas, strategic segmentation, maintaining simple product line and feature structures, breaking an IDS region into several nearly self-contained healthcare markets, burning your brand into every customer interaction to establish value, continuing to push costs beyond hospitals and physicians to their lowest effective denominator, continuing the information technology transition, and preparing for "service quality" not "clinical quality" as the most common competitive dimension pursued. As an IDS becomes structured and lean, the playing field will level and the true competition will begin.

With a sense of future to direct ourselves, we must accept that there is additional infrastructure to be built.

NOTES

1. Word® 7.0, Excel® 7.0, and Windows® 95 are registered products of Microsoft Corporation. Neither the authors nor McGraw-Hill are affiliated with Microsoft Corporation.
2. See also Oren Harari, "Ten Reasons Why TQM Doesn't Work," *Management Review,* January 1993, pp. 33–38 and Oren Harari, "The Eleventh Reason Why TQM Doesn't Work," *Management Review,* May 1993, pp. 31, 34–36.
3. Quoted in Jeremiah L. Sullivan, "Japanese Management Philosophies: From the Vacuous to the Brilliant," *California Management Review 34,* Winter (1992), no. 2, pp. 66–87.
4. J. Philip Lathrop, "Competitive Strategies for the Next Generation of Managed Care," *Healthcare Forum Journal,* March–April 1996, pp. 36–38, 52–55.

I

THE ROOTS OF
HEALTHCARE DELIVERY

1

DELIVERY OF HEALTHCARE IN A CHANGING ENVIRONMENT

THE CHANGING ENVIRONMENT

To virtually any observer the healthcare environment is changing rapidly. The most talented physicians, hospital administrators, and insurers cannot predict the level of payments or services that a given population of people may require. While this will always be a static concept, how to model the change, and even defining the appropriateness of change remains an issue. This argument alone has thrown the U. S. healthcare system into such turmoil that every participant from provider to patient feels its influence. These outcomes were inevitable given the financing and delivery system that grew out of the immediate post-Medicare era, from 1966 to the present. The shift from hospital and inpatient focus to covered life and outpatient focus are understood by all, yet making the change has proved to be a difficult one. Since everyone involved in the healthcare industry is aware of these fundamental occurrences, by their observation of changing patterns of care delivery and financing models, this chapter will focus broadly on the evolutionary changes in the U. S. healthcare system from approximately 1980 to

1996. The remainder of this text will address recent developments and strategies for moving organizations beyond their current level.

Healthcare Delivery and Financing

Major reorganization was necessary in the established healthcare delivery system. The traditional fee-for-service system was generating incentives driving the overall cost of care so high that the federal government was forced to overhaul financing for the Medicare program. Beyond the move to diagnosis-related groups, which was difficult enough, changes needed to be made on the physician and ancillary services components of healthcare spending driven higher and higher by a system rewarding the provision of services, not the outcomes of care processes. Recognizing that the vast majority of healthcare spending is physician directed, incentives to overutilize services needed to be eliminated, at least for Medicare beneficiaries. The earliest attempts in fee reduction for Medicare physician fee schedules caused many physicians to close their practices to new Medicare patients while reduction in hospital reimbursement increased its growing emphasis in cost accounting, utilization review, and quality assurance, the original causes of system change.

While changes in Medicare, and in many cases, Medicaid financing were occurring, employers and insurance companies were growing concerned with increasing volume of medical claims. The finest healthcare system in the world had created access to higher and higher intensity of care while it yet had an open checkbook. Adding to that was the expectation of its public to believe that access to and provision of healthcare services was a "right" of U.S. citizens, what followed was a system of increasing use and cost that would be difficult to slow down, never mind stop altogether. This fundamental shift in public opinion from healthcare as a privilege to a basic right occurred during the mid- to late 1980s as HMOs and the roles of physician extenders reached broader acceptance. While the adoption and growth of the early HMOs were not a causative factor, it augmented a growing social conscience regarding a society caring for its people. Legislators accepted the condition that the government had a responsibility for the health of its people. Access to health services increased while hospital emergency rooms became busier and busier with the uninsured using them for emergent and nonemergent primary care, a trend that continues in all metropolitan areas. Arguments that millions did not have access to the healthcare system were countered that in reality, these millions of medically indigent had the nation's emergency rooms as their primary care offices. But this came at an extreme expense and without any focus on prevention. One unidentified hospital administrator shared his feelings:

> Over the last two years we have had the same individual show up in our ER four times with gunshot wounds and no insurance. Each time he required hospitalization for 4 to 6 days. How do you deal with that?

An answer came from the crowd: "a better shot." Stories like this are yet another example of the stresses placed on the nation's trauma centers. The growing use of specialty physicians and the open checkbook mentality directed more types of patient care to specialists which today, are considered vital services for many primary care physicians. Primary care physicians became accustomed to referring out far too many routine cases, opting to handle only the bread and butter of limited services.

The desire of payors to shift risk to providers began as a turning point when insurance companies began increasing healthcare premiums to employer groups, who in turn, passed some of the increase on to their employees. The initial backlash spawned the development of Preferred Provider Organizations (PPOs) or panels of physicians who, under more restrictive health plans, were the sole providers of care for plan enrollees. Most PPO plans had out-of-network options but it marked the beginning of the restriction of patient choice in favor of controlling employer healthcare expenditures. Employers were not satisfied with the relatively minor cost savings in the face of ever-increasing premiums. Insurance companies continued to control the risk, which is where all the money is in healthcare. Reluctant to give up control, insurance companies increased premiums, and patient utilization of services continued to rise, magnifying employer exposure.

The emergence of employer coalitions seeking to leverage their joint buying power to cover costs and the actions of large self-funded employers began the era of direct contracting, initially with hospital inpatient and ancillary services, then with outpatient physician services. The predominant method was a discount off the standard fee schedule with wide variations based on local market conditions including volume and overall fee rates. On the hospital side, contracting moved to negotiated per diem rates or per case rates similar to DRG-based reimbursement. On the physician side, discounted FFS remained the method of choice.

Employers continued their demand on healthcare providers as the concepts of Total Quality Management (TQM), and subsequently, Continuous Quality Improvement (CQI) became popular in the 1980s. Employers began influencing the actual provision of certain healthcare services through strict utilization review and hospital admission precertifications. Employers demanded access to their network or participating physicians so patients would be able to see them as needed and they began insisting on quality improvement and outcomes measurement to document the scope, amount, appropriateness, and quality of treatment. In effect, employers began demanding accountability from physicians and made it clear that they would seek other providers if they were not satisfied. The extent to which the payors exerted control over providers was based largely on the options available in each market.

Fee structure changes in the form of withholds from physician fees became more prevalent in certain types of health plans. Payors exacted more and more from physicians under the fee-for-service system by making them more responsible for patient utilization of services. Abuse in the form of restriction of healthcare services to patients developed as some physicians sought to maximize the revenue potential from payor plans while desperately holding onto what indemnity insurance remained in their practice. Concurrently, capitated physician contracts emerged, which sought to place the physician, generally primary care physicians, at risk for either all healthcare expenses incurred by the enrolled patient, or for all of the physician component of care. While these changes spread throughout the U. S. gradually, certain markets developed more rapidly than others, most notably the major metropolitan areas of Albuquerque, San Diego, Los Angeles, San Francisco, and Minneapolis. It should be noted that the spread of payor payment models is yet under way; many parts of the U. S. are not yet capitated, although it is expected that virtually all markets will have some degree of capitated reimbursement by the end of 1998 (see Exhibit 1–1).

EXHIBIT 1–1

Stages and Evolution of Managed Care

Stage 1 Unstructured	Stage 2 Loose Organization	Stage 3 Consolidation	Stage 4 Managed Competition	Stage 5 Final Stages
◆ FFS	◆ Loose FFS	◆ Limited FFS	◆ Market Definition	◆ Regionally Defined Markets and Payors
◆ PPOs	◆ PPO Plans	◆ Restricted PPO Panels	◆ Compression	◆ Markedly Fewer Providers
◆ HMOs	◆ Medium Discounting	◆ Capitation	◆ Risk Contracting	◆ High-Risk Contracting
◆ IPAs	◆ Affiliations	◆ POS Plans		◆ Low Margins
◆ Minor Discounting	◆ PHOs	◆ Heavy Discounting		
	◆ MSOs	◆ Hospital and Physician Network Formation		

Changes on the Horizon

The concept of managing care is not new. In 1697 Daniel Defoe suggested that the concept of life insurance be applied to healthcare; in 1714 John Bellers suggested a detailed plan for a national health service in England. In 1754 in France, de Chamousset proposed a plan for hospital insurance. Although these early thinkers were more concerned about improving social conditions and the public's health in general, their counterparts some 250 years later began to realize the enormous cost of caring for specific, identified populations of people.

Insurance companies expecting huge profits on healthcare premiums and employers expecting reasonable payments for healthcare insurance began to see profits dwindling and expenses increasing rapidly. The insurgence of HMOs in the 1970s flourished with the passage of Nixon's HMO Act of 1974 as well as the growth of the Kaiser model and Permanente Medical Group (from the 1960s). This spawned other staff model HMOs around the country. The parallel development of PPO panels by insurance companies began to raise the issue of patient choice for the first time. The 1980s grew as both a decade of expanding incomes for physicians and hospitals and increasing concern of employers paying the lion's share of the expenses of their health plan enrollees. Beginning in the western U. S. and selected areas of the Midwest, most notably Minneapolis/St. Paul, employers began seeking more and more aggressive means to control healthcare expenditures. Contracting models arose which placed increasing levels of risk and co-payments on the shoulders of patients and physicians. Toward the end of the decade, employers had clearly established their desire to move towards provider measurements of quality of care, though this desire was, for most plans, secondary to price. Warnings began to come from Capitol Hill that the Medicare Trust Fund was on the road to bankruptcy somewhere between the years 2002 and 2005. The concept of managed competition was espoused as a market-based response to the healthcare financing crisis. The blue ribbon commission headed by First Lady Hillary Clinton developed a plan of national health reform in isolation of the industry, which allowed political forces the opportunity to attack. The plan was probably never seen as the antidote to the nation's woes, but that the discussion of the next stage of healthcare financing had begun.

At the same time, discussion began among the more progressive organizations including the American Hospital Association, the American Medical Association, and the American College of Healthcare Executives about the need to focus on the health status of a community, or at least a defined population of people (enrollees?). With the mission of securing the public's health and ending the scourge of the un- and underinsured, a.k.a. the medically indigent, political forces began guiding the healthcare system's collective moral conscience toward the need to take responsibility for the health status of its enrollees. Hospitals with and without capitation experience envisioned the quality report card from hell as they began discussions of how to sustain healthy behaviors in their future enrolled populations. As federal health reform fervor died down, so did the urgency to transform a given population's health overnight. While one goal of healthy integrated systems must include the imperative to educate and modify the health behaviors of those for whom they are responsible, current levels of contracting for groups of covered lives are creating this impact in few markets, if any.

KEY PLAYERS: HOSPITALS, PHYSICIANS, COMMUNITY CARE PROVIDERS, THE BUSINESS COMMUNITY, AND INSURERS

The healthcare industry is evolving and the survivors of this transition will need to be lean, flexible, and responsive. Technological changes, new drug therapies, the provision of patient services, information systems, financing, and delivery mechanisms all comprise key elements of the new order of business. The current state of the art in healthcare integration spans the continuum of like organizations linking together to form a horizontally integrated system that is further linked vertically through the corporate and contractual relationships with other community-based providers. A review of the healthcare literature reveals a consistent trend: The integration of *hospitals, physicians, community care providers, the business community*, and *healthcare insurers* are the five key elements of the healthcare provider complement. This is evidenced by increasing developments in telemedicine, the proliferation of home health agencies and services, increased responsibility and funding of public/county health departments (for research and patient care activities), and community health information networks (CHINs).

The roles and relationships between hospitals, physicians, and other community providers continue to expand as their historic activities have moved beyond their traditional roles. Increasingly these entities are exploring how they fit together and the operating efficiencies they can produce as an integrated system. The roles played by home health agencies, long-term care facilities, public health departments, physical, occupational, and other rehabilitation therapists, and other direct care providers will help shape the future integrated healthcare environment.

The interactions of market changes brought about by managed care and the new system players including health maintenance organizations, third-party payors, preferred provider organizations, integrated delivery systems and networks, physician-hospital organizations, physician organizations, independent practice associations, management services organizations, foundations, and the developing community care corporations further affect system changes. Companies are rapidly recognizing that they must consolidate in order to survive. This is especially true in the areas of postacute care: subacute care, long-term care, home healthcare, and rehabilitation services.

The structure and system goals of these entities vary considerably. Many of these entities previously operated either in a discrete healthcare delivery capacity or in a financing role. With the
advent of managed care, institutional providers (e.g., hospitals)
began taking control of larger aspects of the healthcare delivery
component, most notably ambulatory and posthospital (home) care.
The proliferation of durable medical equipment companies as subsidiary, nonhospital operating units created significant contribution
to margin for hospital investors. Private physicians developed
imaging centers, surgical centers, dialysis centers, and reference
laboratories as their contribution. The marriage of insurance risk
took HMOs into the provider/payor arena and PPOs tied physician
groups to employers (and vice versa).

Increasing emphasis on cost control (and outright seizure of
the healthcare delivery system) by employers is ever-increasing. On
the financing end, large employer groups are moving rapidly beyond demands for fixing cost increases, strict utilization review,
and coinsurance sharing in favor of capitated payments, which
allow them to project more accurately their costs and benefit structure. On the delivery end, employers have moved beyond provider
recruitment to actual acquisition and operation of medical practices
as a means of controlling self-insuring ambulatory medical care
costs.

The trends in integration are clear; one needs only to read any
issue of *Modern Healthcare* to see plans on merging, acquiring,
partnering, or dissolving in order to grow into a sustaining player
in healthcare. We see hospitals, insurers, and integrated delivery
systems/networks (IDS/IDN) continually buying, building, or
expanding nursing homes, rehabilitation hospitals and facilities,
clinical laboratories, pharmacies, psychiatric hospitals, ambulatory
centers, and many other kinds of subacute care and geriatric care.
Activity was brisk in healthcare mergers and acquisitions in 1994
and 1995, with over 500 mergers and acquisitions each year as
reported by Irving Levin Associates, Inc.[1,2] A total of 504 business
combinations were announced in 1994, and 623 in 1995, up 20.3%.
Hospital deals dominated the markets followed closely by rehabilitation centers, home health, and long-term care. Market trends
identified included continued acquisition of hospitals and other
provider entities, and acquisition of medical groups. Nonprofits

entered the arena tending to use mergers as a vehicle to reduce the number of operating beds, a requirement in time of decreasing utilization of inpatient services. Antitrust concerns continue in industry consolidation. In North Carolina, a landmark decision allowed Memorial Mission Medical Center and St. Joseph's Hospital, the only two hospitals in Asheville, to gain a certificate of public advantage (COPA) from the state to avoid near certain federal antitrust activity. Since that decision, COPAs have been approved in Montana and are being sought as one means to achieve procompetitive benefits without the scrutiny of a Federal Trade Commission/Department of Justice antitrust review.

Market reforms have driven responses from all elements of the healthcare system. Many of these strategies have had varying levels of success and some have worked extremely well in some markets and not at all in others. Some have clearly been transitional; rapid change is not often accepted by many parties and incremental, subsequential, or no change has proven to be no better. Hospitals and physicians are likely to classify much of the difficulty in dealing with market reform with the following issues:

+ Fraud and abuse prohibitions
+ Corporate practice of medicine
+ Safe harbors
+ Tort law reform
+ Price fixing
+ Tax exemption status
+ Patient referral prohibitions
+ Malpractice litigation
+ Monopoly/market power
+ External review/second guessing of clinical practice decisions

Success in the new order of business will depend on how well entities align partner incentives. The initial wave of individual provider network development, as we see it currently, began with HMO and PPO groupings of physician providers. This remained the status quo until hospitals progressed into medical care financing and acceptance of risk through partnerships or development of health insurance plans. Hospitals began acquiring medical practices in order to create a sufficient base of providers to compete to handle the needs of large enrolled populations. The acquisition and integration of other healthcare businesses have been slower than medical practices. Many hospitals have expanded into providing durable medical equipment, outpatient pharmaceuticals and medical supplies, ambulatory therapies and home health services including physical and occupational therapy, home health nursing, infusion, chemotherapy, nutrition, and hydration therapy. Traditionally, hospitals have expanded in-house services to the marketplace; however, in markets with established private services, hospitals are beginning to acquire businesses to complete the array of services and further their vertical integration. We see that several notable outcomes have arisen from these early integration activities.

The historical outcomes of these early and ongoing integration activities have yielded, at best, mixed results. Any hospital or managed care organization (MCO) that has purchased a medical practice or that employs physicians understands the issues in maintaining provider productivity. The earliest indicators of rapidly decreasing physician production have not yet convinced all buyers of medical practices and other healthcare provider businesses to require productivity benchmarks in compensation plans. Anecdotal information suggests that over 95% of all hospitals who have purchased medical practices have lost money *on practice operations alone.* Complicating matters further is the increasing effect of capitation on physician compensation and productivity. In more advanced managed care markets with significant amounts of capitation, traditional methods of maintaining productivity are not appropriate. Creating physician incentives to maintain costs and quality, while striving to make productivity targets, sends mixed messages if targets are not attainable. Some medical groups have been able to work out incentive programs, although most acknowledge that these models must change to keep pace with the market.

The following sections discuss some of the early stages of market-driven changes or responses and some of the outcomes experienced by these groups.

Hospital-Hospital Relationships

Hospitals responded to the changing patterns in healthcare financing and delivery through focusing on the reduction of operating expenses. In the early stages of increasing fee discounts, hospitals began seeking discounts from suppliers and expanding product lines beyond hospital services. Durable medical equipment and pharmacy services were the most prevalent diversification strategies to bring nonoperating sources of revenue into the hospital setting. Hospitals solicited their hospital neighbors, national and state hospital associations, and began forming purchasing alliances to maximize economies of scale and share ideas for cost containment and revenue enhancement. Many supply purchasing networks diversified to serve their constituent hospital members in areas like hospital consulting, strategic planning, quality assurance, and hospital equipment lease, purchase, and refurbishment. These alliances, such as SunHealth and Voluntary Hospitals of America, moved rapidly into providing or coordinating quality management initiatives like TQM, CQI, clinical pathways, and physician integration/medical staff services demanded by hospital members.

Alliances began developing between hospitals, most often neighboring facilities of differing complexity such as a suburban or rural primary care hospital and a tertiary facility. These affiliations came to mean any of a number of things, most varying so widely as to make the term *affiliation* meaningless for all but marketing purposes. Some affiliations meant that hospital administrators formally agreed to meet on a regular basis to identify areas of potential sharing of information. Other affiliations identified specific activities, a plan of action to be pursued. Affiliations were developing most rapidly in areas consistent with managed care penetration. Hospitals with foresight sought to partner based on specific parameters that included typically quality referral relationships, a win-win philosophy for both institutions, a perception of benefit, noncompetitive clinical services, and regular forums or dialogue on the strength of the relationship (see Exhibit 1–2).

Hospital management relationships continued to flourish as organizations like SunHealth, Quorum, Hospital Corporation of America, HealthTrust, Brim, and others provided contract management services to predominantly small and mid-sized rural and suburban hospitals. Acquisition of community hospitals by investor-owned entities and continued growth of managed care expanded hospital management activities, and many large and medium-sized hospitals began experimenting with managing hospitals in their referral areas. Hospitals quickly learned that effectively managing

EXHIBIT 1–2

Hospital–Hospital Relationships
Traditional Hub-Spoke Alignment

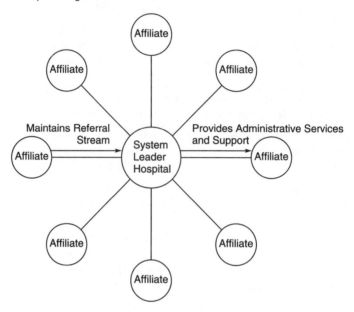

a satellite facility took considerable effort and, in many cases, required more attention than initially presumed. Many satellite facilities could be made to break even on paper, but only after considerable personnel expense from the parent organization. As a result, many local hospitals as well as regional and national management companies scaled back operations such that by 1995 only a handful of national hospital management firms existed.

Hospitals began developing a vertically integrated profile to be competitive in winning managed care and direct contracts. Organizations needed to control the inpatient and outpatient chain of custody of the patient in order to exact the most control over operating expenses. This concept is still generally true. Early stages of vertical integration led hospitals to develop or acquire nursing homes, outpatient surgical centers, and home healthcare as the first steps. True vertical integration, supporting the payors' desire to

EXHIBIT 1–3

Vertical and Horizontal Integration

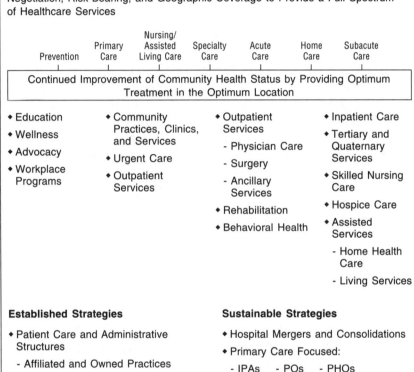

Physician and Organizational Linkages That Allow Centralized Contracting, Negotiation, Risk Bearing, and Geographic Coverage to Provide a Full Spectrum of Healthcare Services

| Prevention | Primary Care | Nursing/ Assisted Living Care | Specialty Care | Acute Care | Home Care | Subacute Care |

Continued Improvement of Community Health Status by Providing Optimum Treatment in the Optimum Location

◆ Education	◆ Community Practices, Clinics, and Services	◆ Outpatient Services	◆ Inpatient Care
◆ Wellness		- Physician Care	◆ Tertiary and Quaternary Services
◆ Advocacy	◆ Urgent Care	- Surgery	
◆ Workplace Programs	◆ Outpatient Services	- Ancillary Services	◆ Skilled Nursing Care
		◆ Rehabilitation	◆ Hospice Care
		◆ Behavioral Health	◆ Assisted Services
			- Home Health Care
			- Living Services

Established Strategies

◆ Patient Care and Administrative Structures

- Affiliated and Owned Practices
- IPA   - MSO   - PHO   - PO
- Foundations
- Joint Ventures
- Physician Equity Models
- Integrated Provider Network

Sustainable Strategies

◆ Hospital Mergers and Consolidations

◆ Primary Care Focused:

- IPAs   - POs   - PHOs
- Group Practices

◆ Physician-Driven Delivery Systems

contract with one party for a broad continuum of care over a defined geographic area, required the addition of medical group services as well as the remaining components of patient care services (see Exhibit 1–3).

Physician-Physician Relationships

As a tradition, hospital medical staffs united on common causes in order to better their fare from the local hospital. What was always a tenuous relationship, that of the physicians controlling much of the destiny of the hospital, physician groups attempted to leverage hospital management into providing them with a better working environment. Access to technology, appearance and conditions of the facilities, quality of the nursing and support staff, better parking, ER operations, and so on, were the areas commonly addressed. The early days of managed care began a trend of physicians beginning to talk to one another about the payor demands being requested of them and of the hospital facility. The outgrowth of Independent Practice (or physician) Associations (IPAs) created a forum for discussion among physicians. Membership was often based upon the reason for developing the IPA. In more forward-thinking communities, physicians banded together as a basis for launching their own health plans, or to partner on an equity basis to form a plan. Specialists participated in these types of IPAs most frequently, for they were the physicians with discretionary income for investment. Few primary care physicians were involved, sometimes because of the specialist perception of themselves as the upper echelon of the medical community, other times based solely on investment criteria.

IPAs, like many other healthcare organizational structures, varied considerably by form, composition, function, administration, goals, and outcomes (see Exhibit 1–4). Most IPAs did not have long life spans due principally to the lack of vision of their organizers, inability to quantify and qualify the goals of the group, inadequate capitalization, and competent and appropriate leadership. Successful IPAs garnered support from the majority of the medical community (or major constituency of physicians in the same IPA market) and expanded their interests into tracking and becoming involved directly in managed care activities. IPAs bargained for and negotiated direct employer and managed care contracts for member physicians taking a small percentage for administration and functioned as technical assistance (ad hoc consulting) to medical groups for existing payor relationships. They developed strong market presence in many markets and became tough competitors for solo practitioners and smaller medical practices. For the first time, nonparticipating physicians were seeing existing patients leave their practice. Numerous examples of medical groups losing 20% of their patients through the loss of one contract were appearing across the country. It marked the first time physicians were at risk for being locked out of the market for new managed care contracts because the IPA networks were controlling the market. From an antitrust perspective, there was still plenty of Medicare and Medicaid business to be had; losing physicians began eating less and getting hungrier. The multiyear phase-in of HCFA's Resource-Based Relative Value Scale (RBRVS) was not the windfall that primary care physicians were led to expect; however, it had a major impact on certain specialty fee schedules. Ophthalmology fees for cataract extraction plummeted about 65% from $3,600 to approximately $800. These changes further impacted the earning profile and value of all specialties.

Physician organizations continued to evolve as managed care increased. In some markets, primary care networks formed to represent the interests of the previously less desirable primary care physicians who now were becoming in demand from managed care organizations. These gatekeepers held significant potential to help

EXHIBIT 1–4

Independent Physician Association

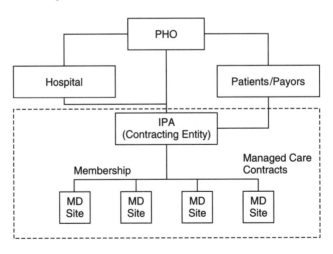

curb the rising cost of healthcare and could actually influence the decision to seek expensive specialty care. More than that, payors and employers found that they could dictate, by contract, that certain criteria be met before a variety of healthcare services could be provided. Physician organizations negotiated terms and conditions as best they could but the payor began controlling more and more of the type of care that would be reimbursed by the plan.

Employer-and-Payor Relationships

Insurance companies found they could be more ruthless in requiring second opinions and precertifications for admission, limiting the amount of a particular service for a given condition, or paying only based on DRGs or an established trim point by condition. Regional payors sought to contract regionally with hospitals, physician organizations (where they existed) and later, systems of care for primary, secondary, tertiary, and quaternary services. It was not unusual to "carve out" specific services such as long-term care, behavioral health, pharmacy, or home health services, nor was it unusual to carve out subspecialty services such as cardiothoracic and neurosurgery, oncology, or radiation therapy, even when such services may be available at a given location (later on, with the assumption of global risk, carve-outs became necessary to obtain the most cost effective arrangement for care). The healthcare rate wars were beginning. Discounting off published room rates and physician standard fee schedules were sought at 15%–25% off market prices. In some cases hospitals and physicians simply refused and the payor capitulated. Most often some discount was given in consideration of volume of patients. In some markets, payors sought other providers and massive shifts occurred crippling hospitals and physicians at the same time. Toward the early to mid-1990s, many geographically dependent hospitals were forced to close due to the shift in patient contracts and drastically changing reimbursement patterns.

Capitation emerged as the model of choice during the late 1980s and became well established in the 1990s. The idea of laying off the risk for excessive services became attractive to payors who already understood the actuarial relationship between risk and the premium dollar. Early capitated contracts with medical groups and hospitals were based on extremely limited information about the fixed and variable costs of each organization to produce its services and the utilization rates of the contracted patients. Few organizations had the skill or data to make reasonable decisions on early capitated agreements. For one, the incentives for providing medical care under a capitated system of payment were completely reversed from a FFS system (see Exhibit 1–5). The shift was from a revenue mentality under the FFS system to a cost mentality when operating under the assumption of risk (see also Chapter 2). Secondly, physicians underestimated their own productivity and spent either far too much time with patients that they lost time for other revenue generating activity, or they began denying care as a means of reducing the amount of their time spent. Under a completely prepaid plan, the best patient for a physician is one that is never seen and has a massive heart attack at age 65. The potential for abuse was certain and employers were slow to respond to their employees' concerns of the management of the new health plans and the conditions the plans were placing on their enrollees.

EXHIBIT 1–5

Capitation vs. Fee for Service
Relationship Between Income Streams Under Fee for Service and Capitation

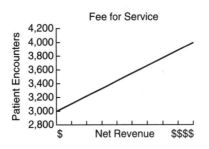

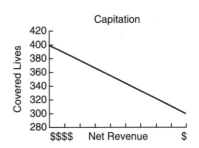

Revenue Increases with Number of Encounters

Gross Revenue Increases by Number of Covered Lives
Net Revenue Decreases by Number of Encounters

Reversal of Incentives under Capitation
◆ Reward for efficient use of resources
- Fewer patient contacts
- Fewer referrals to specialists
- Less intensive care
- Fewer admissions/shorter LOS

Shifting of Focus of Control
◆ Primary care directed
◆ Outpatient focused
◆ Prevention and wellness orientation
◆ Contract-based planning
◆ Decreased recidivism

Through aggressive direct contracting, large employers teamed up with third-party administrators and indemnity insurers to examine new ways to contain costs. Physicians in many markets found that patient loyalty was only skin deep. Anecdotal information suggests that patients will change their physician for as little as a $5 copay per visit. To combine this fact with the provider networks that were developing, the changes effected on the physician side were monumental. On the hospital side, fewer and fewer patients were directed to the facility based on referrals from physicians; they were directed to hospitals who were participating in their health plan. Several national organizations including Delta Airlines sought to establish national contracts for subspecialty care such as cardiac surgery and oncology treatment.

Looking a bit forward, futurist Jeff Goldsmith foresees an interesting concept of "virtual integration" that works like a system, but without the bricks and mortar base. Key components include an operating system of agreements and protocols for managing patients and a framework of incentives that governs how physicians and hospitals are paid. The principal assets of the system are information systems and capital to construct network relationships, HMO licenses, physician organizations, and managed care software.[3] This virtual integration is cited as an example in City of Hope's national cancer network, which, in late 1995 commanded contracts for one million lives through carve-outs and center of excellence agreements with insurers across the country. Despite the attractiveness of a non-asset-based system, Jack Bernard, vice president of American Health Systems, indicates, "Loose affiliations of hospitals in managed care networks are transitional models. The future is systems with directly controlled groups of hospitals and physicians with shared control."[4] As we will see in later chapters, somewhere in between will lie the most effective way of maintaining control of costs and destiny.

THE STAGE IS SET

When one views the long-term evolution of the U.S. healthcare system, it is clear that institutional providers (e.g., hospitals, long-term care centers) are continuing to become aligned with individual providers of care, which, beyond physicians, include mid-level

providers such as physician assistants, nurse practitioners, chiropractors, physical, occupational, speech and language therapists,
counselors, technicians, and other health-related practitioners (mas-
sage therapy, holistic health, etc.). Many analysts believe that third-
party reimbursement for some of these mid-level providers is about
to explode, as insurers and employers seek ways of reducing
healthcare expenditures.

We should be reminded of the words of Michael K. Jhin,
president and CEO of St. Luke's Episcopal Hospital in Houston:

> Consumers and payors want both low cost and accessibility. When
> cost and convenience have been satisfied, then consumers will
> demand quality. Simply stated, they will ultimately seek value. A
> major transformation of the industry is inevitable. We must expand
> our product beyond ill care to include well care, and we must retool
> our care processes for greater efficiency and effectiveness. We are
> challenged not only to bring costs in line, but also to rethink how
> healthcare should be organized and delivered. Effecting this trans-
> formation will define the quality of our stewardship in this new
> frontier. As stewards, healthcare leaders have a societal responsibil-
> ity to manage change for community benefit, specifically the en-
> hancement of health status. Good intentions are not enough. True
> stewardship means we have the responsibility not just for today, but
> also for tomorrow. We must ensure that the resources will be safe-
> guarded to meet the needs of generations to come.[5]

NOTES

1. Eleanor B. Meredith and Sanford B. Steever, "Mergers and
   Acquisitions: What's Going On?" *Healthcare Financial Management
   Association Resource Guide* (Westchester, IL, 1995)
2. Sandy Lutz, "Study Documents Brisk Merger-Acquisition Pace,"
   Modern Healthcare, Feb. 26, 1996, p. 2.
3. Jeff C. Goldsmith, "The Illusive Logic of Integration," *Healthcare
   Forum Journal*, Sept./Oct. 1994, pp. 26–31.
4. Jay Greene, "Alliances Have a New Strategy," *Modern Healthcare*,
   July 10, 1995, p. 48.
5. Michael K. Jhin, "Healthcare Is a Business, Even for Not-for-
   Profits," *Modern Healthcare*, July 22, 1996, p. 28.

PART

II

INTEGRATED COMMUNITY HEALTHCARE

2

CREATING INTEGRATED DELIVERY SYSTEMS

In the developed world, we entrust our safekeeping to complex systems so intangible that most of us cannot begin to comprehend them—air traffic control, electronic banking, managed healthcare, commodities markets, the Federal Reserve. Even if we can master one of them, the others inevitably elude our understanding and control. . . Survival forces a mastery of numerous practical details. Survival is an act of dependence. Although we celebrate individual strength, it is symbiosis at which our species most excels. We are, after all, colony creatures at heart, and inside every cell of our bodies we carry the ancestral signature of cooperative arrangements.[1]

Robert Lee Hotz

WHY AN INTEGRATED DELIVERY SYSTEM?

Transition in the healthcare marketplace is occurring so rapidly that many healthcare providers are simply reacting to pressure to do something that seems to be consistent with the majority direction. This reaction is not necessarily inappropriate, but in the process of rapid response many participants are losing sight of the reasons for moving toward establishing integrated delivery systems. In addition, the building blocks that are being chosen for the foundation of an integrated system often need to be manufactured themselves. Today we are taking healthcare off the foundation that has supported it since the 1940s and supporting it on temporary structures until we can construct a new foundation.

Why does healthcare delivery in the United States need a new foundation? The answer for many appears to rest with the complexity of today's healthcare industry that can be tied to its lock-step functionalism, specialization, and individualism that have made healthcare cost, quality, and access ineffective. At the same time the U. S. healthcare industry continues to be sought out by people around the world who want the best and are able to pay for it. It is important to establish at this point that there is more that is good about our healthcare system than not. However, money, cost, and value for the dollar invested are some of the basic elements that create market-driven expectations. As an industry, healthcare had lost touch with these realities. In part this is because traditional indemnity insurance shielded many consumers from the true cost of healthcare. The costs of healthcare have become so burdensome that end users have been asked for the last 10 years to assume more of the cost burden themselves. This pass-through of cost sharing from employers to employees, from the government to beneficiaries, has become a growing source of irritation between the healthcare industry and the public. Healthcare needs to get back into sync with the market (market is defined here as the purchasers of goods and services). Healthcare has been so insular that it has established an inbred complexity that frustrates everyone inside and outside its structure. There have been pockets of visionary change that go back a number of years, but overall the industry is in need of a significant rebuilding of its foundation and infrastructure.

Business has applied a significant number of techniques to improve its performance, bottom line, and responsiveness to its share holds. They have improved their operating systems and use of their most important asset—their employees. Adoption of the quality programs of Deming, Juran, and Crosby, Total Quality Management (TQM), Market-Driven Management, Strategic Alliances, and Reengineering have become the order of the day for business. As business and industry began to see the benefits of these initiatives they turned to those outside their organization from whom they buy products and services that were significantly impacting their costs and basically demanded that these suppliers become more efficient in their operations or other sources of service and products would be found that could meet their requirements. In like manner, business and industry focused on healthcare and began to ask for the same type of response and in concert with their insurance carriers, began to create leverage situations in those communities that have multiple providers by finding those hospitals and physicians who would work with the employer/insurer to reduce costs.

The pressures that business was feeling to be competitive worldwide and national concerns with the increasing costs of healthcare all came to a boiling point with the proposed Clinton health plan. The plan (though never enacted) became the launching pad for accelerated change on the part of healthcare providers. Healthcare turned to the experience of other business sectors to benchmark best practices that could expedite the rapid learning curve that would support quick and effective reconstruction of the foundations of the healthcare industry. Healthcare has gone back to basics. In this process of comparison, the industry quickly adopted the techniques of Continuous Quality Improvement (CQI), TQM, and Process Improvement, as drawn from the teachings and consulting work of Juran, Deming, and Crosby. These techniques have in turn been linked to the concepts of "value chains" and horizontal and vertical integration, as described by Michael Porter in his books *Competitive Advantage*[2] and *The Competitive Advantage of Nations*.[3]

Porter establishes a basis for integrated delivery systems by laying out an approach that begins with a *value chain analysis*. Simply stated, this approach breaks an organization into its strategically relevant activities and evaluates each activity for its cost behavior, the potential for creating differentiation, and how these activities are interdependent or linked. The linkages represent cost and performance relationships between activities that can be optimized and coordinated to produce cost and operating efficiencies that in turn can establish a competitive edge for an organization or group of linked organizations. According to Porter, these linkages develop from a number of causes such as similar functions being performed across a number of activities or services, cost and performance improvement in direct service due to coordination and optimizing of indirect support services, improvement in the organization, delivery of service that reduces the need for repeat service, and establishment of quality assurance at the front end of service development to produce enhanced outcomes at the back end.

The reader should be able to recognize that value chain linkages exist within healthcare provider organizations and among the different suppliers and channels of the healthcare industry. The linkages within the elements of the value chain of an organization or similar organizations represent horizontal integration while the linkages among other suppliers and channels of healthcare delivery represent vertical integration, thus an integrated system. Therefore, the answer to the question, Why an integrated systems approach? is found in operating efficiency, cost advantage, and positive competitive positioning for offering goods and services in the marketplace (see Exhibit 2–1).

Peter Drucker set the parameters for the purpose of any business in his 1954 book *The Practice of Management*.[4] Drucker indicated that it is the customer who determines what a business is. What a business thinks it produces is not of first importance. What the customer thinks he is buying, what he considers "value" is decisive (we discuss the concept of organizational value in greater depth in Chapter 3). As the customers of healthcare services, employers, insurance companies, and the government are pushing for operating efficiency, cost effectiveness, and quality outcomes without compromising access.

PHYSICIAN-HOSPITAL INTEGRATION AND BEYOND

The response to current pressures on the healthcare industry has initially taken the form of physician and hospital linkages, as discussed in Chapter 1. Over the last 5 years the most dominant form of integrated delivery system development continues to be hospital networks, physician independent practice (or physician) associations (IPAs) and physician-hospital organizations (PHOs). Initially there was a great deal of interest in Physician-Hospital Organizations (PHOs). With few exceptions this linkage did not come about

EXHIBIT 2–1

Integration for Community Health Improvement

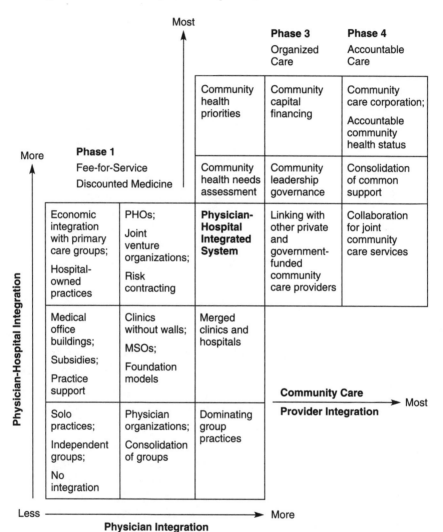

easily. There then followed a shift with hospitals continuing to link with other hospitals to establish regional networks. The formation of these networks has come both from top-down activities by large regional tertiary hospitals as well as bottom-up by community hospitals seeking tertiary hospital partners. Paralleling the hospital activity, physicians continued efforts to organize themselves into primary, specialty, and mixed IPA structures. All of this organizing is being done to level the playing field with managed care providers who has been pressuring independent hospitals and physicians into, at times, unreasonable discounts that would result in future patient steerage to participating providers. The volume needed to offset the discounts have not always occurred with the result that the contracted providers are left to absorb the impact of the lost revenue. However, as more hospital networks have established themselves and local IPAs have become operational, a more mature form of the PHO has surfaced and therefore increased the potential for each of these organizations to provide their participants with more of an ability to control their own destiny, as we shall see.

PHYSICIAN AND HOSPITAL ORGANIZATIONS AND SUPPORTING SERVICES

An Overview of Integration Models

Hospital and physician integration, as discussed in Chapter 1, has occurred in a variety of settings and styles, some more inclined to success than others (see Exhibits 2–2–2–5). Throughout the remainder of this text, numerous examples will be shared on different models of hospital and physician integration, many of which are continuing to evolve in the face of changes in market dynamics and the regulatory environment. The following discussion provides some overview of the prevalent models of physician and hospital integration and networking. The reader is advised to refer to Chapter 6, *Legal Issues in the Formation and Operation of IDS Organizations*, for additional commentary on the organizational and functional structures of these entities from a regulatory perspective.

EXHIBIT 2–2

Integration Strategies—Vertical and Horizontal Integration
Hospital-Affiliated Group Practice

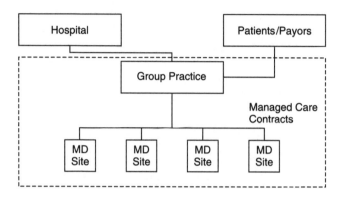

EXHIBIT 2–3

Integration Strategies—Vertical and Horizontal Integration
Group Practice Without Walls

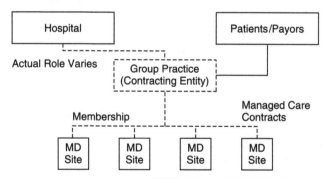

EXHIBIT 2–4

Integration Strategies—Vertical and Horizontal Integration
Foundation Model

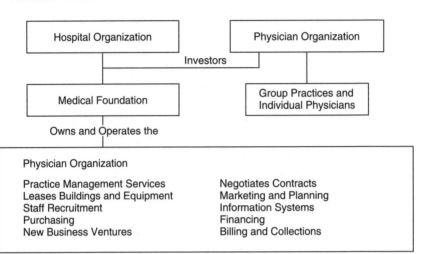

EXHIBIT 2–5

Integration Strategies—Vertical and Horizontal Integration
Fully Integrated Provider Organization

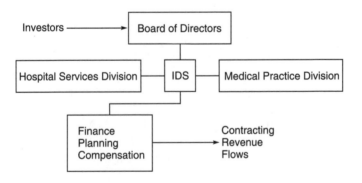

The Complete Transition to Risk Assumption

Recall from Chapter 1 that the beginning of risk assumption on the part of hospitals and physicians was not as smooth as initially expected. The movement to risk (see also Exhibit 1–5) affected not only the income streams but the opportunity to sustain unlimited losses on the parties bearing the risk. As workload units (total encounters) increased, variable costs increased. When the sum total of variable costs exceeds the amounts paid by capitation, loss is sustained. If loss is sustained by September 1 of the calendar year, potential significant loss may accrue before the end of the payment cycle.

Contracting mechanisms have developed to profile the risk assumed by hospitals, physicians, and networks when contracting for global capitation. An example appears in Exhibit 2–6. Here we see the increasing assumption of risk for system components including those commonly carved out and those commonly reinsured. Exhibit 2–7 describes the shifting of risk from types of insurance and contracting mechanisms.[5] The early and still prevalent view of risk

---

EXHIBIT 2–6

Contract Risk Components
Continuum of Risk

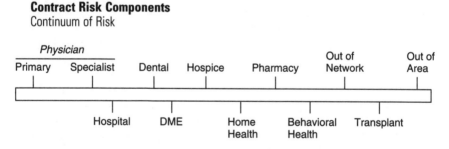

Commonly Carved Out:
Behavioral Health, Pharmacy, Home Health, DME, Dental

Commonly Reinsured:
Transplant, Out of Network, Out of Area

Source: Provider Risk, Inc.—Miami, FL
        Stephen C. George

EXHIBIT 2-7

Risk Shifting
For Health Insurers and Providers

Insurance Types

Indemnity	PPO	EPO	HMO	IDS (PHO/IPA/ MSO)	Provider	Provider/ Insurer

No Risk ──► **Full Risk**

FFS	Disc. FFS	Disc. FFS	Capitation:	Combination	Capitation:	Salaried
	DRG	Combination	PCP and	Contracts,	PCP	*Shareholder*
	Case Rates	Contracts	Specialist	Capitated	Specialist	*Stockholder*
				PCPs	Hospital	

Contracting Types

└──── Direct Contracting ────┘

True Integration

Source: Provider Risk, Inc.—Miami, FL
        Stephen C. George

assumption has led many to believe that the strict control of patient activity through narrow channels of low-cost providers is the dominant and only sustaining form of managed care response. There seems to be growing evidence that less restrictive managed care formats including IPA-model HMOs, PPOs, and point of service (POS) plans may be equally effective. Consider the following excerpt from a release of The Healthcare Advisory Board:

Healthcare Advisory Board 1996: Appraising Financing and Delivery Systems—A Bias for Choice and Virtual Integration

The expert argument of the last decade has been that restrictive HMO plans reliant upon narrow channeling of consumers to low-cost physicians and hospitals stand at a permanent competitive advantage against less restrictive managed care alternatives—PPOs, IPA-model HMOs and, more recently, POS plans. The logic ran that only by channeling patients to a narrow set of low-cost, closely managed physicians and hospitals could HMOs achieve serious reductions in utilization, cost, and eventually, price. As of this writing, that argument appears in doubt. There is gathering evidence at the frontier of broad-panel HMO plans matching narrow-plan costs while still including as many as one-half to three-quarters of all physicians and hospitals in their networks. What no one could have foreseen was the sudden emergence of three new technologies—physician IPAs, capitation, and specialty capitation—that now allow insurers to offer consumers both broad access and low price. The Healthcare Advisory Board believes that the striking early success of these broad-gated plans in advanced markets presages the future of managed care elsewhere in the nation. . .[6]

Given this statement, The Healthcare Advisory Board has speculated on *The End State for Managed Care.*[7] They believe that between 1988 and 1998, the *Zone of Maximum Channeling* occurs where the following has been occurring:

1. Employers channel patients to low-cost health plans.
2. Insurers channel patients to low-cost physicians and hospitals.
3. Insurers micromanage utilization with a heavy hand.
4. Insurers and providers form exclusive partnerships.

As a result of these actions they speculate on how the future might bear out: the elimination of consumer choice, broad insurer authority over healthcare decisions, insurer ownership of proprietary delivery systems, a majority of providers locked out of contracts (in given markets) and the painful loss of freedom for providers in contracts. The Advisory Board view of where the healthcare financing and delivery system might go if early indicators bear out is:

1. Consumers choose from expanded set of health plans.
2. Plans offer broad choice of physicians and hospitals.
3. Insurers retreat from utilization management.
4. Physicians and hospitals retain access to contracts.
5. Exclusive contracts break down.

How and under what circumstances will all these positive changes occur? If in fact the IPA model HMOs, PPOs, and POS plans effectively partner with physicians and hospitals, turning over utilization management, and each side negotiates fair globally capitated rates, gain sharing will exist for each party (see also Chapter 7, *Health Plans Must Serve the Physician*).

Readers should be advised that the assumption of global risk contracting brings with it significant financial challenges. Systems should establish close working relationships with actuaries and reinsurance specialists to identify as many issues of proper risk bearing as possible. The area of reinsurance is particularly sensitive; small changes in assumptions and populations can result in great system expenditures. Reinsurance is a mechanism which provides actuarially-based risk coverage for insurance plan expenses. It is typically used to offset unpredictable plan expenses for unusually high claims. Reinsurance provides high value for the service it provides, if its needs are recognized and assessed correctly within the health plan. Exhibits A and B graphically depict the effect of reinsurance on health plan claim variability. These examples were derived from a Monte Carlo simulation analysis examining the likelihood of claims from a population of 5,000 plan members. Exhibit A, Annual Aggregate Claims, depicts the plan expense

EXHIBIT A

Annual Aggregate Claims
(5,000 Members)

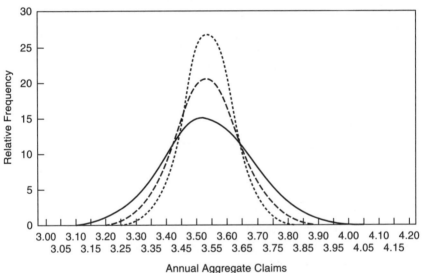

Annual Aggregate Claims
(millions $)

——— Without reinsurance

– – – – With reinsurance at $10,000 deductible

······ With reinsurance at $5,000 deductible

Source: Provider Risk, Inc.—Miami, FL
    Stephen C. George

profiles of the relative frequency of claims with and without reinsurance. According to Stephen George of Provider Risk, Inc., a reinsurance specialist, reinsurance provides the following critical elements in a successfully managed health plan:

1. Reinsurance removes the possibility of claims reaching catastrophic levels but cutting off the tail of high end claims;

2. Reinsurance reduces the probability of exceeding a plan's budget through impact of losses;

3. Reinsurance increases the probability of meeting goals and achieving profits by reducing the overall frequency of high expense claims and narrowing the risk profit; and

4. Reinsurance turns an unknown loss into a known cost.

Exhibit B, Reinsurance Profile of Claim Variability, summarizes these points.

EXHIBIT B

Reinsurance Profile of Claim Variability

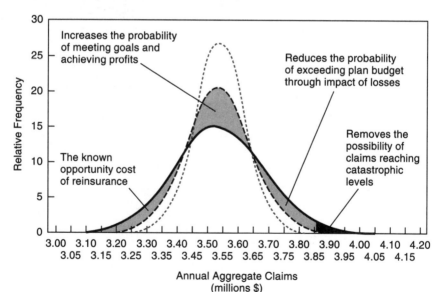

Source: Provider Risk, Inc.—Miami, FL
       Stephen C. George

Some health plans use reinsurance and stop-loss coverage to facilitate physician compensation systems within their plans to reduce the likelihood that any given physician panel's expenses will exceed a certain maximum amount. These sub-system strategies are often found in point of service payment plans.

Physician-Hospital Organizations and Relationships

PHOs have existed for many years, functioning with greater and lesser degrees of effectiveness, in order to counter the effects of managed care (see Exhibit 2–8). While PHOs intended to be a collaborative activity, many were hospital driven and were seen as the hospital's strategy for survival, which happened to require the physicians to come along. When driven by physicians, many PHOs still served to do little more than educate their members about managed care but were marginally successful in obtaining contracts.

PHOs are essentially joint ventures between hospitals and physicians. Recall that a "joint venture" is defined as an integration of operations between two or more separate firms, in which the following conditions are present: (1) the enterprise is under the joint control of the parent firms, which are not under related control; (2) each parent makes a significant contribution to the joint enterprise; (3) the enterprise exists as a business entity separate from its parents; and (4) the joint venture creates significant new enterprise

---

EXHIBIT 2–8

Integration Strategies—Vertical and Horizontal Integration
Physician-Hospital Organization

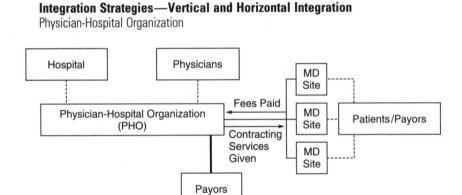

capability in terms of new productive capacity, new technology, a new product, or entry into a new market.[8] Contracting, collaboration, and capitation are the primary reasons providers form PHOs. They typically divide their marketing and contract acquisition effort between retail markets, which include healthcare plans, which are then marketed to employers, or wholesale markets, the employers themselves, often beginning with modest goals. Key goals for establishing the PHO often include contracting with managed care organizations and directly with employers, collaboration and improved relationships with medical staffs, enhancing quality of care, and sharing financial risk. PHO performance is often based less on profitability of the PHO itself and more on securing new revenue streams for participants. The immediate problem for many PHOs is overcoming state laws regarding insurance risk that are forcing many PHOs to contract for limited capitation and fee schedule based, discounted fee for service, or be required to become, essentially, an HMO (insurance company) under state law (see also Chapter 6, *Legal Issues in the Formation and Operation of IDS Organizations*).

Structurally, PHOs seem to either view themselves as being merged with other healthcare organizations or developing into health plans within a few years. Their current focus has been more on gaining direct access to covered lives rather than in building the infrastructure to support integrated care delivery, although recent successes may well be positioning the PHO, along with the IPA, into being a sustainable model for network development. Peter Friend discusses the development of Highland Park HealthCare, Inc., an Illinois PHO, and outlines the following PHO Success Factors from its first 5 years of operations:[9]

1. Strong physician leadership with a vision for the future.
2. Effective governance with strong primary care physician representation.
3. An incentive system that rewards high-quality, cost-effective providers.
4. Strong, full-time management with the ability to balance the needs of the hospital organization and the physician group.

5. An effective information system for claims processing, utilization management, case management, customer satisfaction measurement, quality improvement, and eventually, outcome measurement.

6. A geographically disperse, appropriately sized provider panel with a desirable mix of primary care physicians and specialists.

7. Competitive market pricing.

8. Contracting policies that cover issues such as exclusivity, pricing, and patient volume.

9. Joint ownership between the hospital and physicians.

10. An ability to negotiate capitated contracts and accept managed care risk.

"Super" or Regional PHOs are beginning to form as transitional models of physician-hospital integration expanding the geographic range of hospitals and physicians to attract larger, dispersed, enrolled populations. Marian C. Jennings describes the conditions necessary to form a super PHO:[10]

Market Conditions

♦ Moderate (<30%) managed care penetration.

♦ Few "mergers" already in effect; minimal system development.

Provider Organization's Characteristics

♦ Financially strong and stable.

♦ Strong position in local market.

♦ Attractive to HMOs because of quality, cost, and area served.

♦ Adequate primary care base in place.

♦ Strong, functioning PHO in place.

♦ Physician and management commitment to common vision, including need to accept capitation.

♦ Committed board of directors.

Partner's Characteristics

♦ Little or no service area mix overlap.

- Shared vision of the future, including commitment to integrated delivery systems.
- Common or compatible culture and values.
- Strong, functioning PHOs in place with similar policies, adequate primary care bases, and committed boards.

Antitrust issues continue to loom as recent Department of Justice settlements have delineated contracting restrictions. Under the proposed decrees, certain types of contracting activity that have the net effect of restricting trade among competitors, create unfair bargaining positions, or unfairly motivate physicians to participate have been deemed inappropriate (see Chapter 6-*Antitrust Laws*). The issue has not been unexpected; proscriptions reported are consistent with published guidelines on PHO and contracting activities as they relate to fraud and abuse and antitrust guidance. PHOs, POs, and IPAs, as joint ventures, are risk-sharing relationships. Participants must share substantial risk in the forms of capitation or discounted fee-for-service agreements with significant (20%) risk pool withholds focusing on utilization targets to improve efficiency (using a fact-specific analysis). To put it in other words, when the physician group bears substantial economic risk, each member of the group has a direct stake in the success of the group as a whole, and therefore has an incentive to assure that all physicians practice high-quality medicine and avoid unnecessary utilization of services. The result: if you are not at risk, you can't fix prices; hence, the development of "messenger" models of contracting. Further consideration should be given to contracting arrangements, incentives to participating physicians, and overall regulatory standing of contracting activities to assure compliance within acceptable limits.

Independent Practice/Physician Associations

The IPA is an unusual entity in that it began as a forum for physicians to air their concerns about working with local hospitals and insurers and, for the longest time, most IPAs served no useful function. The IPA has come into greater prominence given the continuing success of the model to control costs and compete in highly managed markets. Consider the following statement from The Healthcare Advisory Board:

Healthcare Advisory Board 1995: The Rise of the IPA—Getting It Wrong

The expert argument across the past three years had been that the looser physician models, such as the IPA, stand at a permanent (terminal) competitive disadvantage against the more completely integrated group practices and staff models. The logic ran that the fierce independence of the member physicians, and concomitant weak central governance, could never yield serious cost reduction and utilization control. At best, the looser affiliations served as a transition stage, a migratory way station along the path to full integration.

As of this writing, the expert argument is wrong. At least as to current competitive success, IPAs are proving the equal of other physician models in managing costs and attracting lives. Nor can the Governance Committee distance itself from the error. Our earlier research reported, at that time correctly, on the relative failure of loose physician affiliations. What we neither had sensed nor foreseen was the sudden market discipline displayed by some IPAs and their member physicians. Across a governance by fiat, reduced hospital utilization by 40%, decreased specialist utilization by 60% and trebled their enrolled lives.

The debate in the West now has turned to whether the IPA is sustainable across the long term. The majority view, even among some IPA administrators, probably is "no." Meanwhile, IPAs continue to multiply and grow, with health systems and groups among the most aggressive investors.

The Governance Committee now believes the IPA, well managed, can be (astonishingly) competitive and remain so across some relevant time frame. Without weighing in at this writing on the "end state," it is easy to recommend that the IPA model be a first, a committed and continuing endeavor for health systems earnest about vertical integration.[11]

Multispecialty IPAs, in an amazing variety of organizational forms, are the most prevalent model (Exhibits 2–9 and 2–10). As primarily a contracting mechanism, IPAs provide the forum for physicians to compete for capitated contracts as a group, sharing in the upside (gain sharing) and downside (deficit coverage), depending on how well care of the enrollees is managed. Physician participants are chiefly independent groups who use the IPA as but one means of patient contracting. As indicated by the previous

EXHIBIT 2–9

Integration Strategies—Vertical and Horizontal Integration
Multispecialty IPA

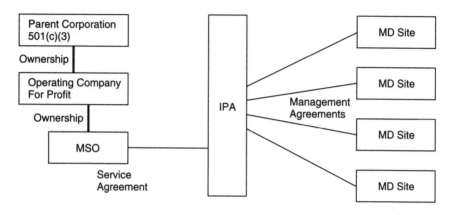

EXHIBIT 2–10

Integration Strategies—Vertical and Horizontal Integration
Multispecialty IPA

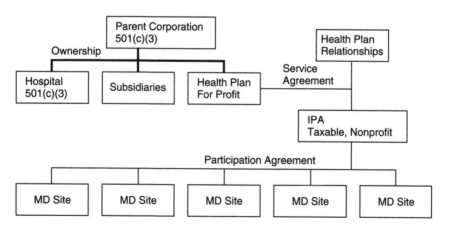

Healthcare Advisory Board statements, IPAs are loosely structured entities that are capable of making the transition from the unrestricted FFS environment to managed care. Like PHOs, IPAs often begin as broad-paneled organizations, which, over time and with increasing contract volume, reduce their ranks through various aspects of utilization management, economic credentialing, or some other means (often done poorly, unjustifiably, and rudely). The logic ran that payors would not contract with organizations comprised of all providers, those cost effective and those not, but would only contract with defined, documented, cost-conscious groups.

IPAs, and in many cases PHOs as well, have proved many markets wrong through their ready assumption of risk and by embracing the philosophy required to compete effectively for covered lives with other organizations. From an organizational standpoint, IPAs are a lower capital alternative to entering the market than other models, although for their advantages they share some inherent challenges as well. IPAs are typically more difficult to manage than a fully integrated group because of the independent nature of the participants. In the earliest stages, like PHOs, they are characterized by relatively weak governance, they are poorly capitalized for the task, and they have minimal systems infrastructure. Utilization management systems must be created in order to assist physician groups in embracing the cost/quality equation (see also Chapter 7, generally). IPA governance is slowly shifting from specialty dominance to larger and larger amounts of primary care recognizing the need for PCP members. Often these governance positions are handled through differing classes of membership or stock, different operating divisions, supermajority or co-majority voting.

Single Specialty IPAs (Exhibit 2–11) are growing in particular local and regional markets in response to market peculiarities, the need for specialty representation, and primary care network development. They focus often on their niche markets where carve-out contracts are available from other systems and networks, including behavioral health, substance abuse, obstetrics, cardiovascular services, rehabilitation, and occupational medicine. These specialty networks contract similarly with their multispecialty brothers under discounted FFS, capitation, subcapitation from PCP or other network, and combination contracting. Capital requirements for market analysis and planning the start-up can run as low as $35,000,

EXHIBIT 2-11

Integration Strategies—Vertical and Horizontal Integration
Single Specialty IPA

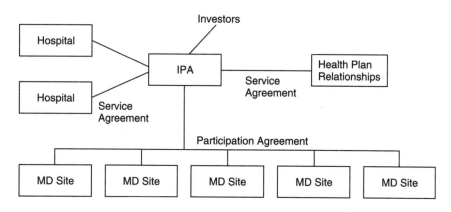

depending on the planned scope of operations and size of the group. As with the creation of any new venture, investigate facilitators and counsel experienced in this form of activity (see also Chapter 5, *Merging Practices, Businesses, and Strategic Business Units*).

Particular financial and operational indicators are similar to any contracting entity. Contract volume and cash flow are always of concern, but red flags should go up when providers experience abnormal or irregular payments, poor communication (specifically, lack of data), and poorly managed operating systems.

Supporting Services: MSOs and Beyond

Management/Medical Services Organizations (Exhibit 2–12) are playing an increasingly greater role as system partner components with HMOs, PHOs, POs, and IPAs in the emerging IDS environments. Their control of daily operations of the owned and operated (corporate) medical practices, as well as the contracted practices spans a prodigious array of services. Patient care delivery, insurance administration, practice and clinical management including medical records, quality of care data, and clinical services integration allow MSOs to wield considerable power in system effectiveness. Simply handling the information services inherent in medical

EXHIBIT 2–12

Integration Strategies—Vertical and Horizontal Integration
Management Services Organization

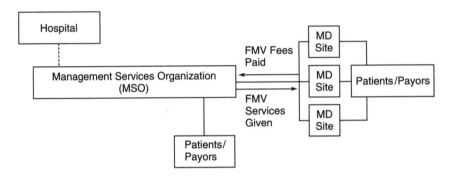

practice operations is daunting. Hospitals are learning rapidly that buying the first practice often opens the floodgates to other opportunities. Buyer organizations that have not planned or established the support infrastructure to manage these businesses have learned business operations the hard way. MSO activity will continue to increase as practice acquisition and network consolidation continues. The specific forms of MSOs may vary slightly, some services being performed by PHOs or IPAs, but the traditional support services entity model should prevail. This is due to the fact that the business operations in MSOs are fairly well defined, and exporting these services or "piggybacking" onto organizations with dissimilar prime functions is likely to be more disrupting than beneficial.

There are opportunities for physician equity positions in MSOs as venture capitalists are moving into the for-profit MSO arena, although the pivotal issue in any equity-based arrangement is liquidity and return on investment. MSO growth must occur in equity models to create the income stream for dividends, or alternatively, to create a system of value for later sale to another entity in the healthcare system.

Investor-owned physician practice management companies (PPMs), such as MedPartners/Mullikin, PhyCor, Caremark, Coastal, InPhyNet, MedCath, and Sterling, are expanding rapidly across the country bringing investment opportunities for physician partners along with experience in physician risk management. Their rapid expansion into areas of medium- to low-managed care penetration is evidence of their desire to become established players. They are organizing physicians in communities much quicker than local hospitals or physicians are doing themselves bringing sophisticated practice management, information systems, treatment protocols and other developed intellectual assets to rapidly become a market force. Once a real darling of Wall Street, PPMs are trading at twice the price to earnings (P/E) ratios of HMOs. They are seen as one of the real competitors in established markets and one of the potential fears in markets they have not yet penetrated.

PPMs are organized similarly to MSOs but are constructed and capitalized to move much quicker than the local MSO. They often acquire assets of primary and multispecialty groups, engaging in long-term (20 to 40 year) employment relationships and leases of facilities. Their gain sharing models frequently involve an equity position through various classes of stock, and incentives are paid through company or stock dividends and actual performance of the local group. As investor-owned organizations, they may be prone to seek specific, aggressive profit margins and create ill feelings among physician "partners" whose opinion on business and healthcare delivery varies significantly from theirs. Although not always the case, physicians should examine their involvement with PPMs as they would any other business transaction (see also Chapter 4 on business transactions and relationships and Chapter 5 on mergers).

Community/Occupational Health Services

Ambulatory surgery, home health, occupational/industrial health, and rehabilitation are among the top ranking services targeted for urban and rural hospitals, immediately behind expansion of family practice/primary care centers. With estimates of hospital-based ambulatory care visits increasing between 4% and 5% annually over the next 5 years, service expansion is anticipated to meet competitive challenges and to provide community services in many markets across the U.S. Community and occupational health services represent an important component of service delivery for provider networks. The most publicized issues include sources of operating revenue, charitable service, and platforms for building community health information and community health needs assessments.

Few medical practices, urgent care centers, or hospital-based primary care clinics make optimum use of industrial accounts as a means to generate revenue. Industrial accounts still pay well in comparison to many other payors in many markets across the country. There are typically few problems with collections and good industrial relationships open doors for direct contracting when the time comes. They are a winning relationship for the employer and can be win-win-win for the practice. Obviously, they are not all superb accounts, but careful consideration should be given to exploring options in local markets.

Community-based stakeholders interested in improving community health status include individual providers, health departments, local government offices, social service agencies, religious organizations, and schools. These entities may provide useful entry points into new areas of business. Contracting with these entities may improve net revenue in advancing markets. In the future integrated environment, it is certain that information networks will include many of these players.

Many hospitals have already developed the capacity to deliver home healthcare services, either through direct provision through a hospital subsidiary, by contract or agreement with public or private sources, or through referral relationships in their markets. In many markets, the optimal time for creating home health agencies, services, infusion therapy, and rehabilitation subsidiaries or product lines has passed. In the emerging integrated environment, these services will be of considerable importance to sustained profitability as they represent opportunity for return on operating margin greater than hospital sources. Building relationships in these areas should be considered if providers value sustained growth.

Other important community providers include chiropractors, optometrists, and podiatrists. The flow of patients in a fee-for-service environment includes patients referred from these independent practitioners, as well as the need for operating a lower-cost setting for providing optimum patient care in response to managed care. Many hospitals privilege podiatrists, recognizing that they provide appropriate patient care within the scope of their specialty and training. Significant links have already developed between podiatry and orthopedics. Chiropractors have developed referral relationships with orthopedics groups although it is not likely that they will be accepted as readily as podiatrists, optometrists, nurse practitioners, or nurse midwives. There exists yet a professional stigma regarding the training and scope of chiropractic and the medical community is still reluctant to accept it.

Physical therapy practices are increasingly approached by a variety of players pursuing integration. Orthopedists, neurologists, skilled nursing facilities, rehabilitation and acute care hospitals, and regional and national physical therapy and rehabilitation chains are in the acquisition mode, although fraud and abuse and anti-referral legislation (Stark Laws) have made a significant impact. Dental care delivery has yet to be absorbed into integrated delivery systems to a great extent beyond staff model IDS groups such as Kaiser-Permanente.

Strategic Partnerships

Creating strategic partnerships is a well-recognized strategy in many areas of the business world. In healthcare, the adage "You don't need to own it all, just be able to control it" is the prevalent view. The caveat of current thought is leaning, however, to *the need to understand it all.* Whether Jeff Goldsmith's "virtual integration," partial integration, or fully integrated models, health networks will need to provide the whole array of services to be competitive, not only on a regional level, but for local sources of business as well.

Strategic partnerships include examining relationships that hospitals and physician groups of all sizes are forming with one another: relationships with insurers (insurance / risk-bearing capacity and third-party payors), physicians and physician delivery networks, ancillary services such as reference labs and pharmacy networks, and for the largest players, purchasing networks. Potential partners are aligning themselves based on historical relations, common vision, goals, and interdependency. Relationships are being strained as business is *not as usual,* and physicians and administrators begin to make hard choices about who may be potential long-term partners.

One problem that is surfacing is hospital-hospital partnering using increased market power to avoid price negotiations, implicating antitrust issues. Key to this issue is the degree to which integrated activities (clinical, administrative, financial, marketing, contracting with managed care plans) are on a risk-sharing basis to avoid antitrust implications. It appears that the FTC is particularly concerned about hospitals forming partnerships without significant financial integration, dividing up services under "centers of excellence" when in reality it is *per se* illegal market allocation.

Along the same lines as strategic partnerships, the IRS indicates in its Exempt Organizations Continuing Professional Education Technical Instruction Textbook (for FY 1996), that they have been receiving ruling requests in three broad areas: the sale of one not-for-profit entity to another not-for-profit entity; a not-for-profit system's sale of one of its hospitals; and the sale of a not-for-profit to a for-profit in which the sales proceeds are used to establish a charitable foundation.[12] The IRS is particularly concerned with the reduction of charitable healthcare services available in the community postsale, suggesting that the amount of annual support should be equivalent to the amount of charitable care provided by the previous hospital annually for at least 3 years.

In assessing organizational readiness and direction, Cathy Sullivan Clark questions in her assessment of ambulatory care planning: Which services should be provided directly or "made" and which should be subcontracted or "bought."[13] Nowhere is this more applicable than in assessing the need for business or service line growth than in strategic partnerships. The following denotes her approach to service line positioning.

Providers can ask themselves the following questions to determine how their ambulatory service line should be positioned over the next 3 to 5 years.

1. How should our market be defined?
2. What role should we play in ambulatory care for our market?
3. What do managed care players require? What are the critical success factors for each component of our ambulatory service line?

4. How can (should) we work with our physicians to provide ambulatory services?
5. Which services should we provide directly? Which services should be provided through subcontracts? What criteria should be used in making the "make versus buy" decision?
6. How will changes in demand impact our ambulatory services? How much should we enhance our services? Are new services needed? Should any be divested?
7. What additional geographic sites are needed?
8. How can we improve the cost effectiveness of our services? The clinical quality? The customer satisfaction?
9. How can we ensure that our ambulatory services function in a coordinated fashion?

Russell Coile points out that cooperation with competitors and strategic business alliances with providers and payors are the paths to success in the transitional healthcare economy of 1996–2000.[14] Indeed, hospital and healthcare alliances including American Healthcare Systems, Premier Health Alliance/SunHealth, and Voluntary Hospitals of America are helping hospitals build voluntary provider networks, negotiate contracts, and manage patient care.[15] Kaiser-Permanente has recently joined the HMO Group, an alliance of 16 group-model HMOs, which allows them to offer out-of-area coverage. Kaiser has further allied with California's State Compensation Insurance Fund to treat injured state employees. This type of expansion paves the way for larger organizations to take a firm position to become a sustaining player in their markets.

A partial listing of strategic business alliances includes the following options, particularly if a system does not currently have the capacity or does not plan to create the capacity:

1. Primary care centers—large, independent groups.
2. HMOs/health insurance plans.
3. Ancillary services including laboratory, outpatient services such as ambulatory surgery, diagnostic and imaging centers, and home infusion.

4. Home health and rehabilitation services.
5. Community health/screening centers—especially good for public awareness and education.
6. Physician ventures including MSOs, PHOs, and IPAs.
7. Occupational health centers/walk-in and urgent care centers.

Community Health Information Networks (CHINs)

The development of Community Health Information Networks is one of the most important operational aspects of healthcare delivery in a managed care environment. As reimbursement declines and the capitated healthcare dollar represents more output of the system, redundancy in all aspects of the financing and delivery system must be eliminated. The contributions of the whole array of community care providers are maximized through state-of-the-art communications on direct patient care, ancillary healthcare services and diagnostic testing, and eligibility verification, among others, and the ease of patient entry into the system becomes the method of tracking patient flow and geographic expansion. These systems are more than just patient scheduling; they include patient episode-specific procedures, visits, hospitalizations, tests, pharmacy information, medical records, and all components of financial and administrative records. Systems must be totally integrated—not just selected component or panels—and disparate systems are destined to wreak havoc.

Healthcare systems are not simply interested in the concept of linking together all service providers from an internal perspective; they truly see the benefits in integrating private providers of healthcare. Although not focusing directly on linking various community healthcare providers, three major systems in California are investing enormous amounts of capital into information networks. Reported recently in several journals are Kaiser-Permanente's Northern California Region: $1 billion over 7 years; Mercy Healthcare Sacramento: $27.5 million over 5 years; and Sutter Health: $150 million over the next 7 years.[16] The majority of these expenses are for internal information networks although they will undoubtedly expand to key community health providers as competition increases further, and as the need to maximize every dollar becomes critical. It is estimated that over 40% of U. S. hospitals are forming CHINs or plan to join one.

As these networks are forming, some states require hospitals and freestanding healthcare centers, such as ambulatory surgery centers, to submit claims-related data to the state government. In North Carolina, the NC Health Information Network (NCHIN), with 106 participating hospitals, feeds information to a central data bank through contracted data processors. Whether state information systems like this simply report utilization data, which is important in its own right, or whether they are able to make the leap to integrated information systems tracking individual episodes of care will determine the success of such networks. The cornerstone of healthcare delivery and financing will rest on the development of information systems to handle data, which will, in turn, allow providers, insurers, and investors to maintain operations in competitive environments.

The problems emerging in the development of these information systems fall into two broad categories. Large healthcare systems like Kaiser, Sutter Health, and Mercy face total system integration issues right now. In advanced managed care markets, competition for patient lives and the systems of service delivery to manage that care are being pushed to new limits on a monthly basis. These advanced markets, including the twin cities, Chicagoland, and selected other areas of the country, are climbing the learning curve for the rest of the nation to follow. Staff model systems, as previously mentioned, are devoting huge sums of capital to system development, which almost requires complete information system overhaul for each component of the delivery network.

At the other end of the spectrum, CHIN development in less advanced markets or in rural areas with fairly strong independent hospitals are experiencing different types of problems. Networking with multiple small and independent providers, and potentially key employer groups, has programmers writing interfaces that are high cost, high maintenance, and of low predictability, from a functional perspective. Smaller CHINs, and particularly those with voluntary subscription, cannot afford system replacement for CHIN members. Integrating disparate systems is a bit like mating different species. The frustrations of the software engineers and the unrealized expectations of phase one participants lead these less developed markets to cautious advancement on the CHIN front. Additionally, research projects or grants integrating healthcare services such as community health information (linking hospital to physician offices to health departments) or telemedicine demonstration projects, as a rule, have not been sustainable by grant dollars. Further development in the use of telemedicine, expansion of fiber optic capacity, and reconciliation of reimbursement for these "transfers" will settle out the finances of how information becomes patient care, and how systems can share resources in appropriate and legal manners.

RELATIONSHIPS PURSUED BY SMALLER HEALTHCARE ENTITIES

From a practical perspective, smaller healthcare entities have everchanging roles in the future integrated environment. The strategies and relationships pursued by small and rural acute care hospitals, specialty hospitals, and ancillary healthcare providers or small healthcare businesses vary significantly. Hospitals, regardless of their size, scope of treatment, and cash reserves or endowment, have three recognized options for continued existence: (1) create risk-bearing capacity to exist as the leader, or hub, of a system; (2) partner, on an equity basis with a risk-bearer/health insurance product; or (3) become a network facility worthy of continued existence through benefiting the network. The only derivation of this concept is the limited scope of care provided by a government-sponsored entity (e.g., rural county hospital) in unusual circumstances. Healthcare businesses such as physical therapy practices, home health agencies, and durable medical equipment firms may have similar options, depending on the size, structure, and geographic coverage of the group.

Smaller hospitals that are still financially viable are looking to partner, typically with a larger hospital or academic center, in efforts to remain as independent as possible, for as long as possible. Hospitals involved in IDS activity continue to partner with other hospitals predominantly. Home care programs, primary care centers, and group practices or clinics are typical alternative partner choices.

Other choices include ambulatory care centers, surgery centers, managed care plans, nursing homes, and insurance companies.

As these hospitals strive to maintain solvency, or are planning for future contingencies, several options exist. The overall goal is to minimize the overhead of hospital operations, eliminate overhead from unused excess capacity, use the physical plant to generate revenue (or at least as the lowest-cost use of space required by other ventures), and to maximize revenue flow from nonhospital operations. Several initiatives that are started by hospitals as wholly owned, or as joint ventures include: Wellness programs, industrial/ occupational health, adult day healthcare, outpatient or inpatient hospice, home health agency or services, and innovative inpatient services such as acute psychiatry, outpatient/short-term surgery, and tertiary hospital admission "swaps."

Improving on services already provided, such as durable medical equipment and outpatient or mail-out pharmacy, many hospitals have moved into home health and outpatient services as additional income sources. In many markets, these services are already saturated by private providers or national chains. A 1995 study by Find/SVP, a New York-based market research and consulting firm, predicted a 12.6% annual rate of growth in home care services through 1999.[17] The same study indicated that during the past five years, home infusion product revenues grew 88.7%, kidney dialysis revenues grew 69.2%, and home medical equipment grew 56%.

These areas rapidly become the professional turf of the ancillary healthcare businesses and entrepreneurial physicians. Independent providers such as physical therapists are being solicited to join regional and national networks as providers, but more often as employees. Physical therapy appears to be the big push at present. Nursing homes and home health services are also important additions for large specialty provider networks.

The strategies for these smaller and, presently, independent providers, lie generally in deciding whether they are large enough to grow into a regional player by accepting risk *to be part of someone else's system of care.* It is unlikely that many large physical therapy chains will become the hubs of integrated systems, but they will likely be acquired by an integrated system. Smaller providers can weather the storm and watch the market for ingress by outside players to decide when it is time to affiliate or sell out.

TOWARD FULLY INTEGRATED REASONING

While all this activity continues there is a segment of an integrated delivery system that is not receiving equal emphasis but yet in essence represents the third leg of a three-legged stool; that is, all other non-hospital/physician community care providers. As indicated earlier this is not an across-the-board fact. There are communities such as San Antonio, Tampa, Rochester, and others across the country that are pursuing collaborative solutions to improving community health status through the involvement of all healthcare and human service providers. These efforts, however, are not as numerous as the organizing of hospitals and physicians. It is important to keep in mind there is more to an IDS than hospitals and physicians. System transition has been studied by numerous individuals and consulting firms around the country including The Health Service Group, BBC Research and Consulting, National Health Advisors, The Advisory Board Company, Voluntary Hospitals of America (VHA), SunHealth, and others indicating the stages of development of a physician-hospital integrated system. Exhibit 2–1 (page 29) extends this typical transitional model to demonstrate the stages of integration through the establishment of a community care corporation that is accountable for community health status.

There is an inherent logic to the unfolding of IDS efforts with hospitals and physicians because of the large dollar volume that is paid out to these two segments of the healthcare industry. The focus on these two segments has produced rapid "up-linking" or "down-linking" as positioning dictates and this is where the danger surfaces. The development of an IDS requires care and attention to detail because so much of the integrated system is based upon service, employment, and managed care contracting as well as acquisition of related healthcare businesses, mergers, and affiliations, and subject to continuous scrutiny by the IRS and DHHS's Office of The Inspector General (OIG). The chapters that follow provide greater detail related to the legalities and financing aspects of developing IDS organizations.

In the midst of this groundswell of activity, Coddington, Moore, and Fischer[18] have referenced a growing level of criticism of IDS's as the right direction, the right solution. But in doing so they balance the criticism with a number of responses to demonstrate that IDS's are not simply in vogue.

For example:

Criticism: Employing physicians doesn't make economic sense.

Response: Established IDSs consider expansion of primary care networks one of the most valuable strategies of the past decade. Indeed, in established highly capitated networks (where you know your costs and income), employment and straight salary may work well under certain conditions.

Criticism: Physicians can't be led.

Response: Look for opportunities for physicians to do the leading (in one sense, why must physicians be led, only?). Physicians need to lead as well as *be guided* by others with the right skills to bring the network together.

Criticism: Vertical integration is nothing more than a strategy to bail out the hospital.

Response: For hospitals that are financially sound, vertical integration is a good tool for maintaining competitive advantage. For most physician networks as well as hospitals, vertical and horizontal integration is important for long-term survival and to maintain competitive market position.

An additional perspective on integrated delivery systems is whether they should be "virtual" or "vertical." The virtual IDS is more informal; vertical integration is the more structured form of IDS. The answer is that both perspectives work together. Not all participants will wish to be irreversibly bound into a given system; other participants may wish to begin on an informal basis to determine fit and appropriateness and then formalize a long term relationship. Lastly, virtual networks based on systems of long-term contractual relationships may work for many organizations as well (see also Chapter 1).

The critical mass of IDS activity is helping the management and boards of hospitals to agree with Drucker's assertion that they are no longer in the business of running a hospital; they are in the business of providing healthcare whatever the environment.[19]

ARE THERE SUCCESSFUL IDS ORGANIZATIONS?

There are many communities where the transition to IDS has yet to begin, and for many who have started, the journey of a thousand days is only one day old. As a result many are continuing to search for examples of successful integrated delivery systems. Unfortunately we are all too early in the game to determine that any particular system is the formula for success. Indeed many presently successful organizations, MedPartners/Mullikin, PhyCor, Columbia/HCA, and others have changed their organizational structure to flex with the changing environment. What we can identify are those factors that are common to integrated systems, which appear to be successful in assembling pieces that produce a continuum of service, demonstrate financial success, and are embracing other care elements in their communities or regions. The identification of common factors was based upon interviews, literature review, participation on a hospital association task force for integrated delivery system development, and experience with supporting regional and local IDS development. The information that follows (see Exhibit 2–13) is not offered with any guarantee that the common elements identified will stand the test of time. There is some safety in numbers when one sees the same elements present in various integrated delivery systems; this should be a strong indicator that they are critical and value-added dimensions for systems that work. In addition, there is no effort to suggest a priority order for bringing IDS elements on-line. Each IDS initiative will have a different starting point in response to the pressures immediately at hand. J. Daniel Beckham[20, 21] has provided some bracketing of what to look for. In 1993 Beckham referenced the work of David Nadler who provided some key elements of the architecture of integration.[22] The organizational model to use is natural systems that lead to biological organizations, based on neobiologic principles or subsumption architecture. Drucker's principles would lead one to believe that IDS size will be a function of its technology, strategy, and market definition.[23]

E X H I B I T 2–13

Creating the Integrated Delivery System
Common Elements

Integrated Delivery Systems	Date of Origin	Market Demographics and Economics	Physicians Participating	Leadership
Lovelace Health System Albuquerque, NM	1922	384,600 population Growing	300	Physicians PCP Led
Intermountain Health Care Salt Lake City, UT	1975	1.2M Growing	300	Management/ Physicians Led
Basset Health Systems Cooperstown, NY	1922	500,000	N.A.	Physicians
Scott & White Temple, TX	1897	900,000	450	Physician
Baptist Health System Birmingham, AL	1921	1.9M Growing	N.A.	Management
The Nalle Clinic Charlotte, NC	1921	1.2M	N.A.	Physician
BJC Health System St. Louis, MO	1993		400	Management/ Specialist Dominated

Organizational Linkages	Managed Care Enrollment System/ Overall	Net Revenue Growth	Information Systems Investment	Challenges
CIGNA	N.A.– 263,000	54% 1990–1994	N.A.	MD Productivity Rightsizing, Cost Reduction
N.A.	415,000	33% 1990–1994	N.A.	MD Productivity Cost Reduction
Community Health Plan	30,000	$2.2M 1994	$25M over 10 years	Growing CHP Enrollment, Information Systems, Cost Reduction
N.A.	109,300– 360,000	N.A.	$1.5M	Cost Reduction, Information Systems, Integration, Quality, Speed, Hospital Viability
Health Partners	72,000– 177,000	50% 1991–1994	$8M 1994–1995	HMO Growth, MD Integration
Multi-Payor Strategy	N.A.	N.A.	N.A.	Expanding PC, Hospital Relationship, Effect of Change
Partners HMO	45,000–			Cost Reduction, Capturing More Managed Care Market

NOTES

1. Robert Lee Hotz, "Lessons on the Ice," *Technology Review* (Boston: Massachusetts Institute of Technology, 1996), p. 5.
2. Michael Porter, *Competitive Advantage* (New York: The Free Press, 1985), pp. 33–61.
3. Michael Porter, "The Competitive Advantage of Nations" (New York: The Free Press, 1990) generally.
4. Peter Drucker, *The Practice of Management* (New York: Harper & Row, 1954), generally.
5. Adapted from Stephen C. George, from "Status of Potential Risk Contracting for Medicare and Medicaid," a presentation given on 10/11/96 at the North Carolina Chapter of The IPA Association of America, in Durham, NC.
6. The Healthcare Advisory Board (The Advisory Board Company, Washington, DC, 1996).
7. Ibid.
8. Joseph Broadly, "Joint Ventures and Antitrust Policy," *Harvard Law Review*, 1526, 1982.
9. Peter M. Friend, "PHO Growing Pains," *Healthcare Executive*, May/June 1996, pp. 12–16.
10. Marian C. Jennings, "Developing a Super PHO," *Healthcare Financial Management*, August/September 1995, pp. 24–25.
11. The Healthcare Advisory Board (The Advisory Board Company, Washington, DC, 1996).
12. Charles F. Kaiser and T. J. Sullivan, "Integrated Delivery Systems and Health Care Update," *Exempt Organizations Technical Instruction Program Textbook*, U. S. Department of Treasury, Internal Revenue Service, 1995, pp. 393–94.
13. Cathy Sullivan Clark, "Planning along the Continuum of Care," *Healthcare Financial Management*, August 1995, pp. 20–24.
14. Russell C. Coile, Jr., "Assessing Healthcare Market Trends and Capital Needs: 1996–2000," *Healthcare Financial Management*, August 1995, pp. 60–65.
15. Jay Greene, "Alliances Have a New Strategy," *Modern Healthcare*, July 10, 1995, pp. 47–50.
16. John Morrissey, "Building Networks to Stay Competitive," *Modern Healthcare*, August 21, 1995, pp. 150–54.

17. "Home-Care Product Revenues on Rise," *Modern Healthcare*, Sept. 4, 1995, p. 34.

18. Dean Coddington, K. Moore, and E. Fisher, "Vertical Integration: Is the Bloom off the Rose?" *Healthcare Forum Journal*, September/October 1996, pp. 42–47.

19. Peter Drucker, *Managing for the Future—The 1990s and Beyond* (New York: Truman Talley Books/Dutton, 1992) generally.

20. Daniel J. Beckham, "The Architecture of Integration," *Healthcare Forum Journal*, September/October 1993, pp. 56–63.

21. J. Daniel Beckham, "The IDS as Moving Target," *Healthcare Forum Journal*, September/October 1996, pp. 48–54.

22. D. Nadler, M. Gerstein, and R. Shaw, *Organizational Architecture*, (San Francisco, California: Jossey-Bass Inc., 1992) generally. This concept of the biologic organization is also described by Francis J. Gouillart and James N. Kelly in their book *Transforming the Organization* (New York: McGraw-Hill, 1995) generally.

23. Peter Drucker, *Managing for the Future*, generally.

3

ESTABLISHING AND BUILDING VALUE

Integrated systems of healthcare derive value through the many functions performed within the system and from their existence in the community as a whole. If one accepts the role of the healthcare provider as serving the health-related needs of the community, then any definition of value must include measures of social and community health as well as the economic health of the integrated system. This chapter begins by establishing the premise of value as traditionally accepted in healthcare business activity and ends with some nontraditional discussion of the value of healthcare services within a community. Economic measures are discussed a bit more deeply than simply an overview; however, a substantial body of knowledge has been published on the subject of business valuation in general. A reference listing of excellent resources on business valuation appears in the appendix of this text.

THE PREMISES OF VALUE IN HEALTHCARE

Ask an art dealer what he means by value and you're likely to get a response based on the buyer's desirability of a particular treasure. Ask a realtor what he means by value and he'll say it's based on the selling price of other properties in the area. Ask a Wall Street investor and he'll say it's a function of return on investment. Ask the IRS about the taxable implications of a healthcare acquisition and they'll say it is the price at which a willing buyer and willing seller would agree, neither being under any compulsion to buy or sell and both having a reasonable knowledge of the relevant facts, a standard definition of *fair market value*.[1] Who's right? They all are depending on your perspective. Taking this concept one step further, the subject of "price" also has a significant impact on value. Is "price" always an issue in discussing value? No. There are many circumstances when the price of a business or venture does not reflect its value, as in the case of a below-market sale. Indeed, businesses or products may have significant value even if "no willing buyer" exists, at least in the traditional sense. In the healthcare environment, value may be any or all of the above in any given situation. A similar question posed by James J. Unland in *The Valuation of Hospitals and Medical Centers* is: What is the value of a highly regulated, capital-intensive business with a high asset book value but a generally gloomy projected financial performance?[2] The answer lies in the specific circumstances detailing the purpose and function of the valuation.

One must begin the process by asking the reason a valuation of a given healthcare entity or component is needed. The most frequent reason for valuation of smaller healthcare businesses such as medical and other professional practices and small service companies is to obtain financing or to determine a price for shares of ownership. Larger entities such as hospitals, nursing homes, and retirement centers utilize valuations almost exclusively for financing purposes. With increasing merger and acquisition activities, the purpose and function of the valuation often changes.

There are several items to keep in mind as we examine the issues of establishing the value of a discrete business or business line:

- All value is the expectation of future benefit.

- ◆ The best indicator of future performance is usually the performance of the immediate past.
- ◆ The seller sells the past while the buyer buys the future.
- ◆ Changes in healthcare delivery and financing may make reliance on historical data somewhat speculative, especially in certain medical subspecialties.
- ◆ The likelihood of realization of benefits must compare with other measures of economic and/or political risk in evaluating acquisition/network initiatives.

The most frequent *standard of value* used in healthcare business valuation is fair market value. Many buyers, however, may consider the value of a given acquisition or merger based on what it might bring to the organization in terms of synergies, positioning, or market power. In most cases, buyers are interested in quantifying the economic benefit based on certain perceptions about the subject business's income, earnings, or benefits stream (see Exhibit 3–1). These instances exemplify the value of a strategic initiative or an

EXHIBIT 3–1

The IVR Pyramid

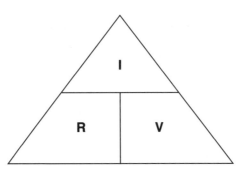

I → Income/earnings/benefit stream as defined by appraiser and appropriate to assignment

R → Risk-adjusted discount rate/cap rate/multiple risk adjusted and applicable to selected income stream

V → VALUE

Robert James Cimasi, CBI, CBC. Health Capital Consultants

investment. In most instances, we are concerned with the economic value of a business entity or business transaction when we examine the value to the healthcare delivery system.

Although value may be in the eye of the beholder, the IRS's Office of Appeals, Office of Appraisal Services, Financial/Engineering Branch considers the value of a business to be a question of fact.[3] The inherent variability in perceptions of value and the potential for fraud and abuse have driven the federal government to establish statutes addressing business valuation as early as 1920 with the U.S. Treasury Department's Appeals and Review Memorandum Number 34 (ARM 34), derived to assist in the determination of intangible value of breweries forced out of business during prohibition (ARM 34 was incorporated into IRS Revenue Ruling 68-609, a.k.a. the Excess Earnings or IRS method). The IRS and OIG have established guidelines for their reviewers in evaluating the potential for private benefit, inurement, and fraud and abuse in the development of healthcare integration activities, discussed later in this chapter and more fully in Chapter 6, *Legal Issues in the Formation and Operation of IDS Organizations.* Exhibit 3–2 indicates a chronology of healthcare regulatory activity affecting the valuation of business entities.

Any buyer's goal is to acquire goods or services at the lowest price; sellers aim to sell at the highest price. These needs usually define the market price, or the price at which a good or service is likely to be sold or purchased. In assessing the motivations of a willing buyer, the classic example of an auction sale comes to mind. The final price is determined when the last willing buyer, the high bidder, exists. Hence, value is also a question of perception. The Principle of Substitution plays a strong role in determining value. This concept states that the value of a given activity or asset (any economic or operational activity) is equal to the cost of acquiring an equally desirable substitute, or one of equivalent utility. The belief is that a purchaser would not pay more for something of equal value or utility, all things held equal. This concept drives much of contemporary thinking on establishing the value of businesses or in assessing the feasibility of alternate scenarios.

We must think also of value in terms of a willing buyer even when no actual transaction may occur. One example includes establishing the value of a professional practice for marital dissolution. Divorce courts seek generally the equitable distribution of marital property. In divorce valuation, no sale actually occurs; however, a willing buyer does exist: it is the current business owner. The standard of value is that which pertains to the marital community, such as the current owner, based on perceptions of risk and other criteria. In strategic investment analysis, discussed later in this chapter, we presume a similar willing buyer.

In Newhouse v. Commissioner, 94 T.C. 193 (1990) the U. S. Tax Court accepted four classes of willing buyers for consideration: a control investor; an active investor; a passive investor and; a public investor. This decision shaped the perception that the value of an asset (or business) may differ significantly based on the classification of the willing buyer. This concept has major impact on the value perceptions in business acquisition and the financial and feasibility analyses of differing healthcare network development strategies.

The term valuation (often synonymous with "appraisal") as used in business valuation, is generally used to mean the process by which an appraiser determines a reasonable approximation of the true economic value of a business, sometimes referred to as business enterprise value (BEV). This basic definition may be augmented or reduced depending upon the degree of precision one ascribes to the concept and the matter at hand. In examining the key issues in a valuation, the issues most often referenced include:

- A description of the property to be valued.
- The purpose of the appraisal.
- The function of the appraisal.
- Any components of the property that are specifically included or excluded, e.g., accounts receivable, personal effects, and artwork.
- The official date of appraisal, e.g., December 31, 1996.
- The applicable standard of value to be used:
  a. Fair Market Value
  b. Investment Value
  c. Book Value
  d. Liquidation Value

EXHIBIT 3–2

Chronology of Key Healthcare Milestones
Pertaining to Business Valuation

1972 Medicare Anti-kickback Statute Section 1128B[b] of Social Security Act (42 U.S.C. 1320 a – 7b[b]) provides felony criminal penalties (5 years/ $25,000.00 fine) to knowingly, willfully offer, pay, solicit or receive remuneration in order to induce business reimbursed under the Medicare or State Healthcare programs.

1986 General Counsel Memorandum (GCM) 39498 – reasonable compensation for physician recruitment – the value of the incentive must bear a discernible direct relationship to the value of the physican to the hospital – 4/24/86.

1987 Medicare & Medicaid Patient & Program Protection Act of 1987 (MMPPA) (Public Law 100-93) – Section 2 – OIG could exclude provider from future Medicare participation as civil alternative to criminal enforcement.

1987 Section 14 of Public Law 100-93 required promulgation of regulations specifying those practices that will not be subject to criminal or civil enforcement of Act—known a "Safe Harbors."

1989 Ethics in Patient Referral Act of 1989 – "Stark Bill."

1989 "Stark Referral Ban" – as part of the Omnibus Budget Reconciliation Act (OBRA) '89 – prohibits a physician from referring Medicare patients to clinical labs in which the physician or a family member has a financial relationship.

1989 Initial proposed "Safe Harbor" regulations published in Federal Register by OIG of HHS – 1/23/89 – solicited comment

1990 OBRA '90 prohibits payment of federal matching funds to state Medicaid programs for physician services unless the physician meets certain requirements and prohibits the unbundling of services by hospitals.

1991 Final "Safe Harbors" regulations published in Federal Register by OIG of HHS 7/29/91.

1991 "Hanlester Decision" – 9/91 – HHS ruled MDs in laboratory limited partnership violated law – barred from future Medicare participation.

1991 IRS General Counsel Memorandum (GCM) 39862 11/22/91 – reversed prior position and ruled that hospital sale of partial income stream jeopardized tax-exempt status, in part because payments were in violation of anti-kickback laws.

1992   OIG releases Special Fraud Alert addressing financial incentives offered by hospitals and other healthcare facilities to recruit and retain physicians – 5/7/92.

1992   Safe Harbors regulation protecting certain limited managed care activities from the reach of the anti-kickback statue was published.

1993   "Comprehensive Physician Ownership and Referral Act of 1993" – Stark II – seeks to extend coverage of present anti-kickback law by prohibiting all self-referral practices and expanding scope of services for self-referral prohibitions. Law to take effect in 1/1/95. Original Stark law applied only to Medicare referrals for clinical lab services – 1/5/93.

1993   D. McCarthy Thornton letter to IRS re: hospital acquisitions of physicians practices dated 12/22/92 is publicly released 3/15/93. Urges IRS to look at payments for: goodwill, value of ongoing business unit, covenants not to compete, exclusive dealing agreements, patient list or patient records – 3/25/93.

1993   Seven (7) new safe harbors provisions – Department of HHS eliminations of 60–40 rule for entities serving rural areas as defined by OMB and used by Office of the Census. Protection for payments/benefits offered by rural entities to recruit protect payments to physican/investors in ambulatory surgical centers group practice protections. Protection for cooperative hospital service organizations (CHSO) – 9/21/93.

1993   Congress expands the Stark law, requiring most healthcare providers to reexamine their financial relationship with physicians ("Stark II") – 8/93. Allows the HCFA to establish additional regulations necessary to protect against program abuse.

1994   Thornton letter of response to AHA Carol Stevens's letter reinforced original 12/22/92 letter.

1995   IRS issues MD recruitment/acquisition guidelines in *Hermann Hospital* case (TX).

1995   Stark II – As of January 1, 1995, prohibited designated services are expanded to include physician and occupational therapy services, durable medical equipment, and inpatient and outpatient hospital services.

1995   As of August 14, 1995, the DHHS issued final regulations interpreting the self-referral prohibitions of Stark I (42 C.F.R. Part 411).

Robert James Cimasi, CBI, CBC.
Health Capital Consultants

The Valuation Assignment: Purpose, Function, and Report Format

Clients use business valuations for many different needs. The *purpose*, or reason a valuation is needed, and the *function*, or how the valuation will be used, dictate several key issues the appraiser needs to begin the valuation. In healthcare, the predominant *standard of value* used is fair market value. Incumbent to this definition is that the property or collection of assets is deemed to have been exposed for sale on the open market for a reasonable period of time, in effect, allowing opportunity for multiple potential buyers to evaluate the offering and make bids. Hence, fair market value assumes *a hypothetical buyer and market* for determining the value of the subject business, in the geographic location of the business on the date of appraisal. Other standards of value such as investment value (used to evaluate investment return) or liquidation value (used often to obtain financing) may also be used depending on the purpose and function of the valuation.

The purpose, function, and standard of value will dictate therefore how the valuation is conducted and the type of reports that are appropriate. It is inappropriate, for example, to use a valuation developed for estate planning purposes to value a partnership interest or to value the business, or any part of its assets for sale, as many of the techniques employed by the appraiser and dictated by appraisal methodology are applied based on differing risk assumptions. Valuations of businesses are either appraisals of the business assets or of the corporate stock of the business.

Independent third-party appraisals are performed on a non-advocacy basis and appraisers must assume an independent position in rendering these opinions. Appraisal fees cannot be based on the amount rendered in the opinion of value and an appraisal engagement cannot be contingent on any additional work from a given client. Hence, appraisal engagements must be individual segments of work; discounts for volume and exclusivity of appraisal work is considered unethical. It is becoming commonplace for hospitals and health networks to utilize a single appraisal or consulting firm for all integration activity. Avoid the temptation to negotiate a fee for multiple appraisals or to restrict the appraiser from working for a competitor; the appraiser would likely be violating any appraisal organization's code of ethics by accepting such an assignment and would certainly be raising a red flag to the regulators. The hint of any impropriety on behalf of the appraiser tarnishes the end product for all parties and the appraisal profession as a whole.

Appraisals must conform with the Uniform Standards of Professional Appraisal Practice (USPAP), and should conform to the American Society of Appraisers (ASA) and the Institute of Business Appraisers (IBA) business appraisal standards and codes of ethics. Qualified appraisers are often bound by their professional associations to adhere to specific guidelines in appraisal practice. Appraisal analysis may also be performed on a consulting basis for the purpose of evaluating or negotiating on behalf of a client, much like a business broker assists clients in the sales of businesses. These analyses are not deemed to be independent appraisals generally and most often include a statement of departure identifying this relationship. Valuation analyses may serve many purposes and functions in:

- ◆ Acquisitions and Mergers
- ◆ Corporate Reorganization
- ◆ Estate/Gift/Tax Planning
- ◆ Financing
- ◆ Partnership Agreements
- ◆ Eminent Domain
- ◆ Buy-Sell Agreements
- ◆ Divorce Settlement
- ◆ Feasibility Studies
- ◆ Litigation Support
- ◆ Physician Recruitment
- ◆ Second Opinions

Business valuations are either limited or complete valuations of the subject business, with the resulting outcome and report format prepared accordingly. Exhibits 3–3 and 3–4 show a checklist of the typical data required to begin the valuation engagement. The following sections summarize the nature of limited and complete business valuations and the types of reports used most frequently.

EXHIBIT 3-3

Medical Practice Valuation
Client Data Checklist

Client:

Practice:

Date of Valuation:

☐ *Profit/Loss Statements* (in detail if possible) and *Balance Sheets* for current fiscal year to date of valuation for 4 previous years.

☐ *Federal Income Tax Returns* (corporate) and *attachments* for 4 previous years.

☐ *Gross charges per provider* (separate professional services and ancillary/technical charges if possible) for current fiscal year to date of valuation and 4 previous years.

☐ *Collections per provider* (preferably, or for the group) for current fiscal year to date of valuation and 4 previous years.

☐ *Patient visits per provider* (office visits only) and *patient treatment only visits* (chemo, IV, hydration, etc.) for current fiscal year to date of valuation and 4 previous years.

☐ *Accounts receivable aging analysis* (a.k.a. aged trial balance), by payor type if possible, as of date of valuation and end of year statements for 4 previous years.

☐ *Sample charge documents* and *practice fee schedule.*

☐ *List of employees by position and salary history* for the current year and previous 4 years.

☐ *Employment, buy/sell and/or stockholder agreements for owners/physicians* including restrictive covenants, if any.

☐ Any *written personnel or office operations policies.*

☐ *Salary and fringe benefits for physicians* for the current year and previous 4 years.

☐ *Annotated list of hard assets* owned by the practice (inventory of equipment and furnishings including nonoperational assets, i.e., autos) with original purchase price and itemized depreciation schedule.

☐ Any *significant contracts* (office lease, equipment, professional services, etc.)

EXHIBIT 3–4

Valuation Questions for Clients

Client name:
Business name:

1. Purpose of valuation: (acquisition, merger, buy-in/pay-out,
                                    divorce, etc.)

2. Function of valuation: (how the report will be used and
                                    distributed)

3. Standard of value: (e.g., fair market, liquidation, investment)

4. Date of valuation established?   (if no, suggest most recent financial
                                    quarter.)

5. Valuation of: Stock   *or*   Assets

6. Type of valuation?   Complete   *or*   Limited

7. Type of report needed: Letter   *or*   Full written
                                    Special format: Oral(?)

8. Specialty/type of business:

9. Number of *income–generating providers*/breakdown:

10. Gross revenues (last full year):

11. Is real estate involved?   Yes   *or*   No

12. Anything excluded?   (real estate, A/R, automobiles,
                                    original art)

13. Tax-exempt buyer?   Yes   *or*   No

14. Full acquisition or other?   (assets only/no employment,
                                    A/R factoring)

15. Employment involved?   Yes   *or*   No

16. Quality of data:

17. Time frame:

        How soon can they send financial data?

Limited Valuation.   Limited valuations or desktop analyses of businesses are based on a preliminary review of business operations, and often without a visit to the business location. The resulting value of these reports may be a single figure or a range of values, depending on the preference of the client. These reports always contain statements regarding the nature of analyses based on such a limited review of data, and that the results of a complete valuation analysis may differ materially from the results of a limited valuation. Limited valuations may be used by owners or buyers to obtain a rough estimate for the value of the business, or to assist clients in evaluating offers. Limited valuations are not "upgraded" generally to complete valuations, as the techniques used in a complete valuation may differ significantly. Limited valuations generally use oral or letter report formats described below.

Complete Valuation.   Complete business valuations are the result of a comprehensive analysis of the operations of the subject business. In the healthcare arena, these analyses must contain specific elements of consideration in arriving at the business enterprise value (BEV) to maintain conformance with guidelines for the use of tax-exempt funds and for issues of potential fraud and abuse. The IRS requires full written reports of complete valuations as documentation of the fair market value of the subject business for acquisition of assets by not-for-profit entities.[4] Investor-owned (for profit) entities may require full written reports for their internal use or as a safeguard against fraud and abuse issues under Stark laws. Complete valuations may be presented as oral, letter or full written reports, though the resulting value does not differ by report format. The main reason for different report formats is to reduce the expense to the client by forgoing the time and effort to produce a formal written document. The appraiser must maintain documentation on all aspects of the assignment. Oral and letter reports are often converted into full written reports in the event that the buyer decides to complete the transaction.

Report Formats.   The three main types of reports are oral, letter (also known as basic narrative or short-form reports) and full written (also known as comprehensive narrative or long-form reports) reports. Oral reports, though quite rare in healthcare, are always documented in writing, typically one to two pages in length. Letter reports may be the result of a limited or complete business valuation, but with an abbreviated report format to reduce the expense of creating a formal report document. Letter reports may range from 5 to 10 pages in length and describe the purpose, function, standard of value, approach to valuation, methods employed, discounts and/or additions to value, valuation conclusion, assumptions, and limiting conditions. Letter reports are often used by buyers to assist in purchase negotiations and are often "upgraded" to full written reports once negotiation on the purchase is completed. Similarly, business owners may use letter reports as evidence of independent appraisal for negotiating with a potential buyer. Full written reports are comprehensive business documents, frequently 70 pages or more (see Exhibit 3–5). Specialty report formats may be developed for given situations dictated by client preference.

Business valuation has made great strides in the past several years, most notably with the delineation of standards of practice in the appraisal field. Consider the following from Shannon P. Pratt, an international authority on business valuation:

> It is absolutely imperative that those responsible for preparing, reviewing, and using business appraisals be aware of both the existing standards and also the development of future standards as they evolve.[5]

The American Society of Appraisers (ASA) and the Institute of Business Appraisers (IBA) have published definitive standards for appraisal practice in the field of business valuation (see Appendix D).

LEGAL AND REGULATORY CONSIDERATIONS
Goodwill

Much of the topic of discussion over the past few years has surrounded the payment or nonpayment of goodwill and the risk of jeopardizing the tax status of the tax-exempt buyer. In light of all the analysis, it is unlikely that anyone considering acquisition is not somewhat familiar with the concept of goodwill. Hence, we will dispense with an elementary discussion and target several key issues.

EXHIBIT 3–5

Full Written Report
Sample Table of Contents

1. INTRODUCTION
   1.1   Subject of the Appraisal
   1.2   Summary Description of the Subject
   1.3   Nature and Purpose of the Appraisal
   1.4   Date of Valuation
   1.5   Ownership and Control
   1.6   Scope of Assignment
   1.7   Definitions
   1.8   Principal Sources of Information
   1.9   Assumptions and Limiting Conditions

2. ECONOMIC CONDITIONS AND INDUSTRY DATA
   2.1   Overview of the National Economy
   2.2   Overview of the State Economy
   2.3   Economic Outlook for the Local Economy
   2.4   State of the Industry
   2.5   Implication for the Subject Business

3. SURVEY OF THE SUBJECT FIRM
   3.1   History
   3.2   Form of Ownership
   3.3   Restrictions on Sale of Subject Interest
   3.4   Prior Ownership Transactions
   3.5   Subsidiaries and Affiliates
   3.6   Management
   3.7   Employees
   3.8   Product Lines
   3.9   Sales and Marketing
   3.10 Customer Base
   3.11 Competition
   3.12 Location
   3.13 Employee Stock Ownership Plan

4. FINANCIAL ANALYSIS
   4.1   Financial Statements
   4.2   Financial Statement Analysis
        4.2.1   Analysis of the Balance Sheet
        4.2.2   Analysis of the Income Statement
        4.2.3   Industry Comparison Analysis
   4.3   Summary of Analysis

The first question to address is generally whether or not good-will exists in a given business. If we define goodwill as the sum total of intangible assets of a business, then any component of total business enterprise value (BEV) that exists beyond the value of the hard assets of the business (equipment and furnishings, inventory, supplies, accounts receivable, plus or minus accruals) is intangible value, or goodwill. Although there are many elements that may suggest the existence of goodwill, the following describes the most prevalent components in the healthcare field:

- Stature of individual provider or provider organization within the industry.
- Extent and nature of referring physicians, hospitals, employers, and health plans.
- Length of time in operation of business and identification in the community.
- Publicized relationships or affiliations with hospitals and other institutions.
- Advertising campaigns, community acceptance, and reputation of the entity.
- Revenue streams.
- Proprietary interests, if any.
- Reimbursement profiles and managed care penetration of the market.
- Employment contracts, favorable leases, and restrictive covenants.
- Patient lists and medical records.

The existence of goodwill is only the first step in identifying and allocating value to goodwill. The U. S. Tax Court enumerated three methods of identifying and valuing business goodwill: the bargain method, the residual method, and the capitalization method. Consider the following excerpt from UFE, Inc. v. Commissioner 92 T.C. 88 (1989):

> The bargain method allows us to recognize the parties' arm's-length bargain as the appropriate measure of intangible value. To use the bargain method, however, the parties must have specifically bar-gained for the various items of intangible value from adverse tax

positions in arm's-length negotiations. . . The second and most well-known method is the residual method. The residual method subtracts the value of cash, cash equivalents, and tangible assets from the purchase price, and the remainder constitutes aggregate intangible value. . . The third method of valuing intangible value is the capitalization method, also labeled the "excess earnings" method. The capitalization method compares the earning potential of the tangible assets to that of an industry average. To the extent that the purchased assets generate greater earnings than the industry average, the difference is considered goodwill.

The residual method is the required method for identifying and valuing goodwill in purchase price allocations for income tax purposes.[6] The excess earnings method, though used extensively, is fraught with problems in application, determination of nominal income levels, appropriate return on net tangible assets, and appropriate capitalization rates for intangible earnings. We will examine this method in greater detail later in this chapter.

The Thornton Letter

In December 1992, Associate General Counsel, Inspector General Division (OIG) of the Department of Health and Human Services, D. McCarty Thornton, responded to an inquiry by T. J. Sullivan from the IRS Office of Employee Benefits, Exempt Organizations, regarding the application of the Medicare and Medicaid anti-kickback statute to certain types of situations involving the acquisition of physician practices.[7] This letter created something of a precedent in opinion of the OIG toward the payment of any amounts for intangible value in the acquisitions of medical practices. The letter response from the OIG questioned how certain arrangements between selling physicians and acquiring tax-exempt hospitals could adversely affect the payment for and amount of services rendered to Medicare (and Medicaid) beneficiaries. The net effect of the letter was to curtail payments of amounts previously identified as goodwill in practice acquisitions by tax-exempt organizations. In subsequent years, the IRS and OIG have softened their position through guidance issued in various internal and external documents.

Despite the threats of the Thornton letter, goodwill can and is paid anytime something is acquired at greater than its hard-asset value. Regulatory guidelines on the content and quality of practice valuations appear to leave a broad path for assigning value to intangibles. More hospitals and other organizations are paying goodwill and other physician incentives with the approval of the IRS, as documented by numerous private letter rulings requested on the integration of providers.

REQUIRED CONTENT OF VALUATIONS

Medical practice valuations must comply with federal fraud and abuse statutes in content, though no strict format has been required. The IRS published recommended elements of a medical practice appraisal in the 1993 (for FY94) Exempt Organizations Continuing Professional Education Technical Instruction Program Textbook (a.k.a. CPE textbook) and updated in its 1995 and 1996 versions. The following elements are specifically prescribed:

- ◆ "Whether the valuation placed on an asset represents fair market value (FMV) depends on the quality of the appraisal."
- ◆ "Applicant (tax exempt organization) represents that all assets acquired will be at or below FMV and will be the result of independent appraisals and arm's-length negotiations" (clarification added).
- ◆ "The business enterprise value (BEV) is defined as the total value of the assembled assets as a going concern (the value of a company's capital structure)."
- ◆ ". . . requested that in all IDS applications that the valuation provide *all recognized approaches* for determining BEV, including *the income approach, the market approach, and cost approach.* The income method is the most often relevant, as it includes the *'excess earnings method'* described in Rev. Rul. 68-609, 1968-2 C.B. 327, and was approved for the valuation of the intangible assets in Rev. Rul. 76-91. . ." (emphasis added).
- ◆ Income approach must include a discounted cash flow analysis.

- Financial statements must be adjusted or "normalized" for extraordinary occurrences.
- "... *reasonable assumptions* are made regarding rates of revenue increase, patient volume, and rates of expense increase based on current market conditions, growth, and best estimates of inflation trends" (emphasis not added).
- Base income for income-based methodologies must be on an *after-tax basis.*
- All three methods (income, market, cost) must be included in appraisal.
- "... the valuation must be based on a discount rate supportable by market transactions."
- "To ensure a correct valuation, the results of the income approach should be tested against other approaches such as market and cost."

Also referenced in the CPE textbooks are the reference to IRS Revenue Ruling 59-60, which prescribes the content for business valuations. This ruling has become a standard by which all business appraisers base their approaches to a specific engagement. Revenue Ruling 59-60 mandates that a thorough analysis of the following areas are required in the content of complete business valuations:[8]

- The nature and history of the practice or business (subject).
- The general economic outlook of the geographic market and the healthcare industry.
- The book value of the subject's stock, hard assets, and financial condition.
- The subject's earning capacity.
- The subject's dividend-paying capacity.
- The estimated value of intangible assets.
- The subject assets (a listing or other wording indicating the assets to be valued/transacted).
- Comparable enterprises and their market value, where applicable.

Appraisers and Valuation Consultants

A large number of consultants have entered the field of healthcare business and medical practice valuation with little or no formal background in valuation methodologies. Their prevalent "Rules of Thumb" in determining business value is based supposedly on market-derived units or industry formulas which prescribe a value by a "best guess" method. With increasing scrutiny by the IRS and the OIG on fraud and abuse, publications such as the OIG's Fraud Alerts and the CPE textbook articles have laid out clearly the methodologies that must be considered. A safe prediction is that all appraisers, accountants, attorneys, and valuation consultants will begin using some form of a number of different valuation methodologies to satisfy IRS/OIG guidelines on medical practice and healthcare business appraisals.

An appraiser or valuation consultant requires knowledge of the applicable standards of appraisal practice, an in-depth knowledge of the healthcare field, and the IRS/OIG guidelines for tax-exempt organizations. Appraisers should not only follow these guidelines strictly to ensure compliance on behalf of the buyer, but should also be experienced in healthcare business valuation using these methodologies to determine a reasonable approximation of the true economic value of the entity. Buyers should interview the appraiser or consultant to ensure adherence to the applicable standards. The risk in using a valuation that does not reflect accurately the BEV is a flawed valuation and the potential exists for civil and criminal sanctions under fraud and abuse laws and the loss of tax-exempt status. It is clear that the IRS and OIG will not look favorably on business valuations that are not based on these standards, given the passage of time and the numerous articles and guidance published. Business appraisers and valuation consultants, by and large, require no certification from state or federal bodies to conduct business appraisals, although professional associations including the American Society of Appraisers, the Institute of Business Appraisers, and the American Institute of Certified Public Accountants have created professional certification programs. State certifications may soon follow.

The most important factors in selecting a practice valuation consultant should include:

- Prior experience in valuing medical practices and healthcare businesses for acquisition or integration purposes.
- Demonstrated understanding of medical practice and healthcare business operations necessary to identify adjustments and assumptions required in various valuation methodologies.
- Adherence to professional standards of appraisal practice including method, presentation of information, and certifications.
- Familiarity with and adherence to regulatory guidance.
- Ability and knowledge to create a supportable opinion of value.

PRACTICAL REALITY IN HEALTHCARE BUSINESS VALUATION

The For-Profit Buyers

It seems sometimes as if the healthcare arena has been divided into those who can pay top dollar and those who can't. This is the cry of the tax-exempt IDS systems bemoaning the idea that they cannot compete with the for-profits because of issues of fair market value and tax status. The reality is that the for-profits may have some leniency from lesser IRS scrutiny; however, fraud and abuse components still exist.

For-profit buyers must be careful about paying inordinate amounts (amounts beyond the reasonable) in asset and stock acquisitions that may reflect a payment for a continued stream of Medicare and Medicaid referrals. Physician employment contracts also may be the subject of scrutiny when total compensation far exceeds the prevailing rate *in the community* for a given specialty. An example might be a medical practice negotiated selling price of $1,500,000 when the FMV appraisal indicates a value of $1,000,000 and a physician employment contract of $175,000 when the prevailing rate for family physicians in the community is $125,000.

Do the for-profits have it easier? Perhaps. Their ability to acquire stock more readily and to include stock as one component of the purchase price allows more opportunity for creative/better physician (seller) deals. Tax implications for sellers are significantly reduced in the sales of corporate stock, currently taxed as capital gains at 28% versus asset sales, which may be taxed as high as 52% including state contributions. Equity arrangements with physicians are easier, generally, given the for-profit's predisposition to investment strategies as compared to the more conservative posture assumed by many of the governing bodies of many tax-exempt organizations.

Does all this mean that the for-profits have a distinct advantage over the tax-exempt organizations, or that the playing field is so far off level that you might as well pick up and go home? Not at all. An overwhelming number of physicians believe that partnering with the for-profits is akin to selling your soul to the corporate devil. The early acquisitions of Caremark, Mullikin (now MedPartners/Mullikin), PhyCor, Pacific Physician Services, and others sent such a wave through the physician ranks that most physicians, all things being equal, would rather partner near home, with folks they know and trust (somewhat). It's the old adage, better the devil you know than the devil you don't. But what about the megaconsolidation of physician practice management companies? MedPartners, based in Birmingham, AL, merged with the Mullikin group to become the largest physician practice management company in the United States, and now has recently acquired Caremark. This consolidation creates a huge organization with estimated 1996 revenues of about $5 billion from its 7,250 physicians, and the ability to cut $15 to $20 million from purchasing and management contracts. That's clout, the kind of neighborhood bully that the local exempt hospital may well have to deal with in its own backyard. Furthermore, the arrangements they make with the selling practices typically include equity, something many developing IDSs haven't yet embraced. The opportunity to offer this type of gainsharing makes sellers think twice before selling off their retirement accounts to a simple paycheck.

VALUATION OF MEDICAL PRACTICES AND HEALTHCARE BUSINESSES

Financial feasibility studies, appraisals, and evaluations normally precede a buyer's decision to purchase a medical group. The IRS documented in the 1993 (for FY94) CPE textbook that in an evaluation for tax-exemption status (and probably fraud and abuse as well), technical documentation in the valuation should answer the following questions:

- What is the amount of the medical group's capital reserve account?
- What is the liquidity ratio (the current assets divided by current liabilities) of the medical group?
- What is the medical group's current working capital to revenue ratio (working capital divided by revenues)?
- What is the medical group's debt-to-assets ratio (total debt divided by total assets)?
- What is the medical group's long-term debt-to-equity ratio (total debt divided by equity)?
- What is the medical group's pretax return on asset ratio (pretax income divided by total assets)?
- What is the medical group's pretax return on equity ratio (pretax income divided by equity)?

The valuation report should, at a minimum, provide the data from which to calculate these ratios. A ratio analysis section, profiled by each year analyzed in the valuation, should be provided. A note of caution: Ratio analysis may serve as a useful tool in some circumstances; however, lack of comparative data may limit its transference to certain geographic areas. Some respected sources of financial and operating ratios include the Robert Morris Associates studies, Financial Research Associates studies, BIZCOMPS, and the IBA Market Data File (available to IBA members only).

Recent IRS Guidance for Medical Practice Valuation

These additional elements were described in the 1996 CPE textbook:

- OBRA requires that valuation appraisals of medical practices do not reflect indirect referral value to hospitals.
- Private benefit and inurement are prohibited.

- It is the organization's burden to establish the facts of a FMV acquisition.
- Organizations must establish that the methodology used to arrive at the price is reasonably likely to result in a final sales price consistent with (exemption).
- The existence of arm's-length bargaining may be questionable when a hospital acquires the practice of a physician on its medical staff.
- Factual assumptions upon which the valuation is based should be reviewed carefully to ensure that they are realistic, and if the valuation uses the income approach, it should be confirmed by the cost and market approaches.
- The "Allocation" process combines the use of cost, market, and income approaches.
- Replacement cost is Fair Market Value in Use (FMVIU).
- Market comparisons of actual sales should be evaluated, adjusted, and applied to operating data of seller's business to arrive at FMV.
- Weighted average cost of capital (WACC) should be used.
- Terminal value is discounted by the capitalization rate.

METHODOLOGIES AND APPROACH TO VALUATION

The following section discusses the prevalent valuation methodologies used to determine the value of medical practices, other professional practices, and small healthcare businesses.

There are three broad theories to valuation: cost, income, and market approaches. The cost theory states the value of a business is directly related to the value of the business assets and the cost to create the business in the marketplace. The income theory states that the value of the business is directly related to the earnings of the business. The market theory states the value of the business is directly related to businesses that have been sold (i.e., comparable sales). Although cost and income methods may stand alone in some cases, it is inappropriate to apply market theory without a reasonable frame of reference of market transactions in the industry being valued. In the healthcare industry, a significant volume of data does exist on the sales of medical practices. It is often difficult to obtain these comparative transactions and disparate operations between these proposed guideline companies and the subject practice often render comparability impossible. There exist few data on the sales of hospitals and medical centers and what little are available are most often anecdotal and incomparable to a given situation.

Value may be recognized also as incremental benefit. Under the Principle of Substitution, the value of a thing tends to be determined by the cost of acquiring an equally desirable substitute, and under the Principle of Alternatives, in any contemplated transaction, each party has alternatives to the transaction.[9] Given this conceptual framework, the value of an entity or collection of assets may be viewed as that which accrues to the assets given comparable alternatives in the marketplace. The incremental benefit possessed by one set of assets (e.g., the subject business) can be said to equal the cost of obtaining an equally desirable substitute, for instance, replicating it from start-up (see Exhibit 3–6). In many cases, market activity may prevent any meaningful analysis using a cost to create (reproduce) approach; reproducing the asset may be impossible

EXHIBIT 3–6

Value as "Incremental Benefit"

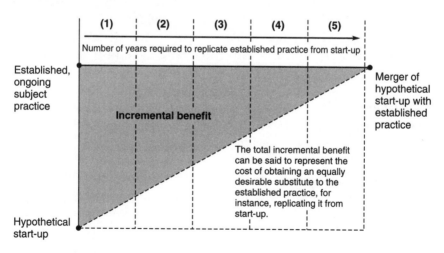

Robert James Cimasi, CBI, CBC. Health Capital Consultants

due to existing competition and other market conditions. In reality, if the market, while real and hypothetical at the same time, cannot support the use of one particular methodology, then other methods are de facto more appropriate.

Comprehensive methods of valuation consider several elements of value in arriving at an overall conclusion. Book value and adjusted book value consider the value of the practice's assets. Income methods that include the capitalization of earnings, the capitalization of excess earnings and discounted future benefits, among others, concentrate on income flows as the principal determinant of value. Valuations should include an extensive review of employment and other covenants that may appear to cause speculation in the valuation of the subject entity (an excellent example is the treatment of income of full- and part-time-employed physicians).

Book Value.   This term indicates the value of the entity as its accounting value and can inflate the value of the business as an economic concern, although it cannot generally consider the FMV of the underlying assets. Book value does not address personal and professional goodwill and may not be an appropriate measure of the value of a given entity.

Adjusted Book Value.   This term should include market values for fixed assets but is strongly affected by forces such as purchasing power and decisions made in a closely held business. Adjusted book value may be a good proxy in some cases, depending on the debt service of the concern, and the intangible and referral nature of the practice.

Liquidation Value.   This term stands for wholesale closure of the business and is typically the lowest value obtained, although not representing FMV necessarily.

Income Methods.   Income methodologies such as the *capitalization of earnings* are best applied in a sole propriety practice or single ownership because of the capability for the owner to exert total control over the growth and direction of the practice from the financial and operational perspectives. This method provides a snapshot of how expected, probable, future earnings of the concern are capitalized into value by a market-derived divisor for return on investment (capitalization rate) of businesses representing similar financial risk. It presumes a steady growth rate into perpetuity.

The *capitalization of excess earnings* (a.k.a. IRS formula method after Revenue Ruling 68-609) is an income approach to valuation wherein the tangible assets and intangible assets of the business are independently valued. The tangible and intangible assets are then combined to determine the total fair market value of the medical practice. Tangible assets are comprised of the fair market value of total operating assets minus total liabilities at the date of valuation. Intangible assets are calculated by capitalizing excess earnings. Excess earnings represent adjusted net income reduced by some reasonable industry return on net assets (i.e., earnings from tangible assets are subtracted from total earnings to arrive at earnings from intangible assets: excess earnings). Similar to a straight income capitalization, the excess earnings method presumes steady growth into perpetuity.

For all the discussion about RR 68-609 by the IRS's Office of Appeals, Office of Appraisal Services, Financial/Engineering Branch (who reviews valuations of medical practices related to acquisitions by integrated delivery systems), consider this excerpt from the IRS Appellate Conferee Valuation Training Program (1980) denouncing the use of the excess earnings method of valuation:

> One of the most frequently encountered errors in appraisal is the use of a formula to determine a question of fact, which on a reasonable basis must be resolved in view of all pertinent circumstances. . . ARM 34 has been applied indiscriminately by tax practitioners and members of the Internal Revenue Service since it was published. On occasion the Tax Court has recognized ARM 34 as a means of arriving at fair market value. The latest and most controlling decisions on valuation, however, relegate the use of a formula to a position of last resort. . . By such a formula (ARM 34) the same value would be found in 1960 as in 1933 although the values per dollar of earnings were very different in those two years. The basic defect is apparent; the rates of return which are applied to tangibles and to intangibles are completely arbitrary and have no foundation in fact. . . All that can be said for ARM 34, or a similar formula method of capitalization using two rates of interest, is that you hope to get a good answer

based upon two bad guesses. It is difficult enough to get one reasonably accurate rate of capitalization using normal appraisal methods. . . To get two fairly accurate rates, one for tangibles and one for intangibles, other than by the use of pure guesswork, is impossible. . . Any capitalization of earnings must take into consideration the economic conditions prevailing at the specific date of appraisal, including those conditions controlling in the industry in this company's area, and even in the national economy.[10]

The basic misconception is that RR 68-609 suggests absurdly low capitalization rates of 8% to 10%. These low rates do not nearly approximate the amount of risk in investing in a closely held business such as a medical practice, home health agency, nursing home, or other investment with questionable liquidity, in a potentially volatile market, in the 1990s. The best adaptation of the excess earnings method is to make two best guesses (documented analyses) on capitalization rates, based upon some foundation of belief of risk and liquidity, and to use this value as a supporting value to be considered along with values determined from other methods.

It is generally recognized that the *discounted cash flows* method is best applied in valuing stable organizations with nonconstant rates of growth. Additionally, this method is considered a good proxy for the upper limit of the fair market value.

Normalizing Income and Expenses

Because the income statements in most professional practices are prepared in a presentation format required for tax reporting rather than to report a true economic picture of the practice performance, adjustments to the statements are generally necessary.

The adjusted income statement assists reviewers in appraising the economic value of the business by establishing guidance on what constitutes expected, probable, historic, and future earnings of the concern. It is by no means, as a rule, the complete baseline from which to form the final opinion of value (see Exhibit 3–7). The adjusted income statement may be manipulated further under specific appraisal methodologies to reflect net income, debt-free income, net free income available for distribution, base income for future cash flows or future earnings, or any of a number of other income streams to be capitalized or discounted.

EXHIBIT 3-7

Reliance on Historical Data

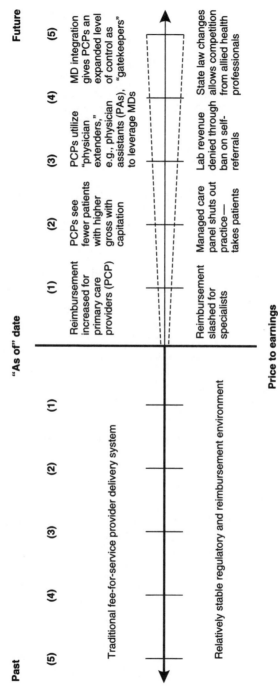

Q: How useful is past in determining value?

Robert James Cimasi, CBI, CBC. Health Capital Consultants

93

Risk Rates of Return–Income Models

As a rate-of-return comparison to other investments, discount and capitalization rates quantify the business owners' efforts. Discount and capitalization rates vary among particular types of professional practices and from one period of time to another. Expressed as a percentage, the more speculative the practice's income stream, the higher the discount rate and the capitalization rate. Conversely, the more stable the income stream the lower the discount rate and the capitalization rate. This stability or instability is typically considered "risk."

One generally accepted risk rate buildup methodology uses a weighted average cost of capital (WACC) as representative of the risk or return for the business. This risk rate is applied typically to *owner's discretionary income* defined as follows:

> Earnings before depreciation, interest, and taxes (EBDIT) adjusted by subtracting depreciation/amortization (= EBT). Then, after applicable taxes and net changes in working capital, reasonable depreciation, amortization, and capital expenditures are added back (if necessary to sustain operations), and Net Free Cash Flow is available for distribution (it should be noted that any straight capitalization of earnings uses adjusted after-tax earnings plus depreciation but not including changes in working capital, amortization, or capital expenditures, which may be adjusted into the income base).

Risk Rate Buildup and Weighted Average Cost of Capital (WACC)

As the income stream to be discounted or capitalized represents return on net free cash flow, the returns are considered to be available to holders of debt and equity of the business. Therefore, a WACC approach is appropriate using the cost of financing for the amounts of equity and debt (for additional reading on WACC, see both of Shannon P. Pratt's books *Valuing Small Businesses and Professional Practices, Second Edition* (Business One Irwin, 1993) and *Valuing a Business, Third Edition,* (Richard D. Irwin, 1996)).

The two basic components of a capitalization rate are the discount rate and a growth factor. The discount rate may be broken down into the risk-free rate of return and a risk premium return. The risk-free rate of return includes the rate of return required by an investor for the "riskless" use of his funds and a factor for expected inflation. The rate of return earned on long-term U. S. Government bonds is considered to be a good proxy for the risk-free rate of return. Let's say at the date of our hypothetical business valuation, the rate of return on a 30-year U. S. Government Treasury Bond was 6.5%. Therefore, for the purpose of building up a discount rate, the risk-free rate of return is 6.5%.

The risk premium return is the additional rate of return required by investors in the market to compensate them for the additional risk in investing in a stock security as compared to a long-term U. S. Government security. In a study published by Ibbotson Associates ("Stocks, Bonds, Bills, and Inflation Yearbook—SBBI"), it was calculated that from 1926, the average total annual returns earned on large corporate stocks (S&P 500) has been approximately 6.9% higher than the total annual returns on long-term U. S. Government bonds (this rate is determined by the most current SBBI yearbook available).[11] Therefore, we have added an additional required return of 6.9% to the risk-free rate of return to compensate investors for this "market equity risk."

In addition to the 6.9% market equity risk, the same Ibbotson Associates' study indicates that the smallest stocks traded on the New York Stock Exchange (defined as the lower 20% of the Standard & Poor's 500 Index) earned an additional 5.3% premium over the larger stocks traded on the Exchange. This "small stock risk premium" has been added to the risk-free rate of return (6.5%) and the equity risk premium (6.9%). Summing the risk-free rate of return with the equity and small stock risk premia equals the average total return required by investors to induce them to invest in the smallest stocks traded on the New York Stock Exchange.

Here is where the professional business appraiser adds his expertise in assessing the appropriate level of risk for the subject business. One school of thought indicates that investing in the stock of a closely held business involves additional elements of risk that must be compensated by offering a higher rate of return. Typically this risk is called *Investment's Beta* and is defined as a measure of systematic risk, the portion of risk that is related to movements in the general market rather than to industry- or company-specific factors.[12] Additional levels of risk may be due to specific risks associated with the industry or the company as compared to the entire marketplace.

The appraiser may choose to sum the risk-free rate of return with the equity and small stock risk premia as the total required return on investment, thereby indicating that the small stock risk premium is sufficient for the risk inherent in the business being valued. The appraiser may choose alternatively to identify and quantify additional depth of risk to be applied to the subject entity. This risk element synthesis is one of the most crucial aspects of the job of the professional business appraiser. The appraiser must identify clearly how he came about their conclusion and why the defined risk rate is consistent with the standard of value under which the appraisal is being conducted. The appraiser cannot simply and arbitrarily state a risk rate to be X amount without support. This is one of the predominant errors in business appraisal by the inexperienced (see Exhibit 3–8).

EXHIBIT 3–8

Investment Risk
Return on Investment Required to Attract Investors

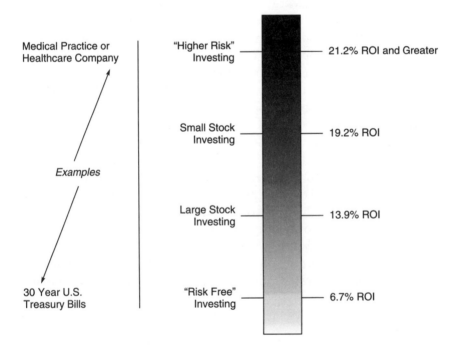

The IRS has detailed its approach in using Investment's Beta for the valuation of medical practices and healthcare concerns in the 1996 CPE textbook:

> Cost of Equity, based on the Capital Asset Pricing Model
> = Risk-Free Premium + (Beta × Market Equity Premium) + Small Stock Premium
> = 6.50 + (1.3 x 6.90) + 5.30 = 20.77
>
> ◆ Note: Beta of 1.3 is assigned by the appraiser based on supportable evidence!

Cost of Debt = Prime Rate at Date of Valuation + 1% = 9.75

> Weighted Average Cost of Capital
> = (Cost of Debt × (1 – tax rate)) × Debt % + (Cost of Equity × Equity %)
> = (9.75 × .65) × .15 + (20.77 × .85)
> = (6.34 x .15) + 17.65 = 18.60 rounded to 19%
>
> ◆ Note: Effective tax rate of 35%. The amount of debt is estimated at 15% as the typical amount of debt in the capital structure of reasonably comparable healthcare practices. This amount may be chosen by the appraiser as actual debt to equity amounts.

It should also be noted that this is only one method for developing a market-based risk rate for a given entity. There are several other acceptable methods that include greater and lesser degrees of subjective analysis. The appropriate assessment of risk must be conducted by an individual trained in investment concepts and with a firm grasp of the operations, financial performance, and geographic conditions of the subject entity as pertains to the investment climate of the economy in general and healthcare industry in particular. Remember, the final outcome of an appraisal is a supportable opinion of value. Other methods may include comprehensive assessments of industry-specific business risk that are supported by the appraiser and are appropriate to the engagement, form of organization, standard of value, and capital structure. As an example, the range of discount rates observed in the healthcare marketplace between 1993 and 1996 for WACC, debt-free analyses has been generally between 18% and 50%.

Capitalization of Earnings—Earnings Growth Method

Base Earnings = expected, probable, future earnings determined from adjusted net free cash flow.

Net free cash flow = Earnings before depreciation, interest, taxes and amortization (EBDITA). Then, after applicable taxes, depreciation is added back yielding the debt free earnings base. The total value of the subject business is then derived by a straight capitalization process using a capitalization rate developed for the business.

Discounted Cash Flows/Discounted Future Benefits

The discounted cash flows analysis is an income approach to valuation, wherein the total value of the business entity is determined by discounting projected cash flows back to the date of valuation. Then, the cash remaining at the end of the projection term flows (a.k.a. residual, terminal value, or reversion) are reduced to present value, summed with the value of the stream of cash flows, and any liabilities are subtracted to indicate total business enterprise value. The theory behind the discounted cash flows method is that an entity is worth the present value of its expected cash flow. The theory of the valuation method is sound, but the application of the approach presents some difficulty. Primarily, it is difficult to project expected levels of cash flows. The steps involved in a discounted cash flows analysis are as follows:

- ◆ Develop a risk-adjusted discount rate.
- ◆ Develop an adjusted pro forma cash flow statement.
- ◆ Discount the projected cash flows by the discount rate.
- ◆ Capitalize the Nth year projected cash flow into a residual value and discount it to the date of valuation (typically 3 to 8 years in healthcare, 10 years in less volatile industries).
- ◆ Sum the discounted cash flows and the discounted residual value to derive the operating value.
- ◆ Add or subtract nonoperating assets and liabilities.

In using the discounted cash flows methodology, the most critical step, beyond the calculation of an appropriate and supportable discount rate, is the projection of the business income and expenses. Although several different means exist for projecting these data including historical average, business regression trend line, industry trend line, percent of revenue, and manual predictions, the best approach requires a detailed understanding of the directions planned of the practice, future revenue growth, provider productivity, and salary expectations (or contractual commitments). Although it is impossible to predict the effect of all forces on healthcare systems, conservative, realizable estimates provide the basis for modeling various outcomes.

Lastly, with continuing change in the healthcare industry itself, and understanding the nature of the healthcare professional practice as a closely held business, it is wise to project future earnings only over 3 to 8 years to account for the many unknown factors that may prevent projections from becoming reality. Most healthcare appraisers would agree that primary care practices are considered more stable than specialty practices, and that companies with short operating histories are less stable than businesses with 5 or more years of experience. The more realistic and accurate the projections, the more likely the discounted cash flows technique represents the true value of the business. Furthermore, the discounted cash flows method is considered by many to be the best proxy for the upper end of fair market value. Exhibit 3–9 shows an example of a discounted cash flows analysis. As a note, the accompanying diskette includes a spreadsheet for performing a discounted cash flows analysis. Please examine the formulas and adjust where necessary. Secondly, the appendix of this text includes a present value table to assist in the calculation of the discounted cash flows.

Market-Based Methods

Market-based methods use capitalization rates and/or comparative multiples that are extrapolated from reported market transactions to derive the fair market value for the subject business. Under the market theory, three methods of valuation are considered generally: (1) actual prior transactions that have occurred within the subject

EXHIBIT 3–9

Anytown Family Practice
Estimation of Value

Discounted Cash Flows Analysis

	Normalized Financial Statement		Twelve Months Ending December 31,				Terminal Year
	1996	1997	1998	1999	2000	2001	
1. Adjusted gross revenue	1,331,968	1,646,456	1,818,823	1,887,028	1,957,792	2,031,208	
2. Total labor costs	867,712	907,920	980,738	1,057,507	1,138,412	1,223,643	
3. Total operating expenses	378,847	394,001	409,761	426,151	443,197	460,925	
4. Earnings before depreciation, interest and taxes (EBDIT)	85,409	344,535	428,324	403,370	376,183	346,640	
5. Depreciation	24,480	24,480	26,000	26,000	28,000	28,000	
6. Earnings before taxes (EBT)	60,929	320,055	402,324	377,370	348,183	318,640	
7. Effective income taxes (40% of earnings)	24,372	128,022	160,930	150,948	139,273	127,456	
8. Debt-free net income	36,557	192,033	241,394	226,422	208,910	191,184	

9. Add: Depreciation		24,480	26,000	26,000	28,000	28,000	
10. Less: Changes in debt-free working capital		40,883	22,408	8,867	9,199	9,544	
11. Less: Capital expenditures		5,000	10,000	10,000	10,000	10,000	
12. Debt-free cash flow available for distribution		170,630	234,986	233,555	217,711	199,640	199,640
13. Terminal exit value multiple							5
14. Terminal value							1,157,332
15. Present value factor @ 20% discount rate		0.83333	0.69444	0.5787	0.48225	0.40188	
16. Present value—Debt-free cash flow/terminal value		142,191	163,184	135,158	104,991	80,231	465,109
17. Sum of present value—5 years	625,755						
18. Add: Present value of terminal year	465,109						
19. Business enterprise value	1,090,864						
20. **Indicated business enterprise value (rounded)**	**1,100,000**						

entity, such as a previous sale of the business or a buy-in or pay-out of owners; (2) comparison with aggregated data of private multiples from comparable business sales; and (3) comparison of private multiples from specific, identified sales of *guideline companies* deemed as reasonably comparable to the subject entity. One word of caution: it is difficult to compare practices or businesses with similar earning histories and locations. There are many tangible and intangible factors that affect these comparisons and in many cases, sufficient data are not available to establish reasonable comparability between businesses. The appropriate application of this technique to a given comparable business requires that the guideline company financial statements be adjusted (as one would normally do with any valuation) and comparisons made to the subject entity. This normalizing of data provides the most substantial basis for comparison. Other methods include utilizing large numbers of market transactions of reasonably comparable businesses to derive multiples for comparison. The large blocks of transactions normalize outliers and provide considerable power to the application of this technique. As an example, the IBA Market Data File has transaction data on over 500 dental practice sales. Even after excluding outlier and obvious incomparable transactions, these data provide considerable insight into the overall market value of dental practices. As one may imagine, many obvious intangible elements may be impossible to compare including patient friendliness, location, years in practice, small town acceptance, and so forth.

Allocation of Purchase Price Technique:
Tangible and Intangible Assets

Business enterprise value (i.e., fair market value) determined under an income approach is often greater than the combined fair market value of equipment, furnishings, and fixtures determined under a cost approach because it includes the intangible value of the business as a going concern, for instance, the goodwill of the business. The value of goodwill can be allocated to the specific intangible assets using the residual method; the value of the latter limited to the value of the former, as calculated under the income approach.[13] Consider the following example:

Clinical Records.   Lakeway Rehabilitation, a fictitious business, maintains an excellent system and complement of clinical records totaling approximately 2,650 records. Of this number, roughly 1,100 records are from patients seen within the last 24 months at both Milford and Salem sites. The remaining records, approximately 1,550, remain on site in Milford. The majority of the records contain typewritten notes transcribed from recorder or entered directly from personal computer. One of the therapists, Kirsten Easley, prefers to hand write clinical notes that appear upon review to be legible and complete. The practice maintains a system for quality assurance in conjunction with their medical director, Dr. Johnson, and is making plans for implementing a more detailed QA monitor regarding the clinical care of patients and medical records. Using a common means of establishing the value of medical and clinical records, the cost approach is applied. This category may also be addressed as custodial rights of medical records.

Assembled Workforce.   An assembled workforce is a valuable asset to any operating business. The time, effort, and lost wages required to train and assemble a staff can be considerable. One estimate of this effort often used is one month's salary of all staff including therapists.

Practice Operating Policies and Procedures.   An operating business was not operating very smoothly on the first day it opened for business. In addition to a trained and assembled workforce, the established business maintains operating policies and procedures that contribute directly to its ability to generate revenue. Many businesses maintain completely developed, tested, and written policies and procedures as well as routine business paperwork such as patient history and encounter forms, invoices, laboratory and clinical forms, and materials that are intangible assets of the business. The replacement cost method is used most often to value these items based on the time spent among clerical, administrative, technical, and professional staff (including physician time) to develop and implement in the current business. A documented and supportable opinion of the value of these items is essential to the correct application of the Asset Accumulation Approach.

Proprietary Tests, Profiles, Treatment Plans, and Clinical Protocols. The average medical or professional healthcare patient care practice does not have a significant investment in the development of specific panels for laboratory tests, disease, or event-specific patient plans of treatment, or clinical protocols. For practices that have developed internal models for enhancing clinical or administrative effectiveness, these models can be of enduring intangible value to the business. Efforts should be made to identify the existence of these items of clinical and administrative guidance and the appraiser should quantify and allocate the value of these items using the replacement cost method.

Covenants. Restrictive covenants of all types are increasingly found in healthcare. Most often included in provider employment agreements, they restrict the competitive practices of sellers from competing in the same or similar lines of business with the buyers of the tangible and intangible assets of their former business. The following outlines several types of restrictive covenants and their applicability to the subject practice.

Covenants between individual employee provider and the selling professional practice (employer) exist between Dr. A and Dr. B as per their shareholders agreement. This sample covenant states:

> *in the event that a shareholder decides to resign from or otherwise is required to terminate his or her affiliation with the corporation and to sell his or her shares of stock in the corporation [as provided herein], then he or she agrees not to compete with the corporation within a 15 mile radius of the City of Milford, Connecticut, in that he or she shall not be employed by or contract with a medical facility or hospital to provide physician services within the aforestated area for a period of one (1) year. The resigning or terminated shareholder agrees not to assist or participate in any way for a three (3) year period in the establishment of a similar or like physician services within the designated area.*

This is a basic covenant that employers often make and that is frequently purchased by buyers who desire to purchase all business assets.

A *covenant between the individual selling provider and the buyer* is more prevalent in the acquisition of a business. This covenant similarly protects the purchasing organization from the effects of an "employee" leaving and creating his own business, taking with him substantial goodwill for which the employer, or buyer, has already paid. It is expected that a covenant of this type will be required of Dr. A and Dr. B in the event they sell their business and are employed as physicians.

Lastly, a *covenant between the selling practice and the buyer* is one where the practice, as a whole, agrees not to compete with the buyer within a specific geographic location for a specific period of time. Typically this type of covenant is superseded by one or both of the above covenants.

Given the referral and personal services nature of medical practices, generally, and of a given practice specifically, it is clear from the tangible asset analysis and the adjusted income statement that significant value derives from the personal goodwill of Dr. A and Dr. B and, to a lesser extent, the professional goodwill of Lakeway Family Practice. Future income flows are affected further by changes in the current and historical payor mix of the practice's patients, which include considerable portions of Medicare, Blue Cross/Blue Shield, and Workers Compensation, the growing self-referral segment in many specialties in Connecticut, the growing managed care environment, the beginning of capitation, new entry into both the Milford and Salem communities, and changes in the referral relationships of physicians.

Trade Name.   The income that flows from the recognition of the trade name of the organization can be an important enduring asset to the business, particularly when the practice has operated in the same geographic area for a reasonable length of time. The premise of value of the trade name of an organization rests upon the ability for patients, and to a lesser extent, referring physicians, to choose to frequent the business. In healthcare, a medical practice or private personal services practice operating under the provider's name, e.g., Marsha Winter, M.D., may have more personal goodwill than business goodwill related to a trade name. The criteria for valuing a trade name typically includes history of patient choice in location of care (which presents immediate difficulties in the area of physical therapy in Connecticut, and other states), individual provider reputation, longevity, history, innovation, rate of acquisition of new patients, and historical advertising of the name.

Valuation Synthesis

Appraisers expect a range of values when applying numerous valuation methodologies. The expected outcome occurs when these amounts fall in a narrow range of values.[14] Outlier estimates do occur for several reasons, each worth examining in its own right, and the reasons for these values should be understood by the appraiser. The following example was taken from a recent appraisal:

> In our evaluation of Lakeway Family Practice we have calculated and analyzed a variety of approaches to valuation. The following is a listing of the specific approaches we have examined:

Book Value	329,195
Adjusted Book Value	218,048
Liquidation Value	113,303
Capitalization of Earnings	1,303,968
Discounted Cash Flows	1,215,214
Market Approach	1,180,210
Initial Conclusion:	1,200,000

Discounts and Premiums for Control and Marketability

The overall value of the business in the specific marketplace may be more or less than initially determined by any individual appraisal method due to factors affecting the marketability of the business. Marketability deals with the liquidity of the asset. Additionally, each owner's individual value may not be directly related to the percentage of ownership due to the existence of, or lack of control.

Minority Discount. The minority discount is a reduction in value of an individual owner's share of the business due to lack of control to direct business decisions such as declaring dividends, liquidating, going public, issuing or buying stock, directing management, and so forth. In many practices and businesses where owners maintain equal positions and control over management decisions, minority share discounts are rare. Minority discounts are seen generally when the purpose of the valuation is to estimate the value of a minority position such as seen in the circumstances of a minority partner buy-in or a financing arrangement.

Control Premium.   A control premium is an addition to value of an individual owner's share of the business for the right to make corporate decisions such as declaring dividends, liquidating, going public, issuing or buying stock, directing management, and so on. Control premiums may also be an issue when a specific position contains the ability to effect a swing vote in the governance of the business. An example might be that when a third partner joins a group and the final ownership will be an equal third of the business, the new partner will have the ability to "team up" with one other to make corporate decisions. Similarly, a 10% or 20% partner may have this swing position, which may increase his overall percentage of value greater than face value.

Marketability Premium or Discount.   The marketability premium is an increase in overall business value due to the attractiveness and ready market of the business. It is reflected most often in initial public offerings of securities, and is rarely seen in the purchase of a closely held business. The healthcare field seems to be a growing exception as hospitals, health networks, provider organizations, and managed care organizations are acquiring provider practices. Marketability premiums are then an additional "bump" in value, often in the range of 10% to 20% for a specific, highly desired business in a very active marketplace. Quantifying, documenting, and supporting marketability premia are very difficult, reflecting the fact that they are seen rarely.

The marketability discount is a reduction in overall business value due to a stock restriction or prohibition such as no ready market, security law restrictions, buy-sell agreements, rights of first refusal restrictions, and shareholder agreements.

There have been numerous studies detailing statistics on lack of marketability that have pertinent bearing on the valuation of medical practices and healthcare businesses (SEC Institutional Investor Study[15]; Milton Gelman[16]; Robert R. Trout[17]; Robert E.

Moroney[18]; J. Michael Maher[19]; and Willamette Management Associates[20]). From these studies, the average discount for lack of marketability for restricted shares of publicly traded companies was 35%. There is strong evidence to suggest that closely held businesses suffer much more from lack of marketability than do publicly traded entities.[21] The vast majority of healthcare business valuations, therefore, will contain some form of a discount for lack of marketability: the liquidity of these types of businesses are not the same as other forms of investment.

In a debt-free calculation, it is inappropriate to apply a full discount for lack of marketability, which we see may be as high as 35% or greater. The preferred approach is to apply the discount on a debt-free basis, although it is generally recognized that no data exist to make this adjustment. Under most circumstances, discounts for lack of marketability range from approximately 10% to 25%. This general statement is not meant to be given lightly. The essence of a proper business appraisal is its ability to convey a supportable opinion of value. An appraiser cannot spend 40, 60, or more hours evaluating a closely held business and simply reduce its value by 25% without substantial justification. On the other hand, it is inconceivable to believe that the marketability of a majority position in a closely held business is equal to that of minority shares of a publicly traded entity. Lastly, given the broad nature of variability in application of valuation techniques and the overall dollars in question, a difference as great as 10% in purchase price may not be a significant issue for buyers or sellers. Most physician-related deals fall apart either for philosophical reasons or because the purchase price perceptions differ by 50% or more.

QUESTIONS AND ANSWERS

Areas of Dispute in Valuation

Business valuation is far from an exact science. The idiosyncrasies of each business, marketplace, and the experience and preferences of the appraiser contribute to the final opinion of value rendered. This discussion addresses each method of traditional valuation and highlights areas subject to dispute and/or abuse in practice and interpretation.

Q   *What are the most important issues in adjusting the balance sheet and income statements?*

A   Place yourself in the shoes of the prudent businessman. To examine the economic operations of a business, the prudent businessman:

- Reduces physician/owner compensation and benefits to FMV for physician professional services only.
- Reduces staff compensation and benefits to local market rates for the classification of employee and job actually performed. Limited consideration is given to years of experience unless increased expense can be objectively demonstrated.
- Adds all "excess" compensation back to income.
- Adjusts any unusual or one-time expenses such as periods of double rent or other expenses charged or categorized not consistent with generally accepted accounting principles (GAAP) to derive representative income.
- Allows expenses typical of the business (automobile, cellular, or computer expenses) deemed to be legal and appropriate as business use only.
- Allows depreciation at rate of economic decline—expect 10 to 15 years for most assets.
- Adjusts all leases to fair market rate (not at favorable rates obtainable by owners or potential buyer) as required.
- Removes nonoperating assets, income, and liabilities from adjusted asset and income statements.
- Adjusts for non-business-related sales or acquisitions (e.g., gain or loss on sale of equipment).

Q   *Mechanically, what types of adjustments should I see under hard assets?*

A   Watch for the following adjustments:

- Cash and other highly liquid assets not typically sold are removed generally.

- Accounts receivable adjustments are appropriate and reasonable; poor A/R aging (a.k.a. aged trial balance) or nonexistent aging schedules are believed to represent "poor A/R" and should be discounted significantly.
- Any booked intangibles are removed.
- Liabilities will likely carry over at full value (except in unusual circumstances where the business has not refinanced an unusually high interest rate on an outstanding note).
- Cost methods are reasonable and any intangible components are supported by revenues.
- Rules of thumb fairly value intangible components and reliance on these methods is not excessive.

Q   *What are the key areas to watch in the methods of valuation themselves?*

A   The following issues are the subject of most of the complaints or scrutiny in business valuation:

Income Methods

- Capitalization and discount rates have demonstrable basis in market transactions reflecting rates of return for similar investments.
- Earnings methods use and appropriately estimate a representative earnings flow number.
- Excess earnings return on equity has basis in fact and is balanced against reasonable liquidity of the existing capital structure.
- Excess earnings premium (often 15% or greater than "normal" capitalization rate) is applied when business is earning in upper 25% of its industry.
- Discounted future benefits methods are often contested because of the numerous component variables; nevertheless, they may be an excellent means to profile future returns.
- Income projections should be realistic and profile the most likely growth scenario for the business.

- Rates of growth of revenue and expenses should be supported by market observations (e.g., medical care component of Consumer Pricing Index) and established plans for expansion or development of the business.
- Income projections must support amortization of purchase price in FMV appraisals. Inability to do so may indicate excessive physician compensation for business income, incorrect budgeting, and/or excessive purchase price.
- Discounted future benefits should only consider future income streams that are reasonably definable (i.e., income beyond 5 years becomes more speculative and a client's insistence on this period may require a risk calculation that obliterates business value).
- The income residual should be capitalized into value *by the capitalization rate—not the discount rate*—before being discounted to present value.

Market Methods

- Prior transactions within previous 5 to 7 years should be considered valid unless highly significant changes in business operations have occurred as evidenced by trend analysis or if intangibles were excluded.
- Market (private) comparisons, if used, should be of similar type businesses (i.e., specialty, geographic locale, population density, size, revenue, or owner compensation).

Adjustments for Control and Marketability

- Discounts for lack of marketability of either owner's shares or of the entity as a whole should be carefully scrutinized under all conditions.
- The presence of multiple potential buyers in a given market in an acquisition valuation may be some evidence against a marketability discount unless previous restrictions exist (e.g., existing right of first refusal to purchase, certain buy-sell and shareholder agreements, security law restrictions).

◆ Stock, ownership, and partnership dissolution valuations may have significant marketability discounts.

Valuation Conclusions

◆ Asset methods should serve as guidelines, especially when the business appears to have no significant intangible value.

◆ Liquidation value should be used in rare cases.

◆ Reliance on Rules of Thumb should be minimized.

◆ Earnings methods (Capitalization of Earnings and Excess Earnings) are used appropriately with the type of business, i.e., sole proprietorship, partnership, etc.

◆ Discounted future benefits are always considered (except when excluded by law) when using the standard of FMV.

◆ Private comparison value derivatives should fairly represent subject practice; out of date comparisons should be discarded.

◆ Valuation synthesis by weighted average may consider all valid approaches for the subject entity, but has no empirical basis in fact.

◆ Final opinion of value using FMV should be supported by postsale, after-tax cash flows with business purchased under market terms, within a reasonable period of time. General rule: business flowing cash from operations independently within 1 to 2 years and payback of amortized expenses within 5 to 7 years (depending on the size of the business).

STRATEGIC INVESTMENT VALUE IN HEALTHCARE

A Model for Quantitative and Qualitative Analysis of Investments

The cost of capital, either debt or equity, varies from one buyer to another. Fair market value dictates that capitalization and discount rates should be representative of market consensus. In healthcare,

Medicare fraud and abuse laws and use of certain tax-exempt funds further dictate that acquisitions use fair market value as the standard for appraising entities for acquisition and other types of integrated activities.

In analyzing the value of an investment, such as acquiring or affiliating with a healthcare provider organization or evaluating a new business product/line or start-up activity, the capitalization and discount rates are based on *the buyer's cost of capital, risk perceptions, and other relevant factors* (interest rate, outlook for business, etc.). The difference between discounting future returns of a business based on market perceptions and the internal cost of capital or investment interests of a large (buyer) organization may be substantial. This difference, combined with an investment risk profile using capitalization and discount rates 10% to 20% less significantly affect the return on investment profile. Please note that choosing to purchase a practice or business solely to acquire a stream of income (which is reimbursed by Medicare/Medicaid) raises serious fraud and abuse issues. Organizations should have sound reasons for pursuing acquisitions, which include community benefit, prior to any strategic investment analysis.

Return on Investment

Equity refers to the owner's interest in a business or property. Most businesses are financed by a combination of equity and debt, which represents the total investment or invested capital. As an example, from a valuation calculated to support a fair market opinion of value:

Return on Equity

Return on equity (ROE) is defined as follows:
Earnings/Equity

Example: A business has pretax earnings of $35,261 and equity of $256,852; the ROE would be

$$\$35,261 \; / \; 256,852 = 14\%$$

Return on Invested Capital

Return on invested capital (ROI) is defined as follows:
EBIT / Investment

Example: A business has $50,000 of interest-bearing debt and $256,852 equity, and it paid $5,000 in interest on the debt and had $35,261 of pretax earnings. The ROI would be

$$\frac{\$5,000 + \$35,261}{\$50,000 + \$256,852} \text{ equals } \frac{\$40,261}{\$306,852} \text{ equals } 13\%$$

To view the investment return as *total cash available from the investment*, that is, including depreciation, we have:

ROI for Total Investment is defined as follows:
EBDIT / Investment

$50,495 + $25,500 = 75,995 / $340,000 = .224 or 22% where $50,495 is pretax net income, $25,500 is depreciation, and $340,000 is the total purchase price

This calculation takes into account total cash available, which dictates an unfunded depreciation account. While most small businesses do not fully fund depreciation, some allowance for replacement should be considered. Note: any unused contingency amounts should also be added back.

Appropriate Rate of Return on Tangible Assets

Consider the following two statements from *Valuing Small Businesses and Professional Practices:*[22]

> There is strong consensus among valuation professionals that the appropriate return rate for tangible assets in the earnings-based methodologies depends on the asset mix in each case. Assets that are highly liquid, low risk, and/or readily acceptable as loan collateral require lower rates of return than assets that are less liquid, more risky, and/or less acceptable as collateral.

This is certainly the case when applying methods such as the capitalization of earnings and excess earnings methods.

> Asset values play a large role in determining collateral. Since loans are not usually made for 100% of collateral, and since there are some costs to borrowing money that are in addition to the basic interest

rate, *the rate of return on net tangible assets used must be at least a few points above the rate at which bank loan money is available to them* (emphasis added).

As we have stated previously, the internal rate of return desired by the buyer for investment purposes varies from buyer to buyer. A company desiring a minimum return on investment of 6% to 8% may choose to project its income targets to reach this goal. They may also choose wisely to tie employment contracts to achieving these minimum thresholds. Capital financing rates may vary accordingly.

An analysis of investments should include profiling both the value of any acquisition or start-up venture, the simple and ultimate cash flow requirements, the purchase terms including cost of financing, amortization of purchase price, and appropriate return on investment desired. This modeling effort is not complicated although it is detailed. Most of the income-based valuation analyses should be recast under various sets of assumptions to obtain the most likely scenario of outcome. The ultimate consideration of strategic investments includes the specific consideration of market activities and the cost of not pursuing a given option (e.g., acquisition, start-up) or of alternative actions.

Internal Strategic Investment Analysis

Reassessing the Value Opinion.   We will recall that a valuation made using the standard of fair market value must be recast to address investment issues. In examining the strategic value of an investment, we take several issues into consideration:

- ◆ Adjusted financial statements are accepted as with FMV standard, or preferably hypothetical post sale *pro forma* cash flow statements are used.
- ◆ The buyer establishes:
  - **a.** The internal rate of return for tangible assets and/or the business as a whole.
  - **b.** The required rate of return (discount rate).
  - **c.** The purchase terms and cost of debt and equity capital (usually internal rate plus hurdle rate, if any).
  - **d.** Details in employment, compensation, capital, and operational budgeting.

In strategic investment analysis, we ask:

- ◆ Could you generate this ROI from other sources?
- ◆ Could you invest these funds elsewhere and get the same ROI?
- ◆ What community benefit results from this acquisition, affiliation, or new venture?
- ◆ Can you afford *not* to pursue this venture due to other network plans?
  - a. Managed care initiatives—preparation or reaction.
  - b. Employees/dependents require more network physicians.
  - c. Physicians leaving community.
  - d. Physicians retiring.
  - e. Counter competitor overtures or ingress into market.
- ◆ Are there alternatives that will yield similar, positive post-sale/affiliation outcomes?
  - a. Other forms of physician integration activities.
  - b. Other forms of community service activities.

Internal Strategic Investment Analysis—Acquisition of a Primary Care Practice. Business: Lakeway Family Medicine
The buyer has established the following:

- ◆ Rate of return for the business based on operating *pro forma*.
- ◆ Required rate of return (discount rate): 12%.
- ◆ Internal cost of capital: 8%.
- ◆ Cash flows examined for 10-year term @ 8% (recognizing speculative nature of years 5 to 10).
- ◆ Taxable or Tax-exempt entity under following scenarios:
  - a. Cash sale.
  - b. 100% internal financing at 8% interest over 12 years.
  - c. 20% downpayment with balance at 8% over 12 years.
  - d. 50% downpayment with balance at 8% over 12 years.
  - e. Recommended level of capitalization profile.
  - f. No changes from *pro forma* employment, compensation, capital, and operational budgeting details.

Changes in Valuation Opinion.   The present value of the future income stream will be calculated by substituting a 12% discount rate as the buyer's required rate of return for this investment. By assuming a 12% discount rate, the buyer believes:

- The *pro forma* performance of this investment is considered to be an in-house operation (for a hospital, another source of nonoperating revenue) and its operational efficiency is evaluated as any other in-house operation is evaluated.
- This investment is worth $X *to the buyer*, based on their justification of how they choose to use internal funds (taking into account the opportunity cost of capital).
- The return on investment profile over the 5-year period, plus the residual value of the business, is satisfactory to pursue this business acquisition. Note: The market value of the business may not change significantly; it does not parallel any internal strategic value.
- The indirect benefit to the organization is consistent with the mission and goals of the institution and good business practice.

Internal Strategic Investment Analysis Results.   Using a 12% discount rate, the present value of the 5-year projected income stream increases from $348,616 to $878,250. To restate this, *the buyer judges the present value of the future stream of income to be worth up to $878,250 in 1996 dollars, based on their own internal needs and expectations for investments,* yet they are purchasing this income stream for only $348,000 (unadjusted for inflation).

Conservative business practice in healthcare would seek total ROI within 5–7 years, due to uncertainties in managed care growth and changes in healthcare in general. In this example, the yield on financing of 8% on the original investment is in addition to overall ROI, any retained earnings of the business, and the residual value of the business at the end of the term.

Importance of Community Benefit in Strategic Investment Analysis

The area of community benefit and the use of certain tax-exempt funds "which contribute directly and substantially" to the purpose for tax exemption should be considered. Healthcare organizations must include these often indirect benefits and weigh them accordingly. These local community issues are as individual as the communities themselves. Some examples include:

+ Improved access to physicians and/or healthcare services.
+ Retention or recruitment of providers.
+ Improvement in treatment modalities.
+ Pooling diverse areas of expertise (e.g., telemedicine/subspecialty consultations in rural areas).
+ Lower cost services for patients.
+ Improved patient convenience.

It is possible to profile many of circumstances to determine the best alternative in any given network venture. The scope of this type of analysis is limited principally by time and effort.

DETERMINING THE VALUE OF HEALTHCARE FACILITIES, NETWORKS, AND IDS COMPONENT ENTITIES

As stated previously, the existence of market data on actual transactions of the sales of hospitals, nursing homes, ambulatory, intermediate, long-term, or assistive living facilities and their holding companies is scarce, at best. We have seen that market comparisons may be made from actual transactions from within the subject entity, or from specific identified guideline companies' adjusted financial and sales multiples. Using these criteria, it is nearly impossible to accurately apply market models of appraisal to the sales of these entities. Yet this appears to be a significant benchmark, if not the predominant method of valuation in the marketplace.

The June 17, 1996, issue of *Modern Healthcare* reported the price/earnings multiple method of valuation used by Wall Street investors when examining the value of hospital companies. The data suggest that the preferred method for valuing Columbia/ HCA, Health Management Associates, OrNda HealthCorp, Tenet Healthcare, Quorum Health Group, Universal Health Services, and Community Health Systems was a multiple of earnings before interest, taxes depreciation, and amortization (EBITDA) ranging from 6.1 times EBITDA to 14.8 times EBITDA. Four companies (Columbia/HCA, OrNda, Tenet and Quorum) ranged from 6.9 to 7.5 EBITDA. Readers may assume correctly that these amounts reflect some belief of investment value in the future earnings of these companies. The question is, how do we evaluate whether or not these amounts are "right"?

Consider the following real example: A hospital sought to purchase a skilled nursing facility (SNF) in a community. SNFs are controlled by most state's Certificate of Need laws, thereby eliminating the "make" option and severely restricting the "buy" option to only those who will sell at fair market value. One SNF facility in the area is interested in selling at 10 times EBDITA ($5,400,000 on earnings of $540,000) because that is what it feels is the selling price for SNFs, and because the owner has signed a long-term management contract for the facility (management needs to buy out the contract upon sale). Breaking down the issue, the appraiser consultant used/determined: (1) $540,000 is expected, probable future earnings; (2) an appropriate risk rate representative of market consensus (FMV standard); (3) an estimated capitalization rate; (4) a market appraisal (guideline company) and/or range of market transactions, nationally and from that state; and (5) an estimate of liabilities, capital expenses, and depreciation. The result was that the appraiser determined that 10 times EBDITA was equivalent to a capitalization rate of 10%. A discounted cash flows analysis with a generous 20% (debt-free) discount rate indicated a BEV of $3,200,000 (recall that the DCF is generally a good proxy for upper end of FMV). The guideline company method indicated a BEV of $3,500,000. The market method using the price-to-earnings ratios and price-per-bed ratios for SNFs across the state (as reported from actual sales by a national trade organization) yielded a BEV of $3,700,000.

From these results, it is likely that the SNF seller is actually basing their value of the facility not on an earnings multiple of 10, but on some predetermined amount plus the buyout of the management contract. From a valuation perspective, FMV determines the value of the entity free and clear of encumbrances or liabilities; the value of the SNF is after owner's reduction of the management agreement buyout. But this raises another issue similar to the statement at the beginning of this chapter: What is the value of a highly regulated, capital-intensive business with a high asset book value *with a generally good projected financial performance?* The difference is: the long-term care market. It is more stable than most other components of the healthcare delivery system, its revenue projections are more stable, its regulation and entry into the marketplace are arguably more stable, and it is a growing industry. The question becomes, is this an industry, and is the subject SNF, a reasonable candidate for a marketability premium? The answer is: maybe so. Working in individual situations, the professional appraiser consultant will guide the client through this understanding and develop a supportable opinion of value based on the circumstances surrounding the subject business, including all aspects of business and market analysis indicated in IRS Revenue Ruling 59-60.

Recall that an investor's decision to pursue may be based on factors other than strict performance of a given entity or group of entities, as in a health system purchase. In the acquisition, merger, partnering, or affiliation of healthcare entities, organization vision and goals dictate the need for embarking on strategies of system growth. From a value perspective, the vision and needs of the healthcare system guide the decisions that determine the options it must take to be successful, be that a local hospital, regional primary care IDN, or regional network of all levels of care. This is the principal reason for the development of taxable lines of business within exempt organizations. As these institutional providers move along the integration continuum, different structures and organizations will emerge that will allow investment strategies broader entry to serve system goals.

One of the most compelling arguments on building value is supported by Richard Normann and Rafael Ramirez: the secret of creating value lies in an organization's ability to build a "value creating system, within which different economic actors—suppliers, business partners, allies, customers—work together to co-produce value."[23] Robert Kaplan and David Norton suggest organizations develop a "balanced scorecard" linking financial perspectives with those of internal business (At what must we excel?), innovation and learning (How can we continue to improve and create value?), and customer perspective (How do customers see us?).[24] The challenge for the rest of us is to make informed decisions based on where we want to go and the means we have to get there.

NOTES

1. U. S. Internal Revenue Code (U. S. Government Printing Office, Washington, DC, Section 20.2031-1(b)).

2. James J. Unland, *The Valuation of Hospitals and Medical Centers* (Chicago: Probus Publishing Co., 1993), p. xi.

3. U. S. Internal Revenue Service, *IRS Appellate Conferee Valuation Training Program* (Chicago: Commerce Clearing House, 1980), pp. 82–86.

4. U. S. Internal Revenue Service, *IRS Exempt Organization Continuing Professional Education Technical Instruction Program Textbook* (Washington, DC, 1993), pp. 235–36.

5. Shannon P. Pratt, et al., *Valuing Small Businesses and Professional Practices, Second Edition* (Burr Ridge, IL: Business One Irwin, 1993), p. 4.

6. U. S. Tax Code 1.338 (b)-2(T).

7. IRS *Exempt Organization Program, 1994*, pp. 185–90.

8. U. S. Internal Revenue Service, *Revenue Ruling 59-60* (Chicago: Commerce Clearing House, 1960).

9. Raymond C. Miles, *Basic Business Appraisal*, (Boynton Beach, FL: Southeast Business Investment Corporation, 1984), p. 22.

10. U. S. Internal Revenue Service, *IRS Appellate Conferee*, pp. 82–86.

11. Ibbotson Associates, *Stocks, Bonds, Bills and Inflation Yearbook* (1996).

12. Shannon P. Pratt, et al., *Valuing a Business, Third Edition*, (Burr Ridge, IL: Richard D. Irwin, 1996), p. 166.

13. IRS Exempt Organization Program, 1996, p. 428.

14. Shannon P. Pratt, et al., *Valuing Small Businesses*, p. 280.

15. "Discounts Involved in Purchases of Common Stock," in U. S. 92nd Congress 1st Session, House, *Institutional Investor Study Report of the Securities and Exchange Commission* (Washington, DC: Government Printing Office, March 10, 1971), 5:2444–56, Document No. 92-64, Part 5.

16. Milton Gelman, "An Economist-Financial Analyst's Approach to Valuing Stock of a Closely Held Company," *Journal of Taxation*, June 1972, pp. 353–54.

17. Robert R. Trout, "Estimation of the Discount Associated with the Transfer of Restricted Securities," *Taxes*, June 1977, pp. 381–85.

18. Robert E. Moroney, "Most Courts Overvalue Closely Held Stocks," *Taxes*, March 1973, pp. 144–54.

19. J. Michael Maher, "Discounts for Lack of Marketability for Closely-Held Business Interests," *Taxes*, September 1976, pp. 562–71.

20. Shannon P. Pratt, et al., *Valuing a Business*, p. 341.

21. Shannon P. Pratt, et al., *Valuing Small Businesses*, p. 280.

22. Shannon P. Pratt, et al., *Valuing Small Businesses*, p. 221.

23. Richard Normann and Rafael Ramirez, "From Value Chain to Value Constellation: Designing Interactive Strategy," *Harvard Business Review* 71, no. 4 (July–August 1993), pp. 65–77.

24. Robert S. Kaplan and David P. Norton, "The Balanced Scorecard—Measures that Drive Performance," *Harvard Business Review* 70, no. 1 (January–February 1992), pp. 71–79.

CHAPTER

4

BUSINESS ACQUISITIONS AND FINANCIAL PLANNING

BUSINESS ACQUISITIONS, TRANSACTIONS, AND RELATIONSHIPS

The nature of the healthcare industry, and industries in general, is that market forces will create change in operation, form, and ownership of many businesses throughout their life span. As members and students of the healthcare industry, we have become quite accustomed to this reality and have seen the growth, consolidation, and demise of many of our neighbor institutions. Business transactions—specifically, business acquisitions and administrative and clinical business transactions—have become part of every administrator's skill set, or should be. Practice managers negotiate managed care contracts while chief financial officers pour over the details of asset purchases and deferred compensation agreements. The following sections describe key issues in handling business acquisitions and transactions, beginning with some topical overviews and moving into acquisition and transaction issues common to the most frequent styles of integration.

Medical Practices

A recent study reported by the Center for Healthcare Industry Performance Studies and Findley, Davies & Co. reported that hospitals paid more for practices with medium managed care penetration (40% to 52% of residents enrolled in an HMO or PPO) with an average sale price of $134,000 per physician, 41% higher than that paid in lower-managed markets and 26% higher than that paid in high-managed-care markets.[1] The study suggests that hospitals pay higher prices as the market is developing; prices then drop off near peak managed care penetration. The study further examined acquisition price and employment terms and found that hospitals are often willing to pay more in purchase price while keeping salary levels modest.

Given this recent history and the state of managed care penetration in the U. S. by early 1997, many markets yet exist where practice acquisitions will occur. Most experienced administrators and consultants have been advising to avoid practice acquisitions if at all possible. Their feelings are clear: physicians stop working when they become employed; almost no incentive exists to maintain productivity. As one example, our consulting group had been working with a medical practice on developing treatment protocols for specific conditions. The physicians could only meet with us at 7:00 A.M. before clinic or at 6:00 P.M., after hours. The project was important to them but only after maintaining their patient load could they devote their time. During the process, the group had been in discussion about selling to the local hospital which transpired about midway through the project, and we continued to work with the group. One small change: after the sale, the physicians could meet with us only between 8:30 A.M. and 4:00 P.M. You see, their working hours had changed and although they were still interested in the project, they would only continue on their employer's time. These stories exist across the country. The earliest wave of practice acquisitions and physician employment offered straight salary agreements to physicians which, in effect, was their retirement plan. The cry of the administrators became "hire is synonymous with retire."

Physician Support Services

One evolving contracting activity in MSOs is at-risk service contracting. In this model, the MSO contracts for multiple years based on a percentage of overhead. For example, if a practice is operating at 63% overhead, and 37% goes to physician compensation (salary + benefits), an at-risk contract for a 3-year term may guarantee overhead at 63% for year one, 60% for year two, and 58% for year three. The MSO is paid a management fee, which comes out of overhead, and the MSO makes the administrative decisions, mostly with input from the physicians. The downside for both parties is how efficiently the practice is run. The MSO is at risk to manage effectively to improve its share of earnings from the practice operations; the physicians share the income in the traditional manner. This method is more like pseudo-equity than true equity. It is difficult for two parties in a relationship to earn substantial returns to consider this a true equity relationship—there is only so far income can be maximized and expenses can get squeezed.

Physician Equity Models

There is only so much income a physician group can generate through clinical activities. Physicians, depending on their stage in professional practice, are often interested in cashing in on the investment they have built up or perhaps would like to hold out for the opportunity for improved return. The result is that many physicians are seeking alternative means to build value in the systems and transfer this gain to themselves, as investors or risk-bearers, bearing the risk of maintaining operations for greater return in the form of revenue streams (dividends) or in the ultimate sale of the business.

As a general principle, equity models divide revenue streams into compensation components and overhead components. Equity models *build* equity by maximizing flow to the equity growing account(s), rather than in disbursements as physician compensation for professional services. Alternatively, equity arrangements with physician groups may mean sharing of retained earnings after expenses, although these types of arrangements, if structured incorrectly, may invite regulatory scrutiny when used for employed physicians.

Equity options are still uncommon in many markets as many physicians still do not know about them. The pivotal issue in any equity-based arrangement is liquidity and return on investment. PhyCor, as one example, doesn't *employ* physicians; it makes them "economic partners." Through buying the hard assets of the medical group, they provide capital and management to the medical group, creating an "economic affiliation." Their idea has been to carve out the bottom line for physician compensation maintaining their entrepreneurial spirit. This equity growth creates value on the management side of medical practice. Through practice growth, total practice expenses, including physician compensation for professional services, are minimized to create a revenue stream for distribution to equity partners, or shareholders. This is the opposite strategy of MSO operation: minimize administrative overhead to increase revenue to the physician practice. The goal of equity models is to create a true investor relationship in an entity that provides a financial return over and above the simple profit margin on operations. There are obvious tax implications for not-for-profit entities as well as relevant fraud and abuse and Stark law implications. One immediate solution arrives in the for-profit hospital, healthcare and managed care organizations, although there are still alternatives for tax-exempt physician equity and gainsharing models to structure joint venture equity arrangements.

As doctors organize in groups, they are looking for capital. The issues for physicians remain the same: independence, control of destiny, clinical autonomy, long-term financial security, and assistance in financing managed care initiatives. Investors are looking for doctors, specifically group practices and physician organizations. There are opportunities for physician equity positions in MSOs as venture capitalists are moving into the for-profit MSO arena. Venture capitalists gave OccuSystems $30 million.[2] In a widely publicized move, the American Medical Association created Physicians Capital Source, assembling nearly 30 investment firms and banks willing to support *physician-led* ventures. Physicians focus then on growth, which must occur in equity models to create the income stream for dividends, or alternatively, to create a system of value for later sale to another entity in the healthcare system. Recent market activities have included PhyCor moving from practice acquisitions to IPAs, American Healthcare Systems operating two venture capital funds that have invested over $45 million in emerging healthcare companies, and several of the large for-profit hospital chains offering equity positions to acquired physicians. The typical options offered to physicians are sales of their practices in exchange for fair market or slightly above fair market employment compensation plus stock and options on the new venture, or in the company as a whole. The obvious risk: whether stock value will increase during the vesting period and liquidity.

According to J. Daniel Beckham, hospitals have two key problems with equity arrangements: (1) equity arrangements are inconsistent with their not-for-profit values, and (2) Medicare fraud and abuse laws and IRS regulations make it difficult to pay physicians the true value of their practices.[3] Beckham points out that as hospitals create or invest in their own for-profit subsidiaries, it sends mixed messages to physicians. He further advises that participation in the bottom line is the most proven of all organizational incentives. In order to create buy-in from the production component of a relationship, incentives must be tangible, desired, and, as a practical matter, place some element of risk of performance to ensure continued production.

Acquisition and Transaction Issues

Organizations face many issues in preparing for a strategy that involves business acquisition and new product line development. Most notably, tax-exempt providers face a number of concerns including a general lack of authoritative guidance, concern over the community benefits accruing to the acquisition, position on private benefit, inurement, and conflict of interest. As a matter of practicality, organizations pursuing physician integration and practice activities should be concerned with rates of utilization of services, productivity, compensation and incentive issues, the classification of the employee, and reporting requirements, as well as the relevant legal issues of fraud and abuse, antitrust, and corporate practice of medicine.

For all of the uncertainty in pursuing these strategies, some guidance is available in the forms of the IRS Audit Guidelines (1990); General Counsel Memoranda (see especially GCM 39862 on community benefit – 1991); the Hermann Hospital closing agreement (1994), which discusses physician recruitment incentives; and the many Department of Justice, Federal Trade Commission, and

IRS private letter and administrative rulings, which tend to set some form of precedent for other networks (see Friendly Hills Healthcare Network, Facey Medical Foundation, Harriman-Jones Medical Foundation, Billings Medical Clinic, and the ongoing cases of the Marshfield Clinic and Hanlester).

Decision to Buy or Sell a Healthcare Business.   Along the same lines as strategic partnerships, the IRS indicates in its 1996 Exempt Organizations Continuing Professional Education Technical Instruction Program Textbook that they have been receiving ruling requests in three broad areas: the sale of one not-for-profit entity to another not-for-profit entity; a not-for-profit system's sale of one of its hospitals; and the sale of a not-for-profit to a for-profit in which the sales proceeds are used to establish a charitable foundation.[4] The IRS is particularly concerned with the reduction of charitable healthcare services available in the community postsale, suggesting that the amount of annual support should be equivalent to the amount of charitable care provided by the previous hospital annually for at least 3 years.

Organizations must assess their readiness and direction in pursuing a strategy of business acquisition, beginning typically with which services should be provided directly or "made" and which should be subcontracted / acquired or "bought."

Providers should clarify the following areas to determine how they should be positioned to respond to market changes:

* How is your market defined?
* Given this market, what are your core competencies within this market and how should you contribute to the healthcare provider community?
* What are the demands for services among your constituency: payor, patient, and employee?
* What are your resources for providing the service: provider, technical, support, equipment, space, and capital?
* Which services or components of the service line should be made and which should be bought, and how is this decided?

It should also be reiterated that recent data suggest that the postsale operations of medical practices have not proven successful.[5] Although the focus has been on the operation of the practice as an individual economic entity, few systems have yet to quantify the synergies, system, or referral value (incremental value) advanced by these practices. Part of the reason for this is that data systems are yet haphazard and are not collecting this information but also that organizations must exercise caution in collecting and reporting these data for fear of regulatory review for fraud and abuse.

Despite these indications, many hospitals believe owning medical practices is a sound long-term strategy. In certain communities health networks are forced into buying medical practices due to actual or perceived market forces. The most sound strategy involves the least resources to effect the desired result. Recall the concept of virtual integration. A system of shared economic incentives, risk, and contractual relationships is likely to be more effective in the long term than a capital- and asset-intensive approach. It is clear that the strengths of the healthcare empires, and indeed empires in virtually all other industries, were built upon large fixed-asset bases and capital. In healthcare as well as in many other industries, large fixed-asset bases are becoming the downfall of corporate balance sheets. Hospitals have continually declining inpatient activity while their physical plants are configured for an inpatient, high-intensity mission. The move to primary care dominance—and mind set—creates a substantially different environment for the delivery of all types of healthcare. In the very near future, the majority of medical decision making will occur in the community primary care area. Buyers should consider closely the reasons for pursuing the acquisition strategy, and once committed, give appropriate attention to ensuring its success.

In evaluating opportunities for business or service line expansion through acquisition, it is helpful to remind ourselves of the common reasons of selling and buying a given business or business line. Among the most common reasons for selling a closely held business are the death of the principal or a partner, dissolution of partnership agreement, poor health of one or more owners/principals, retirement, burnout, lack of capital for growth, continued revenue loss, and fear of loss of security. Among the most common reasons to acquire a business are to retain physicians/providers in community, to recruit new physicians, to build a primary care base/provider network, to satisfy or augment community need for services, and to improve capacity for managed care.

Issues in approaching business sales from the seller's perspective to prompt the sale may include advantageous pricing, relative security through employment, the opportunity to get into a network while the need exists, a selling price at present value dollars, and the overall need to reduce stress from operations. Among the potential advantages to waiting are the chance that greater purchase amounts may be paid in the near future, the opportunity to see how the network grows and how management services function at other practices, the opportunity to improve present operations in hopes of increasing business value and to hear from peers on how their business sales transpired and their level of satisfaction with the process and outcome.

As stated previously, there are several other options for physicians and other healthcare business owners to selling their business, and hospitals and health networks should strive to accommodate these options. Other options to sales include the recruitment of additional providers, providing management services, affiliation (meaningful alignment with tangible value) with hospital or other provider organizations, or the merger with another practice or related business. It may be difficult to change their opinion of their options.

Timing the Sale.   As indicated by Shannon Pratt, businesses seeking the best possible price should consider the following suggestions:[6]

- ◆ Anticipate the sale and prepare accordingly.
- ◆ Make the sale when the timing is good from a financial standpoint.
- ◆ Hold off selling when the seller is convinced that higher profitability is on the immediate horizon, especially if the full potential will not be immediately apparent to an outsider.

As a matter of common business sense, it behooves any business to anticipate a potential sale of the concern so they may employ new operations and investment decisions to improve the financial outlook for the practice. Since many valuation methodologies and assumptions are derived, in part or in whole, from historic financial performance, the business will ultimately prove to be more valuable with strong earnings to equity ratios and a solid capital structure. The ability to "buckle down" and improve operations for even 1 year prior to valuation is enormously helpful for a business that is considering a sale.

It is more difficult to advise a business on the optimum time to sell in a short time frame. There are often too many individual market dynamics to suggest being an early sale in an emerging market or a late sale in a maturing market. It is clear that once the word spreads that practices begin to sell, many of the initial inquiries that come to the buyer are from poorer performing practices. It has been suggested that it is as easy to buy a bad practice as it is to buy a good practice. In reality, it takes much more effort to determine whether an average practice is good, or if average is all you need. In pursuing acquisitions, *be patient,* but be attentive to the market.

Steps in the Acquisition Process

The actual order of activities may vary somewhat between organizations and a number of these issues may occur concurrently (see Exhibit 4–1).

Initial Discussion with Group.   In any potential business transaction one party approaches the other for discussion purposes. In some cases it is to explore potential opportunities or to seek the advice of the other about any of a number of issues. Physicians often approach hospitals to sell simply because they are fed up with the business of medicine. In these simple cases, perhaps an MSO arrangement is what the medical group needs. In the case of discussion of a potential acquisition, the two parties begin with an initial discussion of the needs and expectations of each party. At some point the discussants determine whether or not there is a basis for

EXHIBIT 4–1

Acquisition/Valuation Process Flow Model

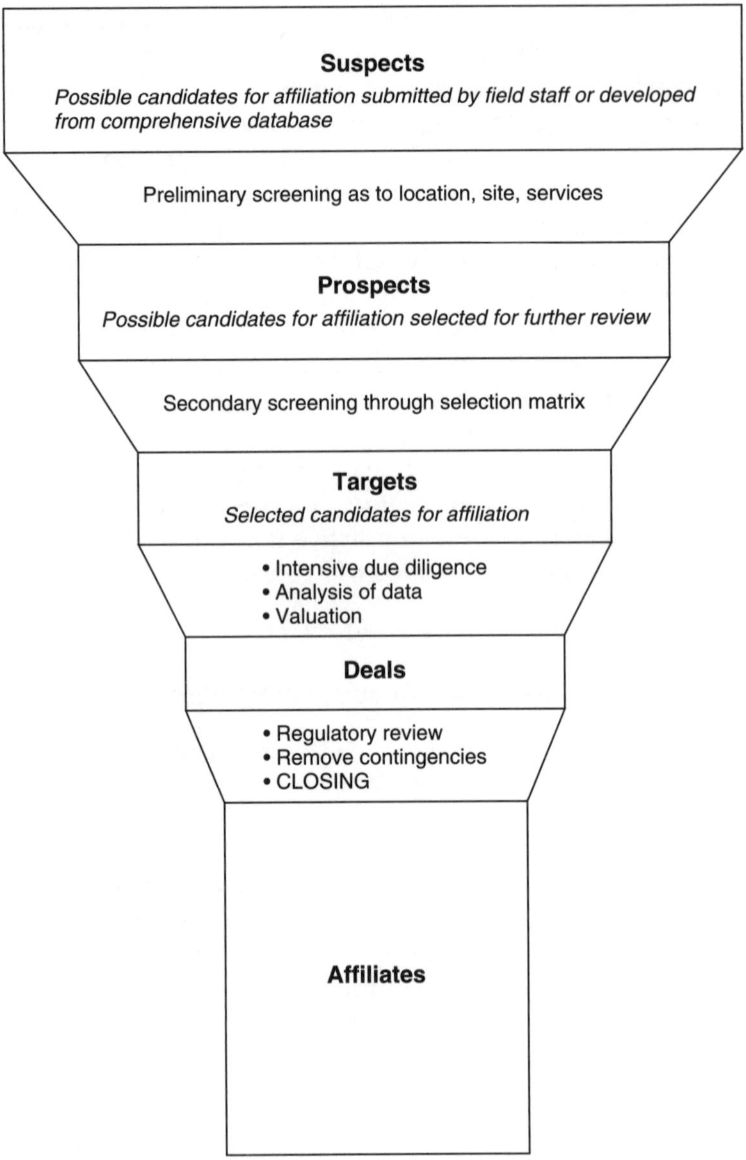

Suspects
Possible candidates for affiliation submitted by field staff or developed from comprehensive database

Preliminary screening as to location, site, services

Prospects
Possible candidates for affiliation selected for further review

Secondary screening through selection matrix

Targets
Selected candidates for affiliation

- Intensive due diligence
- Analysis of data
- Valuation

Deals

- Regulatory review
- Remove contingencies
- CLOSING

Affiliates

Robert James Cimasi, CBI, CBC. Health Capital Consultants

further discussion, a commonality of interest worth pursuing. At this point the parties will begin spending more time looking into the potential relationship and are ready to move to the next phase: confidentiality. One word of note: parties will begin to disclose a variety of information at different points in the process. It is most helpful to use a coordinated approach to gathering information about each other from the early stages to assist in decision making along the way (see Exhibit 4–2).

Confidentiality and Exclusivity Agreements.   Each party will want the content and even existence of discussions between the two to remain confidential (with reasonable exceptions regarding points of law and disclosure). For obvious reasons, hospital buyers do not want physicians spreading information to other physicians or to competitor organizations about the terms, offer, strategies, or other arrangements of any offer discussed or extended. The selling medical group or business is at much less risk for this type of disclosure by the buyer; the buyer has nothing to gain by sharing any of this information with others. Buyers will want to maintain exclusivity in dealing with the seller from the earliest discussions until the deal is made or dies. Sellers would like to maintain options to play buyers off each other. The marketplace however is not an ideal world; buyers will need to negotiate or drop the exclusivity piece. Buyers should aggressively pursue the exclusive dealing clause for a 30- to 90-day period to allow the discussions to mature, but if it is a deal breaker, then go for it without exclusive dealing. Remember that the most successful negotiations will try to maintain a win-win relationship.

Valuation Analysis.   The most frequent next step is the selection of a qualified healthcare business appraiser, as discussed in Chapter 3. Valuation analysis will establish the fair market value of the entity in question. Discussion should occur between the prospective buyer and seller as to the subject property in question: the corporate stock or the assets of the business and what, if anything, may be excluded from the sale (and valuation). Items excluded frequently include automobiles owned by the business, personal property and other sentimental items on site, accounts receivable, and original

EXHIBIT 4-2

What to Disclose and When—A Discussion Checklist

The following list provides some general guidance as to the items of interest to each party and how and when they should be disclosed. It should be noted that this list is not all-inclusive and items should be considered by each party in the transaction as to their level of relative importance.

Physicians/Sellers Should Disclose during Initial Discussions:

_____ Any history of physician and physician extender substance abuse.

_____ Any history of physician malpractice, either for cause or in defense.

_____ Any restrictions or suspensions of privileges, license to practice medicine, or license to prescribe any class of controlled substances.

_____ Any history of felony conviction or incarceration.

_____ Corporate structure of the practice.

_____ Retirement plans, if applicable, during term of agreement planned.

_____ Pending contractual obligations.

_____ Pertinent employee-related information.

Physicians/Sellers Should Disclose during Negotiation:

_____ Unusual circumstances that may impact ability to perform professional actiities in the manner typically expected of physicians and extenders.

_____ Fee, productivity, and cost data.

_____ Listing of managed care activity.

_____ Continuing medical education attended.

_____ Copy of all licenses to practice medicine, and documentation of all professional medical certifications.

_____ A listing of all states where they have held medical licensure.

_____ A listing of all hospitals and clinics where they have held privileges of all types.

_____ A listing of practices or where they may have practiced throughout their professional career (curriculum vitae may suffice).

_____ Capital structure of practice (including debt, equity, and rights to acquire debt or equity).

_____ Preexisting share ownership in practice.

_____ Identity of shareholders (i.e., corporate, individual, tax-exempt).

_____ Basis of shareholders in practice stock.

_____ Holding period of shareholders in practice stock.

_____ Any overlap with acquirer shareholders.

_____ Earnings and profits.

_____ Net operating loss, credit, or other carryovers.

_____ Excess loss accounts.

_____ Deferred gains or losses.

_____ "Built-in" income and deduction items.

_____ Copies of all state and federal tax returns on a legal entity basis for past 5 years.

_____ Protests, litigation, or refund claims by category, tax period, and amount of tax liability on dispute, on a legal entity basis.

_____ Copies of all contracts with payors, services, agencies.

_____ Basis adjustments upon deconsolidation.

_____ Schedule of tangible assets.

_____ Deferred compensation plans (including qualified pension plans).

_____ Employment agreements for physicians and staff including listing of staff and related payroll and benefits information.

_____ Stock option plans.

_____ If available, copies of all existing appraisal reports for property, including real estate (land and buildings) and personal property (equipment, furnishings, etc.).

_____ Personal and professional credit history anomalies.

_____ Tail coverage policy information.

Hospitals/Buyers Should Disclose during Initial Discussions:

_____ Overall financial stability of organization and broad capital structure.

_____ Net operating loss, credit, or other carryovers.

_____ Danger of closing, leasing, merging, or turning hospital over for management contract, or consideration of these options.

_____ Planned CEO turnover.

_____ Imminent changes in patient mix, market share, cost, or fee structure.

_____ Negative changes to its credit rating within last 12 months.

_____ Envisioned relationship to hospital.

_____ Employer-employee, hospital-based physician.

_____ Hospitals at which physician maintains privileges.

_____ Medical management services.

_____ Nonpatient care duties required or desired.

_____ Clarification of referral relationship.

_____ Physician peer relationships.

_____ Practice acquisition/network/managed care strategies.

Hospitals/Buyers Should Disclose during Negotiation:

_____ Immediate plans for administrative/management support services.

_____ Delays in approvals from governing board, financial intermediaries, etc.

_____ Unusual precedent conditions or restrictions in employment or purchase contracts.

_____ Unusual or "Gotcha" clauses in contracts.

_____ Technical provisions in contracts.

artwork. The buyer should decide on the type of report needed for the valuation. As indicated in Chapter 3, a letter report of a complete business appraisal is often sufficient until final negotiations are complete. This format allows the buyer and seller to converse about the results of the appraisal at about 75% of the cost of the full written report. In the event that the discussions progress to fruition, the appraiser may produce the full written report from his notes while making any adjustments based on any changes in assets and liabilities from the date of original appraisal to the date of sale. Often the final appraisal report is not completed until after the day of closing. This report, dated on the day of closing, provides solid documentation of the value of the business at the date of sale, thereby eliminating one source of potential regulatory scrutiny.

Presentation of Findings to Purchaser.   The appraiser presents his results to the purchaser (generally the party who retained the appraiser) who decides whether the business value is sufficient to continue acquisition discussions. Recall that the burden of proof that the business assets are/were acquired at fair market value is on the buyer. Buyers will want to establish the details of compensation, incentive plans, and employment issues such as vacation, CME, and sick time off; professional allotments for education expenses, subscriptions, dues, restrictive covenants; and the administrative arrangements for practice management and retention of practice employees.

Purchaser Board Approval.   In some cases, the governing body of the buyer gives approval for the acquisition before the initial discussions. In other cases, some period of time elapses before final approval is given, often after negotiations and the resolution of the final selling price, compensation arrangements, and other considerations.

Purchaser Presents Offer.   The buyer presents the results of the valuation to the seller, often with the appraiser or consultant present, and discusses the initial offer, which should include details about physician employment and compensation arrangements. Buyers must present the complete package in order for the deal to be received favorably. Reaction from sellers, as expected, ranges from ecstasy to outrage. Most often the seller will want some time to think it over, discuss it among partners, or seek guidance from accountants, attorneys, or consultants. Offers should be presented with time frames for acceptance, typically on the order of 2 to 4 weeks.

Letter of Intent to Purchase. If the presentation of offer is not a complete failure, the buyer and seller should sign a letter of intent signifying their desires to complete discussions on the sale of the business. The letter need not be lengthy but should include the maintenance of the position of exclusivity, confidentiality, nondisclosure, and final acquisition subject toward satisfactory regulatory review and due diligence. The letter may include details of the offer including purchase price, details on employment and compensation, and other administrative arrangements such as dealing with outstanding accounts receivable and prepaid expenses.

Negotiations. Negotiations on any and all of the previously mentioned issues may proceed smoothly or not. This is the time when you begin to learn the most about your potential partner. The attitudes displayed by each side may in fact lead the parties to choose to end discussions (for an excellent treatise on negotiation tactics, see *Getting to Yes*[7]). One item of note, the person negotiating on behalf of the buyer may not be the person the seller deals with after the sale. In many cases the buyer's agent or negotiator may well establish the rapport with the sellers to close the deal, only to have an abrasive, incompetent, or uninformed staff take over the relationship after the sale. Worse yet, the understanding and mutual promises made in negotiation are not upheld with the transition because the parties have changed.

Operational Assessment and Development of Operational Pro Forma.
Detailed analysis of business operations can tell much about the likelihood for continued successful operation or transition into a corporate system. Valuation analysis gets into some of the operational details, but infrequently identifies areas for improvement and is not concerned with operational efficiencies that may be gained

under postsale operating assumptions. The buyer must give some thought to the operations of the business after the sale including the impact of compensation and productivity, patient and managed care contract acquisition, and the simple and ultimate considerations of overhead expenses and amortization of purchase price. It is highly recommended that once a negotiation is leaning toward a reality, an operational assessment is conducted to detail the operational efficiencies to be adopted by other network participants and inefficiencies that warrant correction. Information systems should be evaluated to determine compatibility for corporate reporting and, if necessary, cost estimates obtained to effect system conversion. Similarly, other aspects of postsale operations should be established including allotments for recruitment, capital expenditures, equipment replacement, internal purchase arrangements, and interest rates for amortization. These assumptions should be compiled into a postsale operational pro forma in order to examine the actual impact on the practice under any of a number of scenarios.

Review and Resolution of Regulatory Issues.   In any healthcare business acquisition there is the potential for a variety of legal issues to impact the structure, process, and outcome of the transaction. The buyers should be aware of certain restrictions in negotiating selling price (maintaining fair market value), form of financing (cash sale to avoid Stark law compensation arrangements), valuation risk rates (must reflect market consensus), referral prohibitions (including network and internal, within-group practice referrals), private benefit, inurement, and antitrust concerns. These items, discussed more fully in Chapter 6, must be considered prior to establishing the final selling price and transaction documents.

Due Diligence.   For the purposes of business acquisition, due diligence is the process by which a systematic organizational review is performed by each party to ascertain essential information that may prove vital for the final decision to pursue the transaction. The due diligence is performed typically by each party on the other to determine to the extent possible, among other things, if the representations made in the earlier stages of discussion are truthful or have a reasonable likelihood of occurring (see Due Diligence Check-list in the appendix). The process often includes informal components used in the very earliest stages of the deal, often before the other party is approached to consider the opportunity. This informal "asking around" may include such statements aimed at determining the quality of the medical practice and the physician(s) in particular, and is not unlike the "interviewing" process of checking references. Physicians often have their own sense of the financial stability of the local hospital; however, in urban areas they may be less comfortable with their knowledge base of the prospective partner. The formal review is usually conducted or coordinated by legal counsel on behalf of their clients and often follows a format developed by the respective law firms.

There is the overriding understanding that a buyer has some reasonable right to know the condition of the business they are buying. Indeed the definition of fair market value requires each party to have a reasonable knowledge of the relevant facts. The seller therefore must represent to the buyer, through representations and warranties, that the condition of the business is disclosed prior to the actual transaction of purchase. A business valuation and assessment of the capital structure of the practice is required and should provide the basic elements in representing the overall condition of the business. A valuation, however, is not an operational assessment and cannot begin to identify, in detail, specific day-to-day operations issues or deficiencies that may have an effect on the future value and operations of the business. This level of detail of operations is not required currently by regulatory bodies. One immediate determinant is the overall profitability of the business; it is not likely that a business with significant operational deficiencies will continue to be profitable, or even exist, over several years.

Purchase Agreement/Bill of Sale. The asset or stock purchase agreement is the document that delineates the conditions of the sale of the subject assets (business). These documents can range anywhere from about 7 pages to well over 50 pages, depending on the desires of the clients and style of preparation of the preparing counsel. The major sections included in the purchase agreement include the background of the agreement, the assets (or stock profile) sold and conditions of transfer, the purchase price (including the allocation of purchase price for tax compliance with U. S. Tax Code Section 1060 and IRS Form 8594, Asset Acquisition), terms of closing, contractual obligations and warranties, liabilities of the selling entity, employment and liability for benefits of employees, notices to seller's patients or clients, assignments of name, telephone numbers, and other identifying trade names or logos, representations and warranties, conditions to buyer and seller's performance, survival clauses, indemnification, restrictive covenants, and miscellaneous provisions that may include severability, state law controlling, successors, and early payback provisions. It is advised that the draft purchase agreement be circulated to the sellers well in advance of the anticipated date of closing. Numerous issues may arise, particularly in the allocation of purchase price and in payback provisions, which may require time to work through.

The Bill of Sale and Assignment may be as simple as a single page attachment to the asset purchase agreement with its own attachments of schedules of fixed-asset listing, patient records, contracts, employment agreements, benefit plans, and insurance information (once again, the Due Diligence Checklist covers the vast majority of these topic areas).

Closing.   The closing of a business sale is often a perfunctory duty between parties as all of the issues should be completed and the paperwork needs execution. Each party and their counselors should review the documents prior to the closing so the time spent is limited. Painful closings occur when much yet needs to be negotiated in the documents, pieces are missing, or tension is high between the parties. In the healthcare environment, the goodwill being purchased is far too valuable to be negatively impacted by a poorly orchestrated negotiation and closing transaction.

INTANGIBLE ASSET STRATEGIES

Intangible assets, as we have demonstrated in Chapter 3, comprise in many cases the most substantial component of business assets. Healthcare organizations often desire to pursue market integration strategies short of actual acquisition, ownership, and operations of medical groups or specific healthcare businesses, but must do so within the confines of the regulatory environment. Hospitals and medical groups may seek to establish a relationship with a particular business through an affiliation agreement, but in reality, affiliation often means very little and does not constitute a binding relationship. Provider networks therefore seek to contractually bind targeted groups through other means, most often through purchasing options and rights.

We can begin by defining these agreements and indicate their prevalence and the market conditions conducive to their use. The first area to start in is a review and general description of an intangible asset.

The question we ask is: What *economic* phenomena are necessary for an intangible asset?[8]

1. It must be subject to specific identification and recognizable description.
2. It must be subject to legal existence and protection.
3. It must be subject to the right of private ownership and this private ownership must be legally transferable.
4. There must be some tangible evidence or manifestation of the existence of the intangible asset (e.g., a contract or a license or a registration document).
5. It must have been created or have come into existence at an identifiable time or as the result of an identifiable event.
6. It must be subject to being destroyed or to a termination of existence at an identifiable time or as the result of an identifiable event.

As the result of these requirements, we see that items such as market potential or undefined desirability do not fit the definition of an intangible asset.

The next question we ask is: What economic phenomena are manifest or are indicative of value in an intangible asset?[9]

1. It must generate some measurable amount of economic benefit to its owner; this economic benefit could be in the form of an income increment or of a cost decrement.

2. This economic benefit may be measured in any of several ways, including net income or net operating income or net cash flow, etc.

3. It must enhance the value of other assets with which it is associated; the other assets may include tangible personal property and tangible real estate.

Given this framework, how do the various intangible assets most often considered for purchase in the healthcare environment measure up?

Right of First Refusal

Purchasing the right of first refusal to buy a business is a growing strategy for networks in the early stages of development (although it has been used in more developed network markets). The main reason networks purchase this intangible asset is to stall the acquisition of the group, or in beginning any acquisition activity at all. We have seen in numerous markets that once practices begin to sell, the market transactions intensify: the less desirable groups want to be bought first followed by, in some cases, a purchasing war between competing hospitals, physician practice management companies, and others. Acquiring the right of first refusal for a key group, or several key groups often prevents this from occurring at the beginning of the integration process because these agreements are usually kept quiet.

The right of first refusal (healthcare version) typically includes the following terms:

1. The seller grants the right to first refusal to acquire the business should the owner receive a bona fide offer to purchase from an outside party, which the owner desires to accept.

2. The buyer of the right is offered the option to match the purchase price, which must be established or confirmed by independent appraisal at fair market value, and other terms of the offer, providing, however, that such terms are deemed legal and within regulatory guidelines. In the event that terms cannot be matched in legal form, the right is often extended to include equivalent offers.

3. The right is granted for a particular period of time.

Rights of first refusal often contain other terms and conditions that enhance their value and applicability including provisions for asset versus stock purchase, acquisition of partial assets, assignability, and application of the amounts paid toward purchase price among others.

Understanding and Valuing Rights of First Refusal as an Intangible Asset.
The right of first refusal, much like the option to purchase, is surrounded by a nature unique to other assets frequently purchased in the healthcare industry. The following description defines the nature of the right of first refusal as applies to healthcare transactions:

1. The seller commits to selling to a particular party for a specific period of time, which may or may not be exercised by the seller, for instance, they may not choose to sell during the term of the agreement.

2. The seller is limiting their opportunity, somewhat, to negotiate a greater selling price because the owner of the right is not a bidder. The seller would need to conduct a competitive bidding process prior to presenting the offer to the owner of the right. Such a right, however, is considered a restriction on the sale of the business and any potential buyer would be aware of the existence of the right. One may presume that potential buyers might not expend much effort in negotiating price when subject to the potential loss to the owner of the right. Furthermore, the existence of the right represents a restriction on ownership, which restricts the right of the holder (owner) to transfer the stock (or assets) tending to increase the discount for lack of marketability.[10]

3. The seller, in limiting the opportunity to negotiate a greater selling price, is only limiting it to roughly 10% of the business enterprise value (BEV). This is true for the following reason: A fair market value appraisal is the best estimate of the value of the entity in the healthcare environment. Given that such appraisal is conducted according to generally accepted accounting principles (GAAP) and generally accepted appraisal methodology (USPAP, ASA, and IBA standards), the margin of error should be ± 10% of the final opinion of value. In other words, the final selling price of the business should be no more than about 10% of the appraised value because it is acknowledged that the independent appraisal is reflective of the fair market value of the subject entity in the subject market and while the appraisal is accurate within several significant digits, a significantly greater price cannot be justified. The right of first refusal is therefore directly related to BEV.

4. Related to the appraisal of BEV, limited appraisals yield limited results. The acquisition of the right of first refusal is a legitimate business transaction that is subject to compliance with fraud and abuse, anti-referral prohibitions, and potentially tax exemption statutes under Section 501 (c) (3) of the Internal Revenue Code. Recall from Chapter 3 in the IRS's 1993 (for FY94) Exempt Organizations Continuing Professional Education Technical Instruction Program Textbook: "Whether the valuation placed on an asset represents fair market value (FMV) depends on the quality of the appraisal," and "all assets acquired will be at or below FMV and will be the result of independent appraisals and arm's-length negotiations." The acquisition of the asset then cannot be based upon a limited appraisal. The buyer is responsible for assuring that assets are acquired at FMV. From a practical standpoint, the appraisal must convey a supportable opinion of value of the asset in question, for instance, the right of first refusal. Is a full written appraisal of the business required when only purchasing the right of first refusal? Most counselors would advise no, presuming that the short form report of the business appraisal indicates that a complete appraisal was conducted and conveys a supportable opinion of value. The accompanying intangible asset appraisal, the specific document that values the right of first refusal, should be of sufficient content to convey the necessary components of its appraisal. Remember, the acquisition of intangible assets that are related to BEV must convey a supportable opinion of value.

5. The cost approach to valuation is not viable due to its inability to equate replacement cost (IRS's fair market value in use—FMVIU) to the asset. The market approach is not viable due to a lack of comparative transactions. Rules of Thumb, or industry formulas, have no basis in fact because these agreements are too rare to exhibit an industry trend and secondly, the reliance on rules of thumb is not consistent with generally accepted appraisal methodology. The income approach then becomes the applicable choice to define the economic benefit particular to this type of intangible asset.

As a bit of theoretical discussion, if amounts paid to the owner for the right are applied to the purchase price, in effect, a portion of the purchase price is paid to the group in advance, presuming that a sale does occur during the term, or renewal term of such a contract. If the contract was terminated or allowed to expire, then the payment would belong to the seller and the restriction on the business removed. If, however, the business was then sold to the purchaser of the right of first refusal, or if a new, unrelated right of first refusal was initiated, fraud and abuse issues may be implicated because the transaction begins to look like a payment for favors or continued referrals.

If the seller of the right sells, for a period of years, the potential to accept a lower selling price, what is the value of that right? The right has become an identifiable and quantifiable economic asset. The potential to accept a lower selling price, we have seen, may be as great as 10% of BEV. It may also be $0. The appraiser must make a judgment on what the amount of reduced value might be, which becomes the total amount at risk for selling the right. With nearly all elements defined, the value of the right then becomes a simple function of a market-based return on investment based on the asset mix in question over the period of the agreement.

In summary, the right of first refusal is an identifiable and quantifiable economic asset that is directly related to BEV, and can only be established by complete appraisal. Its existence may decrease the entity's marketability. It can be a desirable asset for developing networks but should be evaluated carefully by a competent independent appraiser familiar with the healthcare environment.

Option to Purchase

The option to purchase a business or collection of assets is related to the right of first refusal with some notable differences. First, the option to purchase often indicates the buyer has the option to initiate the transaction of the business sale. Given that the selling price is likely to be established by independent appraisal at the time of sale, this may have a negative effect on the price received by the seller. These agreements often carry a higher purchase price because the "call" effect of the option is enduring: they are generally not terminated; the business is sold under the option. Because of this, the seller loses considerable control in the timing of the sale, even though timing alone may not have advantaged or disadvantaged the sale; the loss of this asset dimension has value.

The option to purchase often stipulates that the buyer is made aware of significant changes in cash flows and purchase restrictions may reflect any changes in earnings. In addition, the ability of the seller to alter the debt structure of the entity may be limited through this agreement. Regarding marketability, the option to purchase is related to a "Put" right; a contractual agreement that allows the holder *to sell* according to a variety of predetermined criteria. It creates and guarantees a market. The option to purchase, however, does not guarantee a sale; it usually includes provisions similar to the right of first refusal regarding the option to decline purchase. The "Put" option is most often seen in Buy-Sell agreements in efforts to keep shares in the business by requiring the business to purchase shares of departing members. For these reasons, among others, options to purchase are not as common as right of first refusal.

The option to purchase, as it reflects similar restriction on the sale of the business, is valued in a similar manner to the right of first refusal using the income approach.

Clinical Records

Strictly speaking, clinical records are a tangible asset; however, many perceive them as having intangible value. While not legitimizing this misconception, some words regarding clinical record acquisition are important to the subject. Acquiring only the clinical records of a medical group or healthcare business has been a well-worn strategy, although it is generally recognized as a strategy of considerable risk. Fraud and abuse implications abound when an entity acquires only the clinical records while allowing them to remain on site at the practice or business. The payment for the records begins to look like a payment to the medical group for "other" reasons (to buy favor, for continued referrals—a Stark Law violation). Suffice it to say that most advisors strongly urge not purchasing clinical records in this manner, but only as a collection of assets as in the sale of the business.

MAXIMIZING THE TRANSFER OF GOODWILL: TACTFULLY TRANSITIONING PATIENTS, PAYORS, AND STAFF

Goodwill, the intangible but very real and often most substantial component of value in professional practices must be transferred to the new owner or partner upon the sale or merger of the business.[11] If the seller expects to be paid top dollar for the assets, tangible and intangible that they are selling, the owner expects them to exist at the level at which they were appraised. The transfer of goodwill is one of the least orchestrated actions of the purchasing organization and may often result in significant loss in earnings. The following sections suggest the elements of goodwill and how they are derived.

Practice vs. Professional Goodwill

Practice Goodwill = Business Goodwill
- Going concern value generated by physician (usually).
- Name of practice.
- Location.
- Operating systems in place.
- Intact staff.
- Assemblage of assets.
- Patient base.

Professional Goodwill = Personal Goodwill
- Personal reputation.
- Income generated from these "personal patients" who would follow the physician if he left to a competitor practice.

- Client trust.
- Referral relationship with other physicians.

Goodwill Must Be Transferable with Ownership

- Expected future earnings levels to remain the same.
- Marketability of new practice.
- Patient base remaining with practice.
- Referral base remains intact (no ill feelings about sale or town-gown).
- Work habits of physicians remain substantially the same.
- Appropriate fee schedules (no major changes).
- Location remains the same or at least as good/attractive.
- No significant disruption in work flow for extended periods.
- Value maintained by employees.
- Patients accept and perceive change positively.

Transitioning and Maximizing Goodwill Retention

- Maintain a positive relationship with physician(s) preacquisition.
- Keep staff informed and listen to their concerns.
- Plan transition in excruciating detail.
- Settle employee employment agreements and benefits very early.
- Apply for new doctor numbers from payors (8 weeks in advance).
- Set up bank accounts and order checks.
- Retain accountancy firm.
- Coordinate management services.
- Obtain new contracts for all contracts that require changing.
- Design and print forms.
- Survey patients on practice operations, care received, etc.

- Design mail campaign for informing patients of change.
- Arrange insurance (malpractice, business liability, fire/theft/vandalism).
- Arrange bonding of staff.
- Set up computer accounts and add/order hardware/software as necessary.
- Maintain forum for discussion of issues between practice and new owner.
- Resolve problems immediately—medical practices and small businesses operate on a time frame of hours to days, not weeks to months.

Special emphasis should be placed on transitioning practice staff. It has been said that people panic in herds, and recover one by one. Many have attested to the fact that once the word about the business sale gets out, the staff panics. It is extremely important to the ongoing working relationship that the staff is treated with care and respect.

Consider the following guidelines:

- Do not inform the staff about the potential for sale or merger of the practice or business until it has been firmly decided that this is the strategy of choice and, preferably, once the buyer or partner has been selected. Depending on the size of the organization and stature of the individual, you may need to involve the practice administrator early on.
- Decide on which of the staff members, if any, will not remain with the new organization or if they might be transferred to another location or job with the buyer organization.
- Prior to informing the staff, clearly define their roles in respect to the new personnel management structure. Determine whether pay adjustments, positive or negative, will be required. Prepare a comparative analysis of benefits to distribute to the staff.
- Have influential parties (owner physicians and practice managers) inform the staff about the impending change in ownership, why the change was necessary, and what the physicians' administrative relationship will be with the new practice. Be prepared to discuss the new management and reporting structure with the staff.

◆ Arrange for the practice staff to meet with the personnel and/or benefits representative and practice liaison of the new organization *the day after the announcement is made!* It is of critical importance that the employees are given as much information as possible to avoid them stewing over too many what ifs and do you thinks.

◆ If possible, inform the staff at the latest possible date before closing (frequently about 2 to 3 weeks) to allow for on-site transitional and due diligence activities.

◆ Maintain a positive, can do attitude about the transition at all times.

◆ Do not lie or mislead staff about anything.

PRO FORMA FINANCIAL PLANNING

Medical practices and healthcare businesses such as home health agencies, durable medical equipment companies, and physical therapy and rehabilitation firms are all dependent upon patient flows and managed care or direct employer contracts for revenue and business growth. Many factors affect this potential for growth including the decision to add providers or support staff. Adding overhead to any business should be evaluated carefully, especially when overhead may not produce revenue directly. The delicate balance of infrastructure needs provided by support staff and technology can have positive and negative effects on the growth of a business or practice.

Principles of Forecasting in Healthcare Planning

Forecasting business growth in the healthcare industry should be based on the following general principles:

Healthcare is changing rapidly and unevenly across the country as evidenced by:

◆ Continual changes in reimbursement from all payors.
◆ Overall growth, evolution, and dominance of managed care.

- Governmental influence and intervention in reforming healthcare financing and delivery.
- Continuing escalation in uncompensated care, especially for hospitals.
- Decreasing lengths of stay, increasing technological and pharmaceutical development leading to increased outpatient treatment and therapies.
- Increasing competition among all providers on cost first, then on access and quality.

The uncertainty surrounding healthcare delivery and financing dictates that limited, cautious judgment dictate planning efforts:

- *Reasonable assumptions* on rates of increase of income and expenses.
- Conservative growth factors (e.g., medical care component of CPI).
- Neutral or negative growth factors should be considered where appropriate.
- Plan and budget for contingencies (provider turnover, vacancies, and business volumes).

Build checks and balances into each forecast:

- Tie provider compensation to minimum production levels based on historical or national comparative data when appropriate.
- Ensure generation of minimum working capital requirements before entertaining any distributions.
- Create a sense of ownership in operations for all employees and contractors through incentives that are individual, tangible, and attainable, and represent commitment to the organization.
- Profile best, worst, and most likely scenarios for each venture before deciding on forecast (see Exhibit 4–3).
- Expect variations from forecast; revise annual forecast quarterly and multi-year forecast annually.

EXHIBIT 4-3

Lakeway Internal Medicine—Financial Summary
Operating Scenarios

Scenario	Total Net Revenue Years 1–4	Provider Expenses Years 1–4	Operating Expenses Years 1–4	Cumulative Cash Flow (–)	Provider Bonus Dollars Paid Years 1–4	Cumulative Repayment/ Discretionary Funds*
1. Status Quo	625,000	394,800	255,470	(57,869)	24,000	32,599
	646,875	395,160	266,529	(105,281)	24,000	65,198
	669,516	395,542	278,139	(142,045)	24,000	97,797
	693,949	395,946	290,326	(167,968)	24,000	130,396
2. Adding PA/NP	675,000	445,800	267,470	(70,869)	24,000	32,599
	721,875	452,254	277,554	(111,400)	27,328	65,198
	794,516	458,528	289,715	(97,727)	27,680	97,797
	867,949	447,359	322,481	(12,214)	27,827	130,396
3. Locum Tenens/ Physician Recruitment	581,665	446,625	257,470	(155,029)	12,000	32,599
	675,938	372,420	268,629	(152,739)	22,400	65,198
	734,758	398,912	280,344	(129,836)	24,000	97,797
	760,474	399,519	292,642	(94,121)	24,000	130,396
4. Increasing Physician Productivity and Adding PA/NP	750,000	445,800	274,970	(3,369)	24,000	32,599
	875,000	452,254	296,804	89,975	27,328	65,198
	935,000	458,528	311,128	132,745	27,680	97,797
	1,013,350	447,359	325,185	208,207	27,827	130,396
5. **Most Likely** Increasing Physician Productivity, Recruiting, and Adding PA/NP	708,750	467,800	281,970	(73,618)	24,000	32,599
	827,500	428,794	294,548	(2,058)	25,728	65,198
	944,000	461,136	307,888	140,320	27,680	97,797
	1,022,665	464,284	321,684	204,099	27,827	130,396

*Cumulative Discretionary Funds includes Depreciation and Amortization
Cumulative Depreciation over Years 1–4 = 7,321; 14,642; 21,963; and 29,284
Cumulative Amortization of Start-up Costs over Years 1–4 = 25,278; 50,556; 75,814; and 101,112

Summary of Steps in Preparing and Analyzing Pro Forma Statements[12]

1. Analyze the working capital requirements of the business based on industry sources.

2. Analyze the fixed assets of the company to determine whether an additional investment in fixed assets is necessary, or whether any existing assets are above the needs of the business and could be sold without affecting the entity's earning power.

3. Review any contingent liabilities and determine what provision needs to be made for them.

4. Determine the desired structure of long-term liabilities.

5. Summarize a pro forma income statement for the subject company.

Salient Considerations—Providers and Support Staff. Production volume levels should be established as a guideline to financial performance. As previously mentioned, historical volumes will yield some indication of style of practice of the physician and physician extender. It is very difficult to change the practice patterns significantly for physicians and any statements of significantly increasing volume (effort) postsale should be taken with reservation. In such cases, production volume should be addressed contractually with the provider to give each party the clear understanding of how the practice must operate and further, to economically incentivize the provider to maintain production targets. It is easier to increase production levels for midlevel practitioners because they bring little to no intangible value to the business. Given a PA or nurse practitioner who is producing significantly below national comparative standards, the transition plan and pro forma statements should gradually require this individual to attain median production standards as a minimum standard of job performance. In most communities it is far easier to recruit a midlevel practitioner than it is a physician.

The cost of operations is one of the chief considerations in evaluating the financial success of new business ventures. The ability to add providers may become the difference to pursue the arrangement or not. From the physician's standpoint, however, the addition of new providers, especially physicians, dramatically increases overhead and reduces bonus pools. Employment arrangements should address the distribution of bonus dollars in consideration of the addition of new providers and their impact on the financial performance of the practice. This supports the trend for attaching to the physician employment agreement a mutually agreed upon operational pro forma. Once the physicians have agreed to the plan for provider recruitment, base income, and incentive formula, the teeth exist to hold the physicians accountable to the new effort.

Financial rewards for physicians, tangible and intangible, must be derived based on their own system of values. Simply attaching monetary value as an incentive to increase production and net revenues may not be a driving factor for a physician with young children in the home. To paraphrase The Belief System, by Thad Green and Merwyn Hayes, (an employee) must believe that he/she is able to perform the job (capable of achieving/making the effort), and that this successful level of performance will result in an outcome that is tied to this performance, and further, that this outcome is one that is satisfying to that employee, as an individual.[13] Tying these issues together is the goal of the employment and compensation arrangement that must be settled prior to meaningful pro forma analysis.

Business Profiling.   The practice or subject business should be analyzed thoroughly based on its historic operations, its operations in relation to comparative data, documented growth plans for the business prior to sale, and anticipated growth plans postsale. These growth plans should be on a needs-based factor to determine how the subject entity fits into the existing or growing network strategy. The business profile then becomes an excellent tool to coordinate input from various sources.

Content and Implementation.   The pro forma is a typical financial-based model, usually created as an annual, year-end summary of income and expenses or as a monthly cash flow model. It may be created on a cash or accrual basis, although the accrual basis is used more frequently. The creation of the pro forma, for the established operating entity, is a serious annual planning activity which, after initial profile, may be administered in-house. The model must address the existing or proposed governance structure as it impacts general business operations. It may be wise for many organizations to use external sources to develop these documents if in-house expertise is questionable or unavailable. Physician groups may feel more comfortable with external groups coordinating this process, and hospitals may not feel objective enough to consider all the issues.

Forecasting.   The process of forecasting financial performance in the healthcare industry is often conducted over a period of 5 to 10 years and should represent the analysts' most likely scenario for the subject business. The general rule of thumb is to forecast only that which you can reasonably project. In healthcare, therefore, forecasts are most often in the 3- to 8-year range for medical practices, with primary care practices tending to be longer than specialty care practices. Forecasts should include detailed income and expense projections that are documented and have basis in market reality (attention to historical operations, provider productivity expectations, projections on provider recruitment, ingress of managed care, etc.). Growth rates of income and expenses should be reasonable. As one example, our consulting group recently reviewed a valuation (specifically the discounted cash flows analysis) of a primary care/surgery center with two senior physicians very near retirement age performing near the 90th percentile of MGMA production. The growth rates presumed no diminution of effort for the next 10 years and after a period of initial income growth of about 10%, increased revenue approximately 3% per year thereafter. This is one example of inappropriate expectations for income. The underlying assumptions are the basis of any reasonable forecast. Given the serious penalties (fraud and abuse, private inurement and benefit) that may affect both parties, a conservative and reasonable forecast based on attainable goals (and ideally tied to provider per-formance agreements) does indeed portray the most likely scenario.

General Technique. Pro forma analyses begin typically with the creation of a base for income and expenses that derive from the business historical operations. To this base, adjustments are made for unusual occurrences or identified changes in business operations including working capital requirements, fixed-asset analysis, capital expenditures, depreciation, replacement reserve, contingent liabilities, and structure of long-term liabilities (amortization of purchase price, cash advances to sustain operations, etc.). The analyst must evaluate their understanding and basis for growth rates (positive, neutral, or negative) for the projections. The following methods may be employed for any income or expense category: business historical average, percent of revenue, regression trend analysis of the subject business, regression trend of healthcare industry, and manually adjusted rates.

Other data elements to consider, some of which were mentioned previously, are:

- Number of physicians in practice.
- FTE physicians and FTE extenders per population served.
- Severity of illness.
- Risk pools of patients in practice.
- Amount of managed care/capitation.
- Structure of benefits plans.
- Diagnostic clustering of workload:[14]
    a. General medical examination
    b. Acute upper respiratory infection
    c. Prenatal/postnatal care
    d. Hypertension
    e. Nonpsychotic depression
    f. Lacerations/contusions
    g. Ischemic heart disease
    h. Acquired immunodeficiency syndrome

Sources of National Comparative Data.   A number of proprietary data sets exist to assist in pro forma financial analysis. In the healthcare field, the most commonly used are the Medical Group Management Association's Physician Compensation and Production Survey and Cost Survey[15] and the American Medical Association's Physician Marketplace Statistics and Socioeconomic Characteristics of Medical Practices.[16] These references, generally recognized as the industry standard for information on medical practice operations, are available in a variety of formats including standard documents print and electronic media as well as customized reports. Other sources of information include BIZCOMPS, Robert Morris Associates, and the proprietary database of The Institute of Business Appraisers, Inc.

Sample Pro Forma.   Exhibit 4–4 indicates a fairly substantial 5-year operational pro forma for the acquisition of a primary care practice. This exhibit also appears on the diskette ready for customizing to suit your business needs. Please note before modifying the pro forma: examine the cells and the cell pointers to determine which cells calculate automatically and which cells work manually. For the most part, the calculations in year two and beyond calculate automatically. Anyone with basic spreadsheet skills should be able to modify the file as needed. At a minimum, it provides a base for internal pro forma development.

EXHIBIT 4–4a

Financial Analysis—Lakeway Medical Services
Page 1

January 1, 1997   Scenario #1. $275,000 physician salary level; 12-year payback term

Year 1	Month 1	Month 2	Month 3	Month 4	Month 5	Month 6
Income						
Revenue — Dr. A	64,000	64,000	64,000	64,000	64,000	64,000
Revenue — Dr. B	50,417	50,417	50,417	50,417	50,417	50,417
Revenue — Dr. C	30,099	0	0	0	0	0
Revenue — NP: New	0	0	0	3,000	4,000	6,000
Revenue — NP: #1	5,000	8,000	8,000	8,000	6,000	5,500
Revenue — Ancillary & Technical	22,427	18,363	18,363	18,813	18,663	18,888
Revenue — Surgery Center — Net	3,950	3,950	3,950	3,950	3,950	3,950
Total Net Revenue	**175,893**	**144,730**	**144,730**	**148,180**	**147,030**	**148,755**
Physician Expenses						
Direct Compensation — Dr. A	22,917	22,917	22,917	22,917	22,917	22,917
Direct Compensation — Dr. B	22,917	22,917	22,917	22,917	22,917	22,917
Direct Compensation — Dr. C	11,025	0	0	0	0	0
Physician Benefits @ 25%	14,215	11,458	11,458	11,458	11,458	11,458
Malpractice Insurance	20,000	0	0	0	0	0
Subtotal	91,073	57,292	57,292	57,292	57,292	57,292
Expenses as % of Net Revenue	52%	40%	40%	39%	39%	39%
Operating Expenses						
Support Staff Salaries	37,768	37,768	37,768	37,768	37,768	37,768
Staff Benefits @ 25%	9,442	9,442	9,442	9,442	9,442	9,442
Recruitment Expenses — New M.D.	0	0	0	0	0	0
Repairs and Maintenance	2,748	2,748	2,748	2,748	2,748	2,748
Office Supplies and Services	2,500	2,500	2,500	2,500	2,500	2,500
Rent @ $10/sq. ft. x 9,421	7,851	7,851	7,851	7,851	7,851	7,851
Equipment Rental	830	830	830	830	830	830
Telephone and Utilities	3,324	3,324	3,324	3,324	3,324	3,324
Travel, Dues, and Subscriptions	767	767	767	767	767	767
Clinical and Laboratory Supplies	11,667	11,667	11,667	11,667	11,667	11,667
Business Insurance	1,975	0	0	1,975	0	0
Promotion and Marketing	2,000	1,000	6,000	1,000	1,000	2,000
Accounting and Legal Fees	875	875	875	875	875	875
Real Estate Taxes and Insurance	696	696	696	696	696	696
All Other Expenses	8,958	8,958	8,958	8,958	8,958	8,958
Depreciation — Preacquisition	0	0	0	0	0	0
Depreciation — Postacquisition	0	0	0	0	0	0
Capital Expenditures	1,250	1,250	1,250	1,250	1,250	1,250
Amortization of Start-up/Purchase	(11,183)	(11,183)	(11,183)	(11,183)	(11,183)	(11,183)
Subtotal	103,833	100,859	105,859	102,833	100,859	101,859
Expenses as % of Net Revenue	59%	70%	73%	69%	69%	68%
Total All Expenses	**194,906**	**158,150**	**163,150**	**160,125**	**158,150**	**159,150**
Cash Available Minus Expenses	(19,013)	(13,421)	(18,421)	(11,945)	(11,121)	(10,396)
Cash Advances / (Repayment)	**19,013**	**13,421**	**18,421**	**11,945**	**11,121**	**10,396**
Cash Advances Outstanding	**19,013**	**32,433**	**50,854**	**62,799**	**73,920**	**84,316**

	Month 7	Month 8	Month 9	Month 10	Month 11	Month 12	EOY 1	% of Total Revenue	Year 1 Monthly Average
	64,000	64,000	64,000	64,000	64,000	64,000	768,000	42.5%	64,000
	50,417	50,417	50,417	50,417	50,417	50,417	605,000	33.5%	50,417
	0	0	0	0	0	0	30,099	1.7%	5,017
	6,500	6,500	6,500	6,500	7,000	7,000	53,000	2.9%	8,833
	5,500	5,500	5,500	5,500	6,000	6,000	74,500	4.1%	6,208
	18,963	18,963	18,963	18,963	19,113	19,113	229,590	12.7%	19,132
	3,950	3,950	3,950	3,950	3,950	3,950	47,405	2.6%	3,950
	149,330	**149,330**	**149,330**	**149,330**	**150,480**	**150,480**	**1,807,594**	**100%**	**150,633**
								% of Total Expense	
	22,917	22,917	22,917	22,917	22,917	22,917	**275,000**	13.6%	22,917
	22,917	22,917	22,917	22,917	22,917	22,917	**275,000**	13.6%	22,917
	0	0	0	0	0	0	**11,025**	0.5%	1,838
	11,458	11,458	11,458	11,458	11,458	11,458	**140,256**	6.9%	11,688
	15,000	0	0	0	0	0	**35,000**	1.7%	2,917
	72,292	57,292	57,292	57,292	57,292	57,292	**736,281**	36.3%	61,357
	48%	38%	38%	38%	38%	38%	**41%**		
	37,768	37,768	37,768	37,768	37,768	37,768	**453,220**	22.3%	37,768
	9,442	9,442	9,442	9,442	9,442	9,442	**113,305**	5.6%	9,442
	15,000	2,000	2,000	2,000	5,000	4,000	**30,000**	1.5%	NM
	2,748	2,748	2,748	2,748	2,748	2,748	**32,977**	1.6%	2,748
	2,500	2,500	2,500	2,500	2,500	2,500	**30,000**	1.5%	2,500
	7,851	7,851	7,851	7,851	7,851	7,851	**94,210**	4.6%	7,851
	830	830	830	830	830	830	**9,963**	0.5%	830
	3,324	3,324	3,324	3,324	3,324	3,324	**39,882**	2.0%	3,324
	767	767	767	767	767	767	**9,200**	0.5%	767
	11,667	11,667	11,667	11,667	11,667	11,667	**140,000**	6.9%	11,667
	1,975	0	0	1,975	0	0	**7,898**	0.4%	658
	2,000	2,000	2,000	500	500	0	**20,000**	1.0%	1,667
	875	875	875	875	875	875	**10,500**	0.5%	875
	696	696	696	696	696	696	**8,351**	0.4%	696
	8,958	8,958	8,958	8,958	8,958	8,958	**107,500**	5.3%	8,958
	0	0	0	0	0	28,133	**28,133**	1.4%	2,344
	0	0	0	0	0	8,820	**8,820**	0.4%	735
	1,250	1,250	1,250	1,250	1,250	1,250	**15,000**	0.7%	1,250
	(11,183)	(11,183)	(11,183)	(11,183)	(11,183)	(11,183)	**(134,195)**	6.6%	(11,183)
	118,833	103,859	103,859	104,333	105,359	140,812	**1,293,154**	63.7%	
	80%	70%	70%	70%	70%	94%	**72%**		
	191,125	**161,150**	**161,150**	**161,625**	**162,650**	**198,103**	**2,029,436**		
	(41,795)	(11,821)	(11,821)	(12,295)	(12,171)	(47,624)			
	41,795	**11,821**	**11,821**	**12,295**	**12,171**	**47,624**			
	126,111	137,932	149,752	162,047	174,218	221,842	**221,842** EOY 1 Balance Forward		

EXHIBIT 4–4b

Financial Analysis—Lakeway Medical Services
Page 2

January 1, 1997   Scenario #1. $275,000 physician salary level; 12-year payback term

Year 2	Month 1	Month 2	Month 3	Month 4	Month 5	Month 6
Income						
Revenue — Dr. A	65,760	65,760	65,760	65,760	65,760	65,760
Revenue — Dr. B	51,803	51,803	51,803	51,803	51,803	51,803
Revenue — Dr. New	18,000	22,000	26,000	30,000	36,000	38,000
Revenue — NP: New	7,083	7,083	7,083	7,083	7,083	7,083
Revenue — NP: #1	6,829	6,829	6,829	6,829	6,829	6,829
Revenue — Ancillary & Technical	22,421	23,021	23,621	24,221	25,121	25,421
Revenue — Surgery Center — Net	10,144	10,144	10,144	10,144	10,144	10,144
Total Net Revenue	**182,041**	**186,641**	**191,241**	**195,841**	**202,741**	**205,041**
Physician Expenses						
Direct Compensation — Dr. A	22,917	22,917	22,917	22,917	22,917	22,917
Direct Compensation — Dr. B	22,917	22,917	22,917	22,917	22,917	22,917
Direct Compensation — Dr. New	14,167	14,167	14,167	14,167	14,167	14,167
Physician Benefits @ 25%	15,000	15,000	15,000	15,000	15,000	15,000
Physician Bonus @ 15%	0	0	0	0	0	0
Malpractice Insurance	29,000	0	0	0	0	0
Subtotal	104,000	75,000	75,000	75,000	75,000	75,000
Expenses as % of Net Revenue	57%	40%	39%	38%	37%	37%
Operating Expenses						
Support Staff Salaries	40,276	40,276	40,276	40,276	40,276	40,276
Staff Benefits @ 25%	10,069	10,069	10,069	10,069	10,069	10,069
Repairs and Maintenance	2,974	2,974	2,974	2,974	2,974	2,974
Office Supplies and Services	3,000	3,000	3,000	3,000	3,000	3,000
Rent @ $10/sq. ft. x 9,421	8,126	8,126	8,126	8,126	8,126	8,126
Equipment Rental	830	830	830	830	830	830
Telephone and Utilities	3,656	3,656	3,656	3,656	3,656	3,656
Travel, Dues, and Subscriptions	1,025	1,025	1,025	1,025	1,025	1,025
Clinical and Laboratory Supplies	13,125	13,125	13,125	13,125	13,125	13,125
Business Insurance	2,073	0	0	2,073	0	0
Promotion and Marketing	750	750	6,750	750	750	750
Accounting and Legal Fees	919	919	919	919	919	919
Real Estate Taxes and Insurance	720	720	720	720	720	720
All Other Expenses	9,583	9,583	9,583	9,583	9,583	9,583
Depreciation — Preacquisition	0	0	0	0	0	0
Depreciation — Postacquisition	0	0	0	0	0	0
Capital Expenditures	1,294	1,294	1,294	1,294	1,294	1,294
Amortization of Start-up/Purchase	(11,183)	(11,183)	(11,183)	(11,183)	(11,183)	(11,183)
Subtotal	109,603	107,529	113,529	109,603	107,529	107,529
Expenses as % of Net Revenue	60%	58%	59%	58%	53%	52%
Total All Expenses	**213,603**	**182,529**	**188,529**	**184,603**	**182,529**	**182,529**
Cash Available Minus Expenses	(31,561)	4,112	2,712	11,239	20,212	22,512
Cash Advances / (Repayment)	**31,561**	**(4,112)**	**(2,712)**	**(11,239)**	**(20,212)**	**(22,512)**
Cash Advances Outstanding	253,403	249,291	246,580	235,341	215,129	192,617

	Month 7	Month 8	Month 9	Month 10	Month 11	Month 12	EOY 2	% of Total Revenue	Year 2 Monthly Average
	65,760	65,760	65,760	65,760	65,760	65,760	**789,120**	32.5%	65,760
	51,803	51,803	51,803	51,803	51,803	51,803	**621,638**	25.6%	51,803
	40,000	40,000	40,000	45,000	45,000	45,000	**425,000**	17.5%	70,833
	7,083	7,083	7,083	7,083	7,083	7,083	**85,000**	3.5%	7,083
	6,829	6,829	6,829	6,829	6,829	6,829	**81,950**	3.4%	6,829
	25,721	25,721	25,721	26,471	26,471	26,471	**300,406**	12.4%	25,034
	10,144	10,144	10,144	10,144	10,144	10,144	**121,730**	5.0%	10,144
	207,341	**207,341**	**207,341**	**213,091**	**213,091**	**213,091**	**2,424,844**	**100%**	**202,070**
								% of Total Expense	
	22,917	22,917	22,917	22,917	22,917	22,917	**275,000**	11.5%	22,917
	22,917	22,917	22,917	22,917	22,917	22,917	**275,000**	11.5%	22,917
	14,167	14,167	14,167	14,167	14,167	14,167	**170,000**	7.1%	28,333
	15,000	15,000	15,000	15,000	15,000	15,000	**180,000**	7.5%	15,000
	0	0	0	0	0	82,500	**82,500**	3.5%	6,875
	29,000	0	0	0	0	0	**58,000**	2.4%	4,833
	104,000	75,000	75,000	75,000	75,000	157,500	**1,040,000**	43.6%	86,708
	50%	36%	36%	35%	35%	74%	**43%**		
	40,276	40,276	40,276	40,276	40,276	40,276	**483,309**	20.3%	40,276
	10,069	10,069	10,069	10,069	10,069	10,069	**120,827**	5.1%	10,069
	2,974	2,974	2,974	2,974	2,974	2,974	**35,688**	1.5%	2,974
	3,000	3,000	3,000	3,000	3,000	3,000	**36,000**	1.5%	3,000
	8,126	8,126	8,126	8,126	8,126	8,126	**97,507**	4.1%	8,126
	830	830	830	830	830	830	**9,963**	0.4%	830
	3,656	3,656	3,656	3,656	3,656	3,656	**43,870**	1.8%	3,656
	1,025	1,025	1,025	1,025	1,025	1,025	**12,300**	0.5%	1,025
	13,125	13,125	13,125	13,125	13,125	13,125	**157,500**	6.6%	13,125
	2,073	0	0	2,073	0	0	**8,293**	0.3%	691
	750	750	750	750	750	750	**15,000**	0.6%	1,250
	919	919	919	919	919	919	**11,025**	0.5%	919
	720	720	720	720	720	720	**8,643**	0.4%	720
	9,583	9,583	9,583	9,583	9,583	9,583	**115,000**	4.8%	9,583
	0	0	0	0	0	28,133	**28,133**	1.2%	2,344
	0	0	0	0	0	11,925	**11,925**	0.5%	994
	1,294	1,294	1,294	1,294	1,294	1,294	**15,525**	0.7%	1,294
	(11,183)	(11,183)	(11,183)	(11,183)	(11,183)	(11,183)	**(134,195)**	5.6%	(11,183)
	109,603	107,529	107,529	109,603	107,529	147,587	**1,344,702**	56.4%	
	53%	52%	52%	51%	50%	69%	**55%**		
	213,603	**182,529**	**182,529**	**184,603**	**182,529**	**305,087**	**2,385,202**		
	(6,261)	24,812	24,812	28,489	30,562	(91,996)			
	6,261	**(24,812)**	**(24,812)**	**(28,489)**	**(30,582)**	**91,996**			
	198,879	174,067	149,255	120,766	90,204	182,201	**182,201** EOY 2 Balance Forward		

EXHIBIT 4–4c

Financial Analysis—Lakeway Medical Services
Page 3

January 1, 1997   Scenario #1. $275,000 physician salary level; 12-year payback term

Year 3	Month 1	Month 2	Month 3	Month 4	Month 5	Month 6
Income						
Revenue — Dr. A	65,760	65,760	65,760	65,760	65,760	65,760
Revenue — Dr. B	51,803	51,803	51,803	51,803	51,803	51,803
Revenue — Dr. New	45,833	45,833	45,833	45,833	45,833	45,833
Revenue — NP: New	8,333	8,333	8,333	8,333	8,333	8,333
Revenue — NP: #1	7,512	7,512	7,512	7,512	7,512	7,512
Revenue — Ancillary & Technical	26,886	26,886	26,886	26,886	26,886	26,886
Revenue — Surgery Center — Net	13,229	13,229	13,229	13,229	13,229	13,229
Total Net Revenue	**219,357**	**219,357**	**219,357**	**219,357**	**219,357**	**219,357**
Physician Expenses						
Direct Compensation — Dr. A	22,917	22,917	22,917	22,917	22,917	22,917
Direct Compensation — Dr. B	22,917	22,917	22,917	22,917	22,917	22,917
Direct Compensation — Dr. New	15,000	15,000	15,000	15,000	15,000	15,000
Physician Benefits @ 25%	15,208	15,208	15,208	15,208	15,208	15,208
Physician Bonus @ 15%	0	0	0	0	0	0
Malpractice Insurance	30,450	0	0	0	0	0
Subtotal	106,492	76,042	76,042	76,042	76,042	76,042
Expenses as % of Net Revenue	49%	35%	35%	35%	35%	35%
Operating Expenses						
Support Staff Salaries	41,887	41,887	41,887	41,887	41,887	41,887
Staff Benefits @ 25%	10,472	10,472	10,472	10,472	10,472	10,472
Repairs and Maintenance	3,220	3,220	3,220	3,220	3,220	3,220
Office Supplies and Services	3,300	3,300	3,300	3,300	3,300	3,300
Rent @ $10/sq. ft. x 9,421	8,410	8,410	8,410	8,410	8,410	8,410
Equipment Rental	830	830	830	830	830	830
Telephone and Utilities	3,839	3,839	3,839	3,839	3,839	3,839
Travel, Dues, and Subscriptions	1,025	1,025	1,025	1,025	1,025	1,025
Clinical and Laboratory Supplies	14,438	14,438	14,438	14,438	14,438	14,438
Business Insurance	2,177	0	0	2,177	0	0
Promotion and Marketing	813	813	6,813	813	813	813
Accounting and Legal Fees	965	965	965	965	965	965
Real Estate Taxes and Insurance	745	745	745	745	745	745
All Other Expenses	10,063	10,063	10,063	10,063	10,063	10,063
Depreciation — Preacquisition	0	0	0	0	0	0
Depreciation — Postacquisition	0	0	0	0	0	0
Capital Expenditures	1,339	1,339	1,339	1,339	1,339	1,339
Amortization of Start-up/Purchase	(11,183)	(11,183)	(11,183)	(11,183)	(11,183)	(11,183)
Subtotal	114,704	112,527	118,527	114,704	112,527	112,527
Expenses as % of Net Revenue	52%	51%	54%	52%	51%	51%
Total All Expenses	**221,196**	**188,569**	**194,569**	**190,745**	**188,569**	**188,569**
Cash Available Minus Expenses	(1,839)	30,788	24,788	28,611	30,788	30,788
Cash Advances / (Repayment)	**1,839**	**(30,788)**	**(24,788)**	**28,611)**	**(30,788)**	**(30,788)**
Cash Advances Outstanding	184,039	153,251	128,463	99,852	69,064	38,275

Month 7	Month 8	Month 9	Month 10	Month 11	Month 12	EOY 3	% of Total Revenue	Year 3 Monthly Average
65,760	65,760	65,760	65,760	65,760	65,760	**789,120**	30.0%	65,760
51,803	51,803	51,803	51,803	51,803	51,803	**621,638**	23.6%	51,803
45,833	45,833	45,833	45,833	45,833	45,833	**550,000**	20.9%	91,667
8,333	8,333	8,333	8,333	8,333	8,333	**100,000**	3.8%	8,333
7,512	7,512	7,512	7,512	7,512	7,512	**90,145**	3.4%	7,512
26,886	26,886	26,886	26,886	26,886	26,886	**322,635**	12.3%	26,886
13,229	13,229	13,229	13,229	13,229	13,229	**158,746**	6.0%	13,229
219,357	**219,357**	**219,357**	**219,357**	**219,357**	**219,357**	**2,632,284**	**100%**	**219,357**
							% of Total Expense	
22,917	22,917	22,917	22,917	22,917	22,917	**275,000**	11.0%	22,917
22,917	22,917	22,917	22,917	22,917	22,917	**275,000**	11.0%	22,917
15,000	15,000	15,000	15,000	15,000	15,000	**180,000**	7.2%	30,000
15,208	15,208	15,208	15,208	15,208	15,208	**182,500**	7.3%	15,208
0	0	0	0	0	109,500	**109,500**	4.4%	9,125
30,450	0	0	0	0	0	**60,900**	2.4%	5,075
106,492	76,042	76,042	76,042	76,042	185,542	**1,082,900**	43.5%	90,242
49%	35%	35%	35%	35%	85%	**41%**		
41,887	41,887	41,887	41,887	41,887	41,887	**502,641**	20.2%	41,887
10,472	10,472	10,472	10,472	10,472	10,472	**125,660**	5.0%	10,472
3,220	3,220	3,220	3,220	3,220	3,220	**38,636**	1.6%	3,220
3,300	3,300	3,300	3,300	3,300	3,300	**39,600**	1.6%	3,300
8,410	8,410	8,410	8,410	8,410	8,410	**100,920**	4.1%	8,410
830	830	830	830	830	830	**9,963**	0.4%	830
3,839	3,839	3,839	3,839	3,839	3,839	**46,064**	1.8%	3,839
1,025	1,025	1,025	1,025	1,025	1,025	**12,300**	0.5%	1,025
14,438	14,438	14,438	14,438	14,438	14,438	**173,250**	7.0%	14,438
2,177	0	0	2,177	0	0	**8,708**	0.3%	726
813	813	813	813	813	813	**15,756**	0.6%	1,313
965	965	965	965	965	965	**11,576**	0.5%	965
745	745	745	745	745	745	**8,946**	0.4%	745
10,063	10,063	10,063	10,063	10,063	10,063	**120,750**	4.8%	10,063
0	0	0	0	0	28,133	**28,133**	1.1%	2,344
0	0	0	0	0	15,139	**15,139**	0.6%	1,262
1,339	1,339	1,339	1,339	1,339	1,339	**16,068**	0.6%	1,339
(11,183)	(11,183)	(11,183)	(11,183)	(11,183)	(11,183)	**(134,195)**	5.4%	(11,183)
114,704	112,527	112,527	114,704	112,527	155,799	**1,408,306**	56.5%	
52%	51%	51%	52%	51%	71%	**54%**		
221,196	**188,569**	**188,569**	**190,746**	**188,569**	**341,341**	**2,491,208**		
(1,839)	30,788	30,788	28,611	30,788	(121,964)			
1,839	**(30,788)**	**(9,326)**	**0**	**0**	**41,122**			
40,114	9,326	21,462	50,073	80,862	41,122	**41,122**	EOY 3 Balance Forward	

EXHIBIT 4–4d

Financial Analysis—Lakeway Medical Services
Page 4

January 1, 1997   Scenario #1. $275,000 physician salary level; 12-year payback term

Year 4	Month 1	Month 2	Month 3	Month 4	Month 5	Month 6
Income						
Revenue — Dr. A	65,760	65,760	65,760	65,760	65,760	65,760
Revenue — Dr. B	51,803	51,803	51,803	51,803	51,803	51,803
Revenue — Dr. New	47,896	47,896	47,896	47,896	47,896	47,896
Revenue — NP: New	9,167	9,167	9,167	9,167	9,167	9,167
Revenue — NP: #1	8,263	8,263	8,263	8,263	8,263	8,263
Revenue — Ancillary & Technical	27,433	27,433	27,433	27,433	27,433	27,433
Revenue — Surgery Center — Net	13,692	13,692	13,692	13,692	13,692	13,692
Total Net Revenue	**224,014**	**224,014**	**224,014**	**224,014**	**224,014**	**224,014**
Physician Expenses						
Direct Compensation — Dr. A	22,917	22,917	22,917	22,917	22,917	22,917
Direct Compensation — Dr. B	22,917	22,917	22,917	22,917	22,917	22,917
Direct Compensation — Dr. New	15,000	15,000	15,000	15,000	15,000	15,000
Physician Benefits @ 25%	15,208	15,208	15,208	15,208	15,208	15,208
Physician Bonus @ 15%	0	0	0	0	0	0
Malpractice Insurance	31,973	0	0	0	0	0
Subtotal	108,014	76,042	76,042	76,042	76,042	76,042
Expenses as % of Net Revenue	48%	34%	34%	34%	34%	34%
Operating Expenses						
Support Staff Salaries	43,562	43,562	43,562	43,562	43,562	43,562
Staff Benefits @ 25%	10,891	10,891	10,891	10,891	10,891	10,891
Repairs and Maintenance	3,457	3,457	3,457	3,457	3,457	3,457
Office Supplies and Services	3,630	3,630	3,630	3,630	3,630	3,630
Rent @ $10/sq. ft. x 9,421	8,704	8,704	8,704	8,704	8,704	8,704
Equipment Rental	830	830	830	830	830	830
Telephone and Utilities	4,031	4,031	4,031	4,031	4,031	4,031
Travel, Dues, and Subscriptions	1,025	1,025	1,025	1,025	1,025	1,025
Clinical and Laboratory Supplies	15,159	15,159	15,159	15,159	15,159	15,159
Business Insurance	2,286	0	0	2,286	0	0
Promotion and Marketing	879	879	6,879	879	879	879
Accounting and Legal Fees	1,013	1,013	1,013	1,013	1,013	1,013
Real Estate Taxes and Insurance	772	772	772	772	772	772
All Other Expenses	10,566	10,566	10,566	10,566	10,566	10,566
Depreciation — Preacquisition	0	0	0	0	0	0
Depreciation — Postacquisition	0	0	0	0	0	0
Capital Expenditures	1,386	1,386	1,386	1,386	1,386	1,386
Amortization of Start-up/Purchase	(11,183)	(11,183)	(11,183)	(11,183)	(11,183)	(11,183)
Subtotal	119,373	117,087	123,087	119,373	117,087	117,087
Expenses as % of Net Revenue	53%	52%	55%	53%	52%	52%
Total All Expenses	**227,387**	**193,129**	**199,129**	**195,415**	**193,129**	**193,129**
Cash Available Minus Expenses	(3,373)	30,885	24,885	28,599	30,885	30,885
Cash Advances / (Repayment)	**3,373**	**(30,885)**	**(13,610)**	**0**	**0**	**0**
Cash Advances Outstanding	44,495	13,610	0	0	0	0
		Balance	**11,275**	**39,874**	**70,759**	**101,645**

Month 7	Month 8	Month 9	Month 10	Month 11	Month 12	EOY 4	% of Total Revenue	Year 4 Monthly Average
65,760	65,760	65,760	65,760	65,760	65,760	**789,120**	29.4%	65,760
51,803	51,803	51,803	51,803	51,803	51,803	**621,638**	23.1%	51,803
47,896	47,896	47,896	47,896	47,896	47,896	**574,750**	21.4%	95,792
9,167	9,167	9,167	9,167	9,167	9,167	**110,000**	4.1%	9,167
8,263	8,263	8,263	8,263	8,263	8,263	**99,160**	3.7%	8,263
27,433	27,433	27,433	27,433	27,433	27,433	**329,200**	12.2%	27,433
13,692	13,692	13,692	13,692	13,692	13,692	**164,303**	6.1%	13,692
224,014	**224,014**	**224,014**	**224,014**	**224,014**	**224,014**	**2,688,170**	100%	**224,014**
							% of Total Expense	
22,917	22,917	22,917	22,917	22,917	22,917	**275,000**	10.8%	22,917
22,917	22,917	22,917	22,917	22,917	22,917	**275,000**	10.8%	22,917
15,000	15,000	15,000	15,000	15,000	15,000	**180,000**	7.1%	30,000
15,208	15,208	15,208	15,208	15,208	15,208	**182,500**	7.1%	15,208
0	0	0	0	0	109,500	**109,500**	4.3%	9,125
31,973	0	0	0	0	0	**63,945**	2.5%	5,329
108,014	76,042	76,042	76,042	76,042	185,542	**1,085,945**	42.5%	90,495
48%	34%	34%	34%	34%	83%	**40%**		
43,562	43,562	43,562	43,562	43,562	43,562	**522,747**	20.5%	43,562
10,891	10,891	10,891	10,891	10,891	10,891	**130,687**	5.1%	10,891
3,457	3,457	3,457	3,457	3,457	3,457	**41,485**	1.6%	3,457
3,630	3,630	3,630	3,630	3,630	3,630	**43,560**	1.7%	3,630
8,704	8,704	8,704	8,704	8,704	8,704	**104,452**	4.1%	8,704
830	830	830	830	830	830	**9,963**	0.4%	830
4,031	4,031	4,031	4,031	4,031	4,031	**48,367**	1.9%	4,031
1,025	1,025	1,025	1,025	1,025	1,025	**12,300**	0.5%	1,025
15,159	15,159	15,159	15,159	15,159	15,159	**181,913**	7.1%	15,159
2,286	0	0	2,286	0	0	**9,143**	0.4%	762
879	879	879	879	879	879	**16,548**	0.6%	1,379
1,013	1,013	1,013	1,013	1,013	1,013	**12,155**	0.5%	1,013
772	772	772	772	772	772	**9,259**	0.4%	772
10,566	10,566	10,566	10,566	10,566	10,566	**126,788**	5.0%	10,566
0	0	0	0	0	28,133	**28,133**	1.1%	2,344
0	0	0	0	0	18,465	**18,465**	0.7%	1,386
1,386	1,386	1,386	1,386	1,386	1,386	**16,630**	0.7%	1,386
(11,183)	(11,183)	(11,183)	(11,183)	(11,183)	(11,183)	**(134,195)**	5.3%	(11,183)
119,373	117,087	117,087	119,373	117,087	163,685	**1,466,789**	57.5%	
53%	52%	52%	53%	52%	73%	**55%**		
227,387	193,129	193,129	195,415	193,129	349,227	**2,552,734**		
(3,373)	30,885	30,885	28,599	30,885	(125,213)			
0	**0**	**0**	**0**	**0**	**0**			
0	0	0	0	0	0			
98,271	**129,157**	**160,042**	**188,641**	**219,526**	**94,313**	**94,313**	EOY 4 Net for Principal Repayment	

EXHIBIT 4–4e

Financial Analysis—Lakeway Medical Services
Page 5

January 1, 1997   Scenario #1. $275,000 physician salary level; 12-year payback term

Year 5	Month 1	Month 2	Month 3	Month 4	Month 5	Month 6
Income						
Revenue — Dr. A	65,760	65,760	65,760	65,760	65,760	65,760
Revenue — Dr. B	51,803	51,803	51,803	51,803	51,803	51,803
Revenue — Dr. New	50,051	50,051	50,051	50,051	50,051	50,051
Revenue — NP: New	10,083	10,083	10,083	10,083	10,083	10,083
Revenue — NP: #1	9,090	9,090	9,090	9,090	9,090	9,090
Revenue — Ancillary & Technical	28,018	28,018	28,018	28,018	28,018	28,018
Revenue — Surgery Center — Net	14,171	14,171	14,171	14,171	14,171	14,171
Total Net Revenue	**228,976**	**228,976**	**228,976**	**228,976**	**228,976**	**228,976**
Physician Expenses						
Direct Compensation — Dr. A	22,917	22,917	22,917	22,917	22,917	22,917
Direct Compensation — Dr. B	22,917	22,917	22,917	22,917	22,917	22,917
Direct Compensation — Dr. New	15,000	15,000	15,000	15,000	15,000	15,000
Physician Benefits @ 25%	15,208	15,208	15,208	15,208	15,208	15,208
Physician Bonus @ 15%	0	0	0	0	0	0
Malpractice Insurance	33,571	0	0	0	0	0
Subtotal	109,613	76,042	76,042	76,042	76,042	76,042
Expenses as % of Net Revenue	48%	33%	33%	33%	33%	33%
Operating Expenses						
Support Staff Salaries	45,305	45,305	45,305	45,305	45,305	45,305
Staff Benefits @ 25%	11,326	11,326	11,326	11,326	11,326	11,326
Repairs and Maintenance	3,803	3,803	3,803	3,803	3,803	3,803
Office Supplies and Services	3,812	3,812	3,812	3,812	3,812	3,812
Rent @ $10/sq. ft. x 9,421	9,009	9,009	9,009	9,009	9,009	9,009
Equipment Rental	830	830	830	830	830	830
Telephone and Utilities	4,232	4,232	4,232	4,232	4,232	4,232
Travel, Dues, and Subscriptions	1,025	1,025	1,025	1,025	1,025	1,025
Clinical and Laboratory Supplies	15,917	15,917	15,917	15,917	15,917	15,917
Business Insurance	2,400	0	0	2,400	0	0
Promotion and Marketing	948	948	6,879	9,48	948	948
Accounting and Legal Fees	1,064	1,064	1,064	1,064	1,064	1,064
Real Estate Taxes and Insurance	799	799	799	799	799	799
All Other Expenses	11,094	11,094	11,094	11,094	11,094	11,094
Depreciation — Preacquisition	0	0	0	0	0	0
Depreciation — Postacquisition	0	0	0	0	0	0
Capital Expenditures	1,434	1,434	1,434	1,434	1,434	1,434
Amortization of Start-up/Purchase	(11,183)	(11,183)	(11,183)	(11,183)	(11,183)	(11,183)
Subtotal	124,180	121,780	127,711	124,180	121,780	121,780
Expenses as % of Net Revenue	54%	53%	56%	54%	53%	53%
Total All Expenses	**233,793**	**197,822**	**203,753**	**200,222**	**197,822**	**197,822**
Cash Available Minus Expenses	(4,817)	31,155	25,224	28,755	31,155	31,155
Balance	**(4,817)**	**26,338**	**51,561**	**80,316**	**111,471**	**142,625**

Month 7	Month 8	Month 9	Month 10	Month 11	Month 12	EOY 5	% of Total Revenue	Year 5 Monthly Average
65,760	65,760	65,760	65,760	65,760	65,760	**789,120**	28.7%	65,760
51,803	51,803	51,803	51,803	51,803	51,803	**621,638**	22.6%	51,803
50,051	50,051	50,051	50,051	50,051	50,051	**600,614**	21.9%	100,102
10,083	10,083	10,083	10,083	10,083	10,083	**121,000**	4.4%	10,083
9,090	9,090	9,090	9,090	9,090	9,090	**109,075**	4.0%	9,090
28,018	28,018	28,018	28,018	28,018	28,018	**336,217**	12.2%	28,018
14,171	14,171	14,171	14,171	14,171	14,171	**170,054**	6.2%	14,171
228,976	**228,976**	**228,976**	**228,976**	**228,976**	**228,976**	**2,747,717**	**100%**	**228,976**
							% of Total Expense	
22,917	22,917	22,917	22,917	22,917	22,917	**275,000**	10.5%	22,917
22,917	22,917	22,917	22,917	22,917	22,917	**275,000**	10.5%	22,917
15,000	15,000	15,000	15,000	15,000	15,000	**180,000**	6.9%	30,000
15,208	15,208	15,208	15,208	15,208	15,208	**182,500**	7.0%	15,208
0	0	0	0	0	109,500	**109,500**	4.2%	9,125
33,571	0	0	0	0	0	**67,142**	2.6%	5,595
109,613	76,042	76,042	76,042	76,042	185,542	**1,089,142**	41.6%	90,762
48%	33%	33%	33%	33%	81%	**40%**		
45,305	45,305	45,305	45,305	45,305	45,305	**453,657**	20.8%	45,305
11,326	11,326	11,326	11,326	11,326	11,326	**135,914**	5.2%	11,326
3,803	3,803	3,803	3,803	3,803	3,803	**45,634**	1.7%	3,803
3,812	3,812	3,812	3,812	3,812	3,812	**45,738**	1.7%	3,812
9,009	9,009	9,009	9,009	9,009	9,009	**108,108**	4.1%	9,009
830	830	830	830	830	830	**9,963**	0.4%	830
4,232	4,232	4,232	4,232	4,232	4,232	**50,785**	1.9%	4,232
1,025	1,025	1,025	1,025	1,025	1,025	**12,300**	0.5%	1,025
15,917	15,917	15,917	15,917	15,917	15,917	**191,008**	7.3%	15,917
2,400	0	0	2,400	0	0	**9,600**	0.4%	800
948	948	948	948	948	948	**17,375**	0.7%	1,448
1,064	1,064	1,064	1,064	1,064	1,064	**12,763**	0.5%	1,064
799	799	799	799	799	799	**9,583**	0.4%	799
11,094	11,094	11,094	11,094	11,094	11,094	**133,127**	5.1%	11,094
0	0	0	0	0	28,133	**28,133**	1.1%	2,344
0	0	0	0	0	21,907	**21,907**	0.8%	1,826
1,434	1,434	1,434	1,434	1,434	1,434	**17,212**	0.7%	1,434
(11,183)	(11,183)	(11,183)	(11,183)	(11,183)	(11,183)	**(134,195)**	5.1%	(11,183)
124,180	121,780	121,780	124,180	121,780	171,820	**1,527,003**	58.4%	
54%	53%	53%	54%	53%	75%	**58%**		
233,793	**197,822**	**197,822**	**200,222**	**197,822**	**357,362**	**2,616,076**		
(4,817)	31,155	31,155	28,755	31,155	(128,385)			
137,809	**168,963**	**200,118**	**228,872**	**260,027**	**131,641**	**131,641**	EOY 5 Net for Principal Repayment	

NOTES

1. The Center for Healthcare Industry Performance Studies, *Physician Practice Acquisition Resource Book*, (Toledo, OH: Findley-Davies, 1995).

2. Ken Terry, "The Many Pluses of Investing in Your Own MSO," *Medical Economics*, April 10, 1995, p. 136.

3. J. Daniel Beckham, "New Wave Equity," *Modern Healthcare*, July 5, 1995, p. 30.

4. U. S. Internal Revenue Service, *IRS Exempt Organization Continuing Professional Education Technical Instruction Program Textbook* (Washington, DC, 1995), p. 393.

5. Mary Chris Jaklevic, "Buying Doc Practices Often Leads to Red Ink," *Modern Healthcare*, June 3, 1996, p. 39.

6. Shannon P. Pratt, et al., *Valuing Small Businesses and Professional Practices, Second Edition* (Burr Ridge, IL: Business One Irwin, 1993), p. 543.

7. Roger Fisher, et al., *Getting to Yes, Second Edition,* (New York: Penguin Books USA, 1993).

8. Shannon P. Pratt, et al., *Valuing a Business, Third Edition* (Burr Ridge, IL: Richard D. Irwin, 1996), pp. 536–37.

9. Ibid., p. 537.

10. Ibid., p. 359.

11. Ibid., p. 411.

12. Ibid., p. 155.

13. Thad Green and Merwyn Hayes, *The Belief System* (Winston-Salem, NC: Beechwood Press, 1990), generally.

14. Douglas G. Cave, "Analyzing the Content of Physicians' Medical Practices," *Journal of Ambulatory Care Management*, 1994, pp. 15–36.

15. Medical Group Management Association, Englewood, CO, 1996.

16. American Medical Association, Chicago, 1996.

5

MERGING PRACTICES, BUSINESSES, AND STRATEGIC BUSINESS UNITS

MERGING PRACTICES AND STRATEGIC BUSINESS UNITS

Conventional wisdom in merging medical practices and strategic business units seems to indicate that the initial focus should be on addressing the cultural issues of the entities rather than on the benefits gained, such as reduced overhead, operational efficiencies, and better provider call schedules. In small business merger forums, you are likely to hear more about the difficulties involved in bringing two "similar" groups together than the benefits achieved. These difficulties stem from basic human and professional instincts inherent in human nature. The following summary denotes key areas that are the underpinnings of medical practice business, professional, and personal relationships. Although much of the following discussion is presented from a medical practice merger perspective, attention to these detail items are likely to be the only way that a successful merger will occur across any autonomous business unit.

Q Why do separate groups, practices, or businesses entertain a merger?

A The answer must be addressed in the context of small autonomous units such as medical practices and healthcare businesses versus larger organizations such as hospitals, physician groups, and health plans. Small groups or businesses may lack confidence about their ability to compete given the rapidly changing marketplace. Concern over the predomination of group practice, the increasing business aspect of medicine, the burden of forecasting business growth, and the general picture of risk leads most physicians to link up with larger, presumably more stable groups. Sharing calls, relief of isolation in solo practice, having a colleague in the office, and small scale overhead control round out the list of prevalent reasons.

Larger entities seek mergers for some of the same reasons, although mostly on a larger scale. Hospital mergers may stem from immediate or imminent financial loss in one example to the adoption of a proactive position to avoid competitor ingress into an otherwise stable market. In some cases, mergers seem to make sense, given the regulatory approvals, or in the landmark case of Memorial Mission and St. Joseph's Hospital in Asheville, NC., the hospitals found state immunity from federal antitrust review under a state Certificate of Public Advantage (COPA). Many of the investor-owned entities, large and small, use mergers as a means for rapid growth and capital acquisition. Emphasis on service delivery, cost, quality, utilization, and convenience are also driving factors.

Q What are some of the precipitating factors that drive groups to merge?

A Increasing overhead expenses and reduced per-physician earnings are among the most frequently cited reasons. With expenses approaching 70% in some practices, there is not much room left for provider income. High-dollar specialties cannot afford too many inefficiencies in the system and there appears to be no readily apparent change: fees and reimbursement keep dropping and cutting overhead is difficult. Increasing discounted fees and the initial experiences with capitation gives most physicians cause for concern in less developed managed care areas. The need for a partner to weather the storm is also a compelling reason for solo physicians and smaller groups, citing safety in numbers.

Q Why are so many groups finding difficulty with merging?

A There are many reasons for which different groups have difficulties in merging their economic and cultural business components. Economic issues are daunting enough: fee schedules, physician compensation, employment and buy-sell agreements, business and real estate valuation, and financial projections may be extremely sensitive issues to resolve between two different groups. Cultural issues including new practice styles and expectations, personnel management, interpersonal relationships, and the blending of practice patients create tensions that most groups neglect to consider in light of the vast economic benefits perceived. Other difficulties with merging include lack of vision, leadership, and effective governance, choosing the wrong partners, failure to make good on needs of clinical and economic consolidation, working through the tough points between members, and generally not completing the merger details.

Q What are some of the myths of economic savings in mergers?

A The first myth is that the pooling of resources on a small scale is likely to gain significant economic advantages. Bringing less than about 10 physicians into one group (plus several extenders) will not yield much in the way of savings in overhead control. The complexity added with slightly less than this number warrants more practice or business management horsepower than either of the individual groups, and the expense will likely be about the same, if not higher.

The second myth is that capturing and maximizing ancillary services from a larger group will be an ongoing significant revenue source. Although ancillary services will continue to be a strong revenue source, increasing prohibitions are scaling back the potential that groups once enjoyed, and corporate systems may well need to capture these services outside the practice setting. This creates concern for physician bonus pools and requires careful planning. Additionally, physician compensation plans, in private or corporate systems, cannot directly or indirectly tie physician compensation to ancillary revenues (gross distributions of total practice revenues is legal; careful structuring of distribution plan is advised).

The small healthcare business world is significantly different from what it was 5 or 10 years ago. Changing patient volumes and patterns of care, ever increasing regulatory issues, new and emerging (pervasive) lifestyle concerns among physicians, and the power shift to a gatekeeper mentality makes specialists reluctant partners for multispecialty arrangements. Issues on income distribution, especially mixing primary care and specialists, are more difficult in lean times. Topping all of it off is a greater fear of loss of autonomy than ever before.

Q What are the best reasons to consider a merger?

A Among the best reasons are (1) to create a group of substantial size for managed care contracting; (2) to gain or retain a significant market share/geographic coverage or presence; (3) to add primary care (or selected specialty care) building clout for all types of future negotiations (managed care/practice sales); (4) to achieve demonstrable economies through significant overhead reduction; and (5) physical facility consolidation and improvement over inadequate facilities. Most important are the compelling conditions that make a business merger the correct choice. Exhaustive study should precede the go-ahead decision on behalf of each group to ensure a commonality of need, interest, desire, and strength to achieve a successful merger.

Q Does the value of each business automatically increase by merging?

A Automatically increase, no. A successful merger of two strong groups will most likely have a positive impact on the economic value of the entity, although valuation about 1 year postmerger will give the best indication. An unsuccessful merger will be readily apparent to the appraiser and be reflected in the opinion of fair market value. Value is not simply added by creating one large semi-dysfunctional group, or one with significant risk of dissolving. The increased market power of the merged group may neutralize some of this when being pursued by a buyer seeking a group of sufficient mass for vertical integration or strategic partnership, such as in the case of a specialty or multispecialty group partnering with a primary care group. Nonetheless, the fair market value of the entity should reflect the desirability and marketability of the subject group in relation to the universe of comparable entities in the geographic market. All things held equal, a well functioning and strong merged group will be more valuable than a poorly merged group.

FACILITATING A MERGER: PRACTICAL EXPERIENCES AND SELF-ASSESSMENT

Deciding to Merge

Considerations to evaluate include:

+ Why are we considering a merger, i.e., what are our objectives in pursuing this merger? What are the compelling reasons and conditions that would make this the strategy of choice?

+ Are there alternatives? Will they create similar, positive outcomes?

+ Who are the potential partners and why are they being considered? What do they add to this group and will they allow us to achieve our objective?

+ Why are we compatible partners and what potential advantages and impediments are foreseen?

+ Will there be significant governance and management challenges due to dissimilarities (group size, incomes, overhead, practice style, et cetera)?

+ Can we afford to merge ($10,000 per physician or $500,000 to $1,000,000 for medium-sized hospital—external costs only)?

+ Can we afford not to merge? Are there compelling factors in the marketplace that would force you into a negative bargaining position or, at worst, cause your business to fail?

+ Are there anticipated regulatory (chiefly antitrust) and due diligence issues?

+ Time frame: Most practice and small business mergers should be completed in 6 to 12 months after initial conversation with potential partners to avoid changing minds, disillusionment, and disruption. Expect about 3 months for the leading group to discuss, educate, and make the decision to pursue potential partners and an additional 1 to 3 months to evaluate potential partners before approaching them. From here, plan about 3 months to discuss and educate within your group, to evaluate compatibility and practice styles, and discuss governance and management. Only after these issues have been framed should you approach compensation. Larger entities (e.g., large physician networks and hospitals) may require significantly more time to work through community benefit issues (as appropriate), business plan development, due diligence and regulatory review, document preparation, transition planning and preparation, and final implementation.

Merger Planning

Visioning and strategic planning may well be the only ways that organizations can blend economic operations and cultures. As mentioned above, the organization leading the process must develop a clear understanding and imperative that a merger is required as the first step.[1] Once the leading (read: initiating) group decides on the merger path, the next step is to evaluate potential partners. The following section elaborates on merger planning citing examples of do's and don'ts when evaluating the likelihood for merger success with a potential candidate.

Feasibility—Opportunity to Determine Likelihood of Merger

Signing of Letter of Confidentiality and Premerger Discussions

The Letter of Confidentiality creates in each group the understanding that each party can explore, in confidence, the potential relationship. These need not be exhaustive documents but should be executed before formal discussions begin.

Role of Merger Facilitator

The merger facilitator is an outside disinterested perspective to the merger process. The facilitator should be engaged jointly by each party to the merger or in the case of a merger of numerous groups, such as in a large multispecialty organization, the facilitator should be engaged after presentation to an organizing membership of the parties. The facilitator is the main coordinator of effort, keeping people on schedule for accomplishing the tasks each group must perform along the way. This role is vital to the success of the merger. It is difficult for any party with a vested interest, for instance, ownership interest, to not appear overbearing when it comes to coordinating project work. An independent outside professional can ride the issues with practices and physicians without creating personal ill feelings that may negatively affect working relationships after the merger. The merger facilitator is also the main point of contact for all issues in the merger process.

Commitment

Each group must be committed to the group practice environment as the preferred choice of practice. The reason you are considering a merger in the first place is because you do not want to go it alone or sell out and become an employee without control (some of the physician management company equity models are offering aspects of control and investment and while true equity is rare, expect this to increase). Each group needs to realize that they need greater strength to withstand competitor and market conditions than remaining in their current structure. Each group must desire to control costs, utilization, and risk, and maintain a commitment to high quality care. Groups must understand the need to retain capital and reduce expenses, remembering that operating margins are identified in advance and that equity is built through retaining earnings and developing a value-creating organization. Recall Richard Normann and Rafael Ramirez: the secret of creating value lies in an organization's ability to build a "value creating system, within which different economic actors—suppliers, business partners, allies, customers—work together to co-produce value."[2] Each group must realize that a merger will require somewhat less autonomy than in their existing practice, but much more than in any other long-term alternative—you have to give up power to get power. Lastly, each party must agree and sign a statement of purpose or objectives for discussion (not intent). Remember, we are still in the early stages of determining whether partners are right for each other. Groups should begin to outline their objectives as individual physicians, delineating their own personal and professional aspirations before each group comes to a general consensus of the personal and professional issues that are important to them. The facilitator discusses (and assists each group, as necessary) these areas of concern and coordinates discussion of the areas of commitment as they relate to common objectives and potential conflicting objectives.

Negotiation on Key Areas of Concern

Key areas of concern will include common issues in business governance, management, operations, compensation, and other factors as well as unique issues identified in the previous commitment assessment.

Governance

The guiding principle is that you should seek balance in power, authority, and mutual respect of the parties (a merger is where each party retains some facets of their own identity; a takeover or acquisition results in one party being subsumed into the other). Groups should take guidance from their key areas of concern and not seek to covet, but to expand each other's wealth. As the old saying goes, you have to give up something to get something. In the process, not everyone can play the role of the leader. A lead (coordinating) physician or principal from each organization should be elected to represent that group; in the event of larger numbers of shareholders, several members may be worthwhile. That leaders should lead and followers should follow is a good maxim. Once each group has decided on its representative, work through that representative, raising your issues as needed, but don't micromanage the process. Everyone is busy enough with clinical and other duties and the merger process is time-consuming as it is. Groups coming together should create allowances for dissimilar group size. It is natural that a smaller party may feel overwhelmed or undervalued (not from a financial sense, although this applies as well) when partnering with a larger group. Not only does the smaller group sense this disparity, but one can immediately envision the postmerger governance dynamics when the smaller merged group still retains a minority voting position. One way to address this, maintaining parity for the larger group, is to allow some votes based on majority, i.e., greater than 50% of the voters, some votes requiring a supermajority, e.g., greater or equal to 66%, and/or requiring co-majorities among operating boards or divisions of the group. A resourceful facilitator can work with each group and the merger attorney to create a win-win relationship if differing group size is the most significant issue. Lastly, maintain formality in governance without undue burden.

Management and Personnel

How management is envisioned and what level is required depends on group size and complexity. The merging of two medical practices with three physicians each may not significantly increase the complexity of the new group, depending, of course on individual circumstances. The ultimate merging of 30 physicians is another matter entirely. Either existing manager, in the case of two groups merging, or any of the existing managers in the case of a larger merger may not be appropriate for the new group. The groups should work with their merger facilitator to develop the conditions under which the new group would see the management function, and what knowledge, skills, and abilities are important for the administrator of the new group. In bringing two groups with competent administrative staff together, pick one to lead; team management seldom works. Evaluate needs and skills for the role and outplace the departing manager(s) through a qualified outplacement counselor. Regarding major financial operations decisions, identify charitable care issues, write-off and courtesy policies of each group to determine whether they may be in potential conflict. In these times of decreasing reimbursement and increased risk, it is important that everyone understand the implications of charitable contribution. Evaluate capital needs and the strategy for developing a base (remember, equity models build equity, partially by not distributing reserves back to the physicians) or identify the means to acquire capital from outside resources. Identify means and plan for asset depreciation and amounts for replacement reserves. Reevaluate staffing needs (provider and support staff) and supervisory responsibilities for all employees and functional units. Flatten and downsize should be the general idea. Mergers only begin to save real money by eliminating duplicative services, most importantly, duplicative staffing. Identify differences in staff cultures and begin to think of how the merger will necessarily affect changes in operations and in staff culture. Prune and groom should be the goal. Now is the time to create a new organization and leave all the excess baggage behind; leave behind not only staff but outmoded practices and bring in new ones that you've wanted to for years, but couldn't. Now is the ideal time to make all types of positive changes.

Blending of Processes and Cultures

Blending personnel in organizations requires a critical analysis of practice or professional styles, compatibility and autonomy. Individuals who have become accustomed to one style of conducting business may find it difficult to assimilate into the new environment. These issues become one of the greatest obstacles to successful merging, and are one of the most frequent causes for merged organizations to split. These cultural issues should be examined very carefully to ensure that a common understanding is present before moving ahead. Work schedules and habits, especially related to use of personnel, should be discussed. Just because Sadie leaves early on Fridays and has always had 1 hour and 15 minutes or so for lunch doesn't mean that it can continue in the new organization. Similarly, most smaller practices and businesses operate without time clocks, but few organizations over 30 staff do. The technical proficiency of providers should be examined—not only the physicians, but the physician extenders as well. In most professional practice mergers, it is difficult to exclude a given physician (or dentist, counselor, or therapist) on the grounds of lack of technical proficiency. Preferably these issues are identified by each group and dealt with prior to and outside of merger discussions. In the event that one party questions the inclusion of a specific individual, tactful, professional discussion should rule, recognizing that this may become a sticking point. Other technical staff, such as laboratory and radiology, should be evaluated, and appropriate action taken where needed.

The range of expertise within specialties (e.g., GI procedures, minor surgery, urgent/injury care, occupational medicine) should be determined and the groups should jointly decide on a plan of recruitment if a given specialty or technical proficiency is desired. The groups should also analyze referral patterns and hospital privileges, and identify after-hours call coverage concerns, especially as they relate to insurance and managed care participation. Groups who are able to evaluate utilization should do so, although this is typically beyond the scope of most practices and small healthcare businesses. Demand management, the ability to maximize the use of all business resources to their optimum utility, should be embraced, not only for the coordination of administrative and support services, but in scheduling and providing of clinical care. For example, supply inventories should be examined to ensure that adequate amounts are available on site and that replacements are available on short notice (delivered within 48 hours). By reducing the inventory, cash flow is enhanced; by negotiating timely delivery—and many suppliers have geared up to support demand management—overall resource utility is improved. Demand management concepts can extend as well into staff scheduling, administrative processing, patient scheduling (determining historical peak periods), and other areas of business limited only by your imagination.

All types of healthcare businesses should make the commitment to continuing education and quality improvement in all facets of their work. In the new era of differentiation of health services, high quality and high functioning teams are of greater value (to the marketplace and to the ongoing business) than other "me too" businesses. Related to examining and creating a better business environment is the willingness of individuals and groups to modify personal or parochial habits for the good of the group. No one group or person has the monopoly on good ideas and the overall success of the business and satisfaction of its members should require each member to adapt to the activity or style of practice that most benefits the organization. While some accommodation should be expected, not everything can be resolved. Compatibility of personal ethics, lifestyles, and religious affiliation are among the greatest differences to overcome in interpersonal and business relationships. Potential partners should openly discuss any and all of these areas that they believe may cause personal or professional conflict for them.

Name of the Practice or Business

Selecting the new name of the entity is also an area of considerable difficulty (readers might wonder why, but it is). No single group should dominate the discussion or foist their name onto the new entity. At a minimum, groups should evaluate and discuss their beliefs on an appropriate name for the new group. In some circumstances, the groups may know intuitively that they will be selecting one of the existing names, as in the case of a smaller group joining a slightly larger group with better location, name recognition, etc. One method to delay the naming if there is some concern that it may take some time, is to establish a transition period of 6 to 12 months after merging to work on potential names for the new group. This method allows the principals to keep focused on clinical care as well as all the other issues of merging and deal with the name issue last. Culturally, allow the new identity time to develop; do not attempt to create it all at once. Culture shock, an appropriate term, occurs when individuals (principals and staff) are thrown into a new, somewhat unknown environment causing confusion and frustration. Some aspects of business operations can and should be changed immediately, especially those that relate to administrative processes and key areas that the groups agree should change immediately. But don't bite off more than you can chew; change in organizations is similar to the body's prioritization system right after a big meal: after this significant event, you can't jump up and run a marathon. Take your time, but plan your time, and prioritize the actions that need completion first.

Physician Compensation and Employment Agreements

Groups should make a commitment to leveling the income field among providers by some equitable means of distribution (see also *Physician Compensation* in Chapter 7). In the merged environ-ment, a greater likelihood exists for income disparity, especially in multispecialty groups. These groups should make a commitment to supporting primary care development and network participation to ensure the adequate flow of patients into the practice. Groups must be particularly careful in treating ancillary income and should create effective and legal ancillary distribution methods (see also Stark Laws in Chapter 6). Establish a system for mutual respect and reward within appropriate risk sharing. Groups and members should be rewarded for their share of activity and how that activity benefits the group. For example, an otolaryngology group with one member who specializes in pediatrics (read: sees almost all the pediatric cases) has a significantly different pattern from his partners. In the income distribution method, this may prove to be a significant issue. Likewise, the percentage of total income from capitated patients and other payor sources may be different between physicians; these should also be addressed.

Consider effect of ownership on partner recruitment and retirement. Do not create impossible buy-ins and pay-outs for the group or you will not be able to recruit new partners, and exiting partners may seriously impact cash operations, physician salaries, and bonuses. Consider deferred compensation and cash value policies where feasible.

Valuation of Practices

Define tangible and intangible assets of each group and whether significant disparity exists. Should goodwill be considered? Typically it is not included although it may exist in varying degrees between the groups. Frank discussion should be coordinated by the merger facilitator on the handling of intangible assets including a definition, by group, of what each brings and how its importance relates in the marketplace. From here the groups can choose to include all or part of the intangible assets. Further discussion includes what other assets are included or excluded from valuation—for example, automobiles owned by one practice, original or personal artwork, heirloom private furnishings, etc. The main issue is to determine what might stay and what might not, and attach value estimates to the sum of each group's assets. Discuss also the impact or need for real estate usage, purchase, or divestiture. Recognize economic value of each party aside from hard asset value. This may be thought of as the strategic value of merging two or more specific groups (see Strategic Investment Value in Chapter 3). This concept gets back to your earliest premerger internal discussions; who are our potential partners and why? With each step of the merger process, greater and greater validation of the concept is made, for without it reservations exist and the potential for differences to force the merger apart (which may be OK since the decision not to merge with another party may end up being the best decision).

Pension/Retirement Plan (Partially Funded vs. Fully Funded Plans)

Analyze and determine equitable payout or rollover for each party's pension or retirement plan for employees and partners. Each party's accountant should be able to reconcile the statements and guide the principals through the best way to maximize benefit from each plan. In some cases, maintenance of individual plans is possible and works out best for the group, as long as equity is maintained in business contributions to the plan. Stock issues—redemption, dissolution, new values, and taxes—should be coordinated through each group's accounting counsel with assistance from the merger attorney and merger facilitator. In the case of large mergers or the merging of two groups of different sizes, different classes of stock may be issued with defined voting rights to balance the governing decisions of the newly merged organization. As mentioned previously, requiring a majority, supermajority, or co-majority vote on certain issues may obviate the need for different classes of ownership. Again, be careful how ownership is structured and how it affects the ability to recruit new potential partners.

Leasing, Purchasing, and Building Arrangements

Merger planning should include an evaluation on what real property will be required to operate the new organization. Many smaller mergers can be implemented successfully by remaining in existing facilities but larger ones may need to divest one or more buildings, remodel, lease, or build new space to maximize efficient operation. Real estate usage should be examined carefully to identify opportunities for savings and new purchase; building or divestiture should really be based on a unanimous consensus of the partners (in reality this may be impossible; the group has to go with the most sound decision and move on).

Signing of Letter of Intent to Merge

The Letter of Intent to Merge establishes the time frame and confidence among the parties that a strong potential exists for a merger. It establishes the merger schedule and plan (see Exhibit 5–1) and allows each party to clearly see that progress is being made, not simply more discussion. Lastly, it establishes that major issues are already resolved: baseline discussions on governance, operations, facilities, and financial matters. The fine points are yet to come.

DECISION AND IMPLEMENTATION

Role of Merger Attorney

The merger attorney is a neutral participant who processes papers and transactions regarding the merger of the parties. He or she should be a health law specialist with experience in these types of business transactions. The merger attorney advises on matters related to the transaction only, focusing on facilitating the arrangement and explaining each suggested approach to each party's attorney.

EXHIBIT 5–1

Lakeway Pediatrics/Stratford Pediatric Group
Merger Plan

Phase One   Strategic Planning Discussion with Each Group

Methodology: Systematic overview of eace group focusing on:

- Why is a merger being considered?
- Alternatives that will allow similar, positive postmerger outcomes.
- Partner compatibility.
- Merger costs ($5,000 to $10,000 per physician)
- Antitrust, fraud, and abuse issues.
- Benefits vs. detriments inherited by each group.

Outcome: Decision to continue merger process

Time Frame   Month 1–2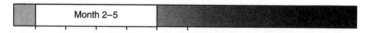

Phase Two   Feasibility Study

Methodology: Financial and operational analysis

- Key concerns of individual physicians and of each group
- Operational assessments of each practice
- Valuation of each practice
- Postmerger financial projections
- Governance, personnel issues
- Pension plans and employment agreements

Outcome: Decision to continue merger process

Time Frame   Month 2–5

Phase Three   Decision and Implementation

Methodology: Open discussion and hands-on activity

- Refinement of issues
- Coordination of legal counsel and accounting
- Document design and completion
- Operations coordination/real property management
- Recruitment/outplacement of staff
- Completion of employment/benefits agreements and issues

Outcome: Completed merger—practice operational

Time Frame   Month 4–6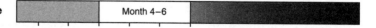

(New) Practice Administrator

The practice administrator is the key individual in creating the new environment (culture) of the merged group. Although practice administrators often move heaven and earth to make sure that everything gets done correctly, they serve three primary functions related to the merger. As facilitators, they assure and encourage all information processing needed by the new group, not limited only to physician, group and business licenses, and regulatory / administrative requirements (new plan numbers, contract changes, etc.), but they also coordinate the numerous pieces of information required by the principals, the merger attorney, merger facilitator, and all external groups. They know where everything is, and without them almost everything would be lost. They serve, therefore, as coordinators before and after the merger. They also serve as confidants for providers and staff to foster discussion about the future, how they will survive, how existing operations will be affected, and how to make the process run tolerably well, if not smoothly.

PREMERGER OPERATIONAL ASSESSMENT

The following areas should be examined in the form of an operational assessment.

Management and Personnel
- Which, if any, employees will be leaving.
- New position descriptions and performance standards.
- Benefits coordination and resolution of disparities.
  a. Listing by name, age distribution, and sex.
  b. Documents on file (I-9, W-4, employment applications, etc.).
  c. Salary histories, benefits records, and sick/vacation time schedules.
  d. Training received and cross training.

Business Operations and Systems
- Patient relations and marketing.
- Formal marketing plans and service area of practice.

- Age/sex distribution of patients and population analysis.
- Scope of accounts (payor mix, industrial accounts, etc.).
- Telephone Operations.
  a. Number of phone lines/extensions/fax.
  b. Answering machine/services.
  c. Emergency procedures/logs/messages/pages.
  d. Patient difficulties/satisfaction.
- Appointment Scheduling.
  a. Day/date/time analysis.
  b. Manual/computerized/method.
  c. Reserved slots, walk-ins, extenders, and follow-up policy.
- Medical Records.
  a. Number of active charts, completeness, and legibility.
  b. Filing system, pull tabs, and outguides.
  c. Office notes, loose filing, and backlogs.
- Insurance.
  a. Frequency of filing.
  b. Manual/electronic, superbill.
  c. Data backup, systematic monitoring, and tracking.
  d. Denials, claim refiling, and time frames.
  e. Third-party participation and contractual adjustments tracking.
- Financial Management.
  a. Prospective operating budget established.
  b. Education/training of staff.
  c. Accountancy services/frequency of reporting.
  d. Cost containment/inventory control.
- Collections.
  a. Written and working policies.
  b. Readability of bills/frequency/time of service.
  c. Phone calls and collections referral service.
  d. Deposits required for procedures/cash collections.

- ◆ Internal Control.
  a. Charge and payments posting and canceling, deposits, and bonding.
  b. Petty cash maintenance and change fund.
  c. Recording disbursements.

Physical Facility

- ◆ Renovations, parking, and updates.
- ◆ Interior/exterior appearance.
- ◆ Ingress/egress.
- ◆ CLIA/OSHA.

Real Estate

- ◆ Owned/leased (how much/fair value rent).
- ◆ Mortgage or lease terms.
- ◆ Leasehold improvements.
- ◆ Immediate improvements required.

DEAL BREAKERS

Deal breaking issues should only occur very early in the process, typically in the feasibility stage where parties are identifying compatibility and likelihood of a similar view of the practice of medicine. In some cases deal breakers surface early in the negotiations of key areas of concern phase, often after governance and into compensation issues. Compensation continues to be one of the most difficult issues to overcome in merging two entities. It is advisable to identify potential deal breakers, for each group, early in the process to decide on whether partnership compatibility exists. Although it sounds somewhat defeatist, the sooner two groups decide they are not suited to each other, the better they both are. Mergers are difficult, time-consuming efforts, and fewer than half of the original negotiations result in completed mergers.[3] Both organizations benefit by identifying incompatibility early so they may continue with their partner searches.

NOTES

1. Thomas L. Kelly, "What It Takes to Consummate a Merger," *Medical Economics*, January 9, 1995, p. 30.

2. Richard Normann and Rafael Ramirez, "From Value Chain to Value Constellation: Designing Interactive Strategy," *Harvard Business Review*, 71, no. 4 (1993), pp. 65–77.

3. Anita J. Slomski, "Got the Urge to Merge? You're Not Alone," *Medical Economics*, April 11, 1994, p. 50.

III

THE LEGAL AND REGULATORY ENVIRONMENT

6

LEGAL ISSUES IN THE FORMATION AND OPERATION OF IDS ORGANIZATIONS

OVERVIEW OF LEGAL AND REGULATORY ISSUES

Fraud and Abuse and Anti-Referral Laws

The primary concern of the fraud and abuse and anti-referral laws is the avoidance of fraud and overutilization in the Medicare and Medicaid reimbursement programs. A 1989 study by the Department of Health and Human Services Office of the Inspector General found that patients of referring physicians who invested in independent clinical laboratories ordered 45% more tests for their patients than Medicare patients in general.[1] This finding became the impetus for enacting the Stark anti-referral laws.

Violation of these statutes incur severe penalties, including criminal charges for violation of the anti-kickback statutes. To compound these severe penalties, many commonplace activities in the healthcare arena would be prohibited by these laws but for the application of statutory and regulatory "safe harbors," which protect these activities from prosecution. Although the federal laws govern only payments for items or services by Medicare and

Medicaid, many state laws have similar prohibitions that apply to all third-party payors, with varying safe harbor protections.

In mid-1996, both houses of Congress passed H.R. 3103, the Health Insurance Portability and Accountability Act of 1996. When signed into law by the president, this new law will provide additional funding for fraud enforcement, and it will also require the Office of the Inspector General to issue advisory opinions on whether certain activities constitute prohibited remuneration under the anti-kickback laws, whether the activity will fall under a safe harbor, and whether the activity is grounds for certain penalties.[2] In addition, many provisions of the new law will apply to private payors as well as to Medicare and Medicaid.[3]

MEDICARE ANTI-KICKBACK LAW
General Rule

The Medicare anti-kickback law[4] generally prohibits the filing of false claims and the payment of illegal remuneration to receive Medicare benefits or payments. The illegal remuneration prohibition specifies that persons in violation of the statute will be found guilty of a felony and fined up to $25,000 and/or will be subject to prison for up to 5 years. Culpable conduct under the statute is:

1. Knowingly and willfully soliciting or receiving *any remuneration* (including kickbacks, bribes, or rebates), directly or indirectly, overtly or covertly, in cash or in kind:

    a. In return for referring an individual to a person for the furnishing or arranging for the furnishing of any item or service for which payment may be made in whole or in part under Medicare or Medicaid.

    b. In return for purchasing, leasing, ordering, or arranging for or recommending purchasing, leasing, or ordering any good, facility, service, or item for which payment may be made in whole or in part by Medicare or Medicaid.

2. Knowingly and willfully offering or paying any remuneration (including any kickback, bribe, or rebate), directly or indirectly, overtly or covertly, in cash or in kind to any person to induce such person:

a. To refer an individual to a person for the furnishing or arranging for the furnishing of any item or service for which payment may be made under Medicare or Medicaid.

b. To purchase, lease, order, recommend, or arrange for purchasing, leasing, or ordering any good, facility, service, or item for which payment may be made in whole or in part by Medicare or Medicaid.

The Medicare anti-kickback law is intended to prohibit "actions in which the defendant intends to exercise influence over the reason or judgment of another in an effort to cause the referral of program-related business."[5] Unlike the Stark II anti-referral law, the anti-kickback law is a criminal statute that requires the defendant to have "knowledge and willfulness"; in other words, the defendant must have "acted with knowledge that his conduct was unlawful."[6] In United States v. Greber,[7] the defendant paid a referral fee of 40% to physicians referring patients to him for diagnostic services, which the defendant called "consulting" fees, even though some of the referring physicians performed no services for him. The court held that the anti-kickback statute was violated if *any* purpose of the payment was to induce referrals. The court reasoned that Congress intended the word "remuneration" to include situations where a service was actually rendered in addition to a referral. Similarly, in United States v. Kats,[8] the defendant owned a 25% share of a clinic that sent specimens to a lab for diagnostic purposes. The defendant's clinic received a 50% kickback of fees for tests that it referred to the lab. The court held that the government need not show that compensation for referrals was the primary purpose of a payment. Even if only one purpose of a payment was to induce referrals, the statute was violated.

The Stark law, in contrast, is a strict liability type of statute, in which the defendant's state of mind is not relevant. Similar to the Stark law, however, the anti-kickback law interprets "remuneration" very broadly and it has several safe harbors.

Safe Harbors

As with the anti-referral statute, the anti-kickback statute also provides safe harbors, many of which are similar to, but not exactly like, the anti-referral safe harbors. These safe harbors protect certain payment and business practices from criminal prosecution or civil sanctions under the statute.

Investment-Interest Safe Harbors.   The anti-kickback law has two safe harbors applicable to investment interests. One is for interests in large entities, and the other is for interests in small entities. These safe harbors define remuneration as not including any payments made to an investor that are a return on investment, such as dividend or interest income, as long as certain criteria are met.

Large-Entity Safe Harbor.   The large-entity safe harbor applies to entities having over $50 million in net assets related to the furnishing of items and services. To fall under the large-entity safe harbor, the following criteria must be met:

1. If the interest is an equity security, it must be registered with the Securities and Exchange Commission.
2. An investment interest held by one in a position to make referrals must be obtained on terms equally available to the public through trading on a national stock exchange.
3. The entity must not market or furnish the entity's items or services to passive investors differently from the way it would market to noninvestors.
4. The entity must not loan funds to, nor guarantee a loan for, an investor who is in a position to refer to the entity if the investor uses any part of that loan to obtain the investment interest.
5. The amount of payment to an investor in return for the investment interest must be directly proportional to the amount of capital investment.

Small-Entity Safe Harbor.   The small-entity safe harbor has slightly different requirements:

1. Less than 40% of the value of the investment interests of each class of investments may be held in the previous fiscal year or past 12-month period by investors in a position to refer.

2. The terms on which an investment is offered to a passive investor who is in a position to refer must be no different from the terms offered to other passive investors.

3. The terms on which an investment interest is offered to an investor who is in a position to refer must not be related to the previous or expected volume of referrals from that investor to the entity.

4. Passive investors must not be required to make referrals to the entity as a condition for remaining as investors.

5. The entity or investor must not market or furnish the entity's items or services to passive investors differently from the way it would market to noninvestors.

6. A maximum of 40% of the entity's gross revenue in the prior fiscal year or past 12-month period may come from referrals.

7. The entity may not loan funds to, nor guarantee a loan for, an investor in a position to refer if the investor uses any part of that loan to obtain the investment interest.

8. The amount of payment to an investor in return for the investment must be directly proportional to the amount of the capital investment of that investor, including the fair market value of any preoperational services rendered.

The regulations define an "investor" as an individual or entity who either directly holds an investment interest in an entity, or one who holds it indirectly, such as by having a family member hold the interest, or by holding a legal or beneficial interest in another entity holding the interest, such as through a trust or holding company. An "investment interest" is defined as a security issued by an entity, such as shares in a corporation, interests or units of a partnership, bonds, debentures, notes, or other debt instruments. An "active investor" is defined as an investor who either (1) is responsible for the day-to-day management of the entity and is a *bona fide* general partner in a partnership; or (2) has agreed in writing to undertake liability for the actions of the entity's agents acting within the scope of their agency. A "passive investor" is an investor who does not fall under the definition of an "active investor," such as a limited partner under the Uniform Partnership Act, a corporate shareholder, or a bondholder or holder of a debt security.

Space and Equipment Rental Safe Harbors.   As with the requirements for the Stark laws, lease payments made by a lessee to a lessor for space or equipment rental will fall under a safe harbor if certain criteria are met. The criteria under this safe harbor are similar to, but not exactly like, the criteria for the safe harbor under the Stark anti-referral statute:

1. The lease must be in writing and signed by the parties.
2. The lease must specify the premises or equipment covered by the lease.
3. If the lease is intended for part-time access, then the lease must specify exactly the schedule of such intervals, their precise length, and the exact rent for such intervals.
4. The term of the lease must be for at least one year.
5. The aggregate rent must be set in advance, it must be consistent with fair market value in an arms'-length transaction, and it must not be determined in a manner that takes into account the volume or value of referrals or other business generated between the parties for which payment may be made under Medicare or Medicaid.

As it relates to space rental, fair market value is defined as the value of the rental property for general commercial purposes, not adjusted to reflect the additional value that either party would attribute to the property due to its proximity or convenience to sources of referrals. As it relates to equipment rental, fair market value is defined as the value of the equipment when it is obtained from a manufacturer or professional distributor, not adjusted to reflect the additional value that either party would attribute to the equipment due to its proximity or convenience to sources of referrals.

Employment Relationships Safe Harbor.   For employer-employee relationships, the safe harbor simply defines remuneration not to include amounts paid by an employer to an employee who has a *bona fide* employment relationship with the employer, for employment in the furnishing of items or services payable by Medicare or Medicaid. This safe harbor has fewer requirements than the related safe harbor under Stark II.

Personal Services Contracts Safe Harbor.   This safe harbor defines remuneration not to include any payments made by a principal to an agent or independent contractor as compensation for the agent's services if the following criteria are met:

1. The agency agreement is in writing and signed by the parties.
2. The agreement specifies the services to be provided by the agent.
3. If the services are to be part-time or sporadic, and not full-time for the term of the agreement, the agreement must specify exactly the schedule of such intervals, their precise length, and the exact charge for such intervals.
4. The term of the agreement is for at least 1 year.
5. The *aggregate* compensation paid over the term of the agreement is:
    a. Set in advance.
    b. Consistent with fair market value in arms'-length transactions.
    c. Not determined in a manner that takes into account the volume or value of referrals or other business generated between the parties for which payment may be made by Medicare or Medicaid.
6. The services to be provided under the contract must not involve the counseling or promotion of a business arrangement or other activity that violates any state or federal law.

It is important to note that the aggregate compensation must be set in advance under this safe harbor, unlike the Stark II safe harbor. Thus, in managed care contracts, the contract must specify the total amount to be paid under the contract for all the services to be performed.

Sale of Practice.   Another safe harbor defines remuneration as not including payments made to one practitioner by another practitioner for the sale of his or her medical practice. The two requirements that must be met under this safe harbor are:

1. The period between the date of the first agreement pertaining to the sale and the completion of the sale is no more than 1 year.
2. The seller will not be in a professional position to make referrals to the buyer of the practice where such services would be paid for by Medicare or Medicaid.

Referral Services.   Remuneration does not include payments, or the exchange of anything of value, between a participant and a referral service if:

1. The referral service does not exclude participants or entities who meet its qualifications.
2. The participant's payments must be:
   a. Assessed equally and collected equally from all participants.
   b. Based only upon the cost of operating the referral service, not on the volume or value of referrals.
3. The referral service cannot impose requirements on the manner in which the participant provides the services to a referred person, but it may require that the participant charge at the same rate it charges nonreferred persons, or it may charge a reduced rate or no fee.
4. The referral service must make five disclosures to each person seeking a referral, which it must maintain in a written record signed by either the referred person or the discloser. These disclosures must address the manner of selecting the group of participants to whom the referrals are made; whether the participant pays a fee to be listed; the manner of selecting a particular participant; the nature of the relationship between the referral services and the group of participants; and the nature of any restrictions that would exclude a person or entity from being a participant.

Warranties.   Any payments or exchanges of anything of value under a warranty given by a manufacturer or supplier of an item to the buyer, whether it be the provider or beneficiary, will be covered under a safe harbor if certain criteria are met. A warranty is generally defined as a manufacturer's or supplier's agreement to replace a defective item on terms equal to the agreement that it replaces. The requirements to be met are:

1. The buyer must fully and accurately report the price reductions and free items obtained as part of the warranty in the cost report or claim for payment that it files with DHHS or the state.

2. The buyer must provide information supplied by the manufacturer or supplier upon request by DHHS or the state.

3. If the reduction amount is unknown, the seller must fully and accurately report the price reduction or free item obtained as part of the warranty on the invoice or statement submitted to the buyer, and it must notify the buyer of its duty to report the reduction.

4. If the reduction is unknown at the time of sale, the manufacturer must fully and accurately report the existence of the warranty on the invoice or statement to the buyer and tell the buyer of its duty to report. Documentation on the calculation of the price reduction must be provided to the buyer when it becomes known.

5. The manufacturer or supplier must not pay any remuneration to any individual, other than a beneficiary, or to an entity for any medical, surgical, or hospital expense incurred by a beneficiary other than for the cost of the item itself.

STARK II ANTI-REFERRAL LAW

The Stark law[9] was enacted in 1989 and is named after its sponsor, Representative Fortney "Pete" Stark. The Stark law generally prohibits referrals by physicians to entities in which they have a financial interest. Stark I originally applied only to payments for clinical laboratory services, where the referring physician owned a financial interest in the referred-to laboratory. Stark II became effective on January 1, 1995, and expanded the prohibitions to 11 "designated health services."

General Rule

The general rule of the anti-referral prohibition provides that physicians or their immediate family members who have a "financial relationship" with an entity cannot make a referral to that entity for the furnishing of designated health services for which payment may be made by Medicare or Medicaid. The referred-to entity cannot bill Medicare, any individual, or other entity or third-party payor for any designated health services provided from a prohibited referral.[10]

Definitions. A "financial relationship" is defined as an ownership or investment interest in the referred-to entity, or a compensation arrangement with the entity. An "ownership or investment interest" can be through equity, debt, or any other means, and it includes an interest in an entity that holds an ownership or investment interest in an entity providing the designated health service. A "compensation arrangement" is any arrangement involving any remuneration between a physician or immediate family member and the referred-to entity, unless it involves only insurance payments, debt forgiveness for inaccurate tests or procedures, or the provision of items or devices used solely to collect, transport, process, or store specimens for the entity providing the item, device, or supply. A compensation arrangement, therefore, normally would include payment of salaries, rental or lease payments, and any other type of remuneration being exchanged.

"Immediate family" is defined in the regulations generally as the range of relatives who could be in a position to influence the pattern of a physician's referrals. More specifically, the definition includes husband or wife; natural or adoptive parent; child or sibling; stepparent, stepchild, stepbrother, or stepsister; father-in-law, mother-in-law, son-in law, daughter-in-law, brother-in-law, or sister-in-law; grandparent or grandchild; and spouse of a grandparent or grandchild.[11]

With regard to physician services, a "referral" is the request by a physician for an item or service payable by Medicare Part B, including a request for a consultation by another physician, and any test or procedure ordered by, or to be performed by or under the supervision of that other physician. With regard to items other than physician services, the request or establishment of a plan of care by a physician that includes the provision of designated health services under Medicare Part A or Part B is also considered to be a referral. An exception to the definition of referral under the statute involves services that are integral to a consultation by certain specialists. If the following services are furnished by or under the supervision of the specialist pursuant to a consultation requested by another physician, then they are not "referrals" by a referring physician: (a) A request by a pathologist for clinical diagnostic lab tests and pathological examination services; (b) A request by a radiologist for diagnostic radiology services; or (c) A request by a radiation oncologist for radiation therapy.

As of January 1, 1995, the referral prohibition applies to 11 "designated health services." Between January 1, 1992, and January 1, 1995, the prohibition only applied to clinical laboratory services, but 10 more services were added effective in 1995. The designated health services to which the referral prohibition currently applies include the following services:

1. Clinical laboratory services.
2. Physical therapy services.
3. Occupational therapy services.
4. Radiology services, including MRI, CAT scans, and ultrasound services.
5. Radiation therapy services and supplies.
6. Durable medical equipment and supplies (iron lungs, oxygen tents, hospital beds, and wheelchairs used in the patient's home).
7. Parenteral and enteral nutrients, equipment, and supplies.
8. Prosthetics, orthotics, and prosthetic devices and supplies.
9. Home health services.
10. Outpatient prescription drugs.
11. Inpatient and outpatient hospital services.

Reporting. Any entity furnishing items or services payable by Medicare must submit information on its financial relationships to the Health Care Financing Administration (HCFA), unless the entity provides 20 or fewer Part A and Part B items or services per calendar year. Information that must be reported includes the names of physicians and their immediate family members who have a financial relationship with an entity, the nature of that financial relationship, and the covered items or services provided by the entity. The information must be filed within 30 days after notification from the carrier or intermediary, and within 60 days after any changes in the submitted information. Entities also must retain documentation of the information submitted and furnish it to HCFA or the Office of Inspector General upon request.

Effective June 1, 1996, HCFA is mandating the use of a single new-provider application form that increases the amount of information required on the applicant's operating locations, ownership, and affiliations.[12] HCFA has also indicated that it has contracted with data verification firms to ensure that information listed on the applications is truthful, and the agency is also increasing its on-site visits to providers to ascertain whether providers are actually providing the services for which they are billing.[13]

Sanctions.   Sanctions for violating the referral prohibition are somewhat severe and include denial of payment for designated health services rendered through a prohibited referral, mandatory refunds of claims paid, civil monetary penalties, and exclusion from the Medicare and Medicaid reimbursement programs. Civil monetary penalties for filing prohibited claims are up to $15,000 for each service billed. Civil monetary penalties for circumvention schemes, such as a cross-referral network, are up to $100,000 for each arrangement. Sanctions also apply for failure to report information, in the form of a civil monetary penalty of $10,000 for each day beyond the deadline that the information remains unreported.

Safe Harbors.   There are several safe harbor provisions that protect common activities in the healthcare industry from sanctions. There are three safe harbors that apply to both types of financial relationships—ownership/investment interests and compensation arrangements. These three safe harbors relate to physicians' services, in-office ancillary services, and prepaid plans. Safe harbors applying only to ownership/investment interests are for publicly traded securities, shares in regulated investment companies, hospitals in Puerto

Rico, rural providers, and hospital ownership. Safe harbors applying only to compensation arrangements are for office space rental, equipment rental, *bona fide* employment relationships, personal service arrangements, unrelated remuneration, physician recruitment, isolated transactions, group practice arrangements with a hospital, and payments by physicians for items and services.

Exceptions to Ownership and Compensation Arrangements

Physician Services.   An important safe harbor protects referrals between physicians in the same group practice. If physician services are provided personally by, or under the personal supervision of, another physician in the same group practice as the referring physician, then the activity does not constitute a prohibited referral.

The statute defines a "group practice" as a group of two or more physicians legally organized as a partnership, professional corporation, foundation, nonprofit corporation, faculty practice plan, or similar association. To qualify as a group practice, the association must meet the following requirements:

1. Each physician member must provide substantially the full range of services that the physician routinely provides, including medical care, consultation, diagnosis, or treatment, through the joint use of shared office space, facilities, equipment, and staff.

2. Substantially all of the services of the physician members are provided through the group and billed under the group's billing number, and amounts received are treated as group receipts. "Substantially all" means at least 75% of the total patient care services of the group practice members.[14]

3. Overhead expenses and income are distributed in accordance with previously determined methods.

4. No physician member receives compensation based directly or indirectly on referrals, unless for a productivity bonus.

5. Group members must conduct personally at least 75% of the physician-patient encounters of the group practice.

6. The arrangement must meet other requirements that may be imposed by the Department of Health and Human Services from time to time.

An important aspect of this definition is that an entity whose individual physicians bill in their own individual names does not qualify as a group practice. The group must attest in writing, on a yearly basis, that it meets the requirements of the group practice definition. The group practice may pay its physician members a productivity bonus or profit sharing if the bonus or share is based upon services personally performed by the physician or services incident to personally performed services, and if the bonus or share is not calculated based upon referrals.

In-Office Ancillary Services.   Another important safe harbor applies to in-office ancillary services. To qualify for this safe harbor, the arrangement must meet the following requirements:

1. The ancillary services must be furnished personally by one of the following:
   a. The referring physician.
   b. A physician in the same group practice (as defined above) of the referring physician.
   c. Individuals directly supervised by the physician or a physician in the same group practice.
2. The services must be furnished in a building in which the referring physician furnishes services unrelated to the designated health services. If a group practice is involved, the services may be furnished in another building used by the group practice for some or all of the group's clinical lab services, or for the centralized provision of the group's designated health services.
3. The services must be billed by one of the following:
   a. The physician performing or supervising the services.
   b. The group practice, through the group's billing number.
   c. An entity wholly owned by the physician or group performing the service.

Services excluded under this safe harbor are for durable medical equipment and supplies, but those included are infusion pumps, and parenteral and enteral nutrients, equipment, and supplies. The final regulations issued for Stark I in August 1995 define "direct supervision" to mean "supervision by a physician who is present in the office suite and immediately available to provide assistance and direction throughout the time that services are being performed."[15]

Prepaid Plans.   Referrals made under managed care plans also are protected by a safe harbor if certain criteria are met. The services must be furnished by an organization having a contract with an enrollee, where the organization is a federally qualified HMO, or where it receives prepaid payments under a federal demonstration project.

Exceptions Limited to Ownership and Investment Interests

Ownership of Publicly Traded Investment Securities.   Ownership of a publicly traded investment in a large company is protected under a safe harbor if certain requirements are met. The ownership may be in the form of shares, bonds, debentures, notes, or other debt instruments. The requirements for this safe harbor are:

1. The terms of the investment must be those that are generally available to the public.
2. The interest must be publicly traded, and must be listed on NASDAQ, AMEX, or a foreign or regional stock exchange publishing daily quotes.
3. The average shareholder equity in the company must be greater than $75 million over the previous 3 years.

Ownership of Shares in a Regulated Investment Company.   This safe harbor protects investment interests in regulated investment companies, as defined in I.R.C. § 851(a). To qualify for this safe harbor, the company must have had average total assets exceeding $75 million over the previous 3 years.

Designated Health Services by Puerto Rican Hospitals.   Designated health services provided by hospitals located in Puerto Rico are also protected by a safe harbor. The designated health services are limited to the 11 services defined above.

Rural Providers.   Another safe harbor protects designated health services that are furnished in a rural area. A rural area is defined as an area located outside of a Metropolitan Statistical Area, or similar urban area, as defined by the federal Office of Management and Budget.[16] In addition to the requirement that the services be furnished in a rural area, substantially all (75%) of the designated health services must be furnished by the rural provider to individuals residing in that rural area. With regard to laboratory services, testing must be performed on the premises of the rural laboratory. If not, the laboratory performing the testing must bill Medicare directly.

Hospital Ownership.   The final safe harbor relating solely to ownership and investment interests is for hospital ownership. Under this safe harbor, for designated health services provided by a hospital, the ownership or investment interest must be in the hospital itself, not in a subdivision of the hospital. In addition, the referring physician must be authorized to perform services at the hospital. If an entity, such as a joint venture, is jointly owned by a hospital and another entity, then this safe harbor will not apply, since there is no ownership interest in the hospital.

Exceptions Limited to Compensation Arrangements

The remaining safe harbors apply only to compensation arrangements and are commonly relied upon to protect many common activities in the healthcare industry.

Space Rental and Equipment Rental Safe Harbors.   The space rental and equipment rental safe harbors are similar and thus are considered together here, although applicable differences are noted. To fall under the office space or equipment rental safe harbors, seven criteria must be met, as follows:

1. There must be a written lease, signed by the parties, that specifies the premises or equipment covered by the lease.
2. The space or equipment rented must not exceed that which is needed for legitimate business purposes.
3. As applied only to the space rental safe harbor, the space must be used exclusively by the lessee when it is

being used by the lessee, but the lessee can pay for common areas based upon its pro rata share owed for the common areas, calculated as a ratio of the lessee's space to the total space.

4. The lease term must be for at least 1 year.
5. The rental charges over the term of the lease must be:
   a. Set in advance.
   b. Consistent with fair market value.
   c. Not determined in a manner that takes into account the volume or value of any referrals or other business generated between the parties.
6. The lease would be commercially reasonable even without any referrals between the parties.
7. The lease complies with any other requirements that may be imposed by new regulations.

"Fair market value" is defined as the value in an arms'-length transaction, which is consistent with the general market value. The value cannot be adjusted to reflect the additional value that either party would attribute to the proximity or convenience to the lessor where the lessor is a potential source of patient referrals.

Bona Fide *Employment Relationships Safe Harbor.* Employer-employee relationships are not considered to be referral arrangements and will fall under a safe harbor if five criteria are met:

1. Amounts are paid by an employer to a physician or family member who has a *bona fide* employment relationship with the employer for the provision of services.
2. Payments are made for identifiable services.
3. The amount of remuneration is:
   a. Consistent with fair market value for the services.
   b. Not based on the value or volume of referrals. A productivity bonus is permitted if it is for services personally performed by the physician or family member.
4. The agreement would be commercially reasonable even without referrals.

5. The arrangement meets any other requirements imposed by new regulations.

This safe harbor is very frequently relied upon and is somewhat easy to comply with. An important consideration is that the payments must be for identifiable services—not a subterfuge disguising payments for referrals.

Personal Services Contracts Safe Harbor.   The personal services contract safe harbor is similar to the employment relationship safe harbor, except that it applies to independent contractor arrangements. Such arrangements will fall under this safe harbor if eight criteria are met:

1. The remuneration must be from an entity under an "arrangement" or a contract.
2. The arrangement must be in writing and signed by the parties, and it must specify the services covered.
3. The arrangement must cover all of the services to be provided by the agent to the entity, such that there are no "side agreements."
4. The aggregate services contracted for must not exceed that which is reasonable and necessary for legitimate business purposes.
5. The term of the arrangement must be for at least 1 year.
6. The compensation to be paid over the term of the arrangement:
   a. Must be set in advance.
   b. Must not exceed fair market value.
   c. Must not be based on referrals.
7. The services to be performed do not involve the counseling or promotion of an illegal business arrangement.
8. Other requirements that may be set forth in new regulations.

Under the Stark laws, the compensation may be specified on a per-service or a per-hour basis, unlike under the comparable anti-kickback safe harbor. A physician incentive plan is permitted, which is defined as any compensation arrangement between a physician and an entity that may have the effect of reducing or limiting the services provided to enrollees of the entity. Compensation can be referral-sensitive, such as with capitation, withholds, bonuses, and the like, if two criteria are met:

1. No specific payment is made to a physician or group to induce them to limit medically necessary services as to a specific individual.
2. If the plan puts the physician or entity at substantial financial risk, as defined in 42 U.S.C. § 1395mm(i)(A)(ii), the plan must comply with any requirements set forth in the regulations.

Unrelated Remuneration.   Another safe harbor protects arrangements where remuneration is provided by a hospital to a physician for services unrelated to the provision of designated health services.

Physician Recruitment.   Incentives provided to physicians to induce them to relocate to a hospital's service area will fall under a safe harbor if certain requirements are met:

1. The remuneration must be provided to the physician to induce him or her to relocate to the hospital's area so that the physician can be on the hospital's medical staff.[17]
2. The physician must not be required to refer patients to the hospital.
3. The remuneration must not be based upon referrals.
4. The incentive must meet other requirements as defined by the Department of Health and Human Services.

In Polk County, Texas v. Peters,[18] the court held that a physician recruitment agreement violated the Stark laws because the physician agreed to refer patients to the hospital in exchange for an interest-free loan, free office space, rent and utility subsidies, and reimbursement for malpractice insurance.

Isolated Transactions.   The Stark law also exempts "isolated transactions" from its coverage if certain criteria are met. Specific isolated transactions include the one-time sale of property or a medical practice. The requirements that must be met are:

1. The remuneration paid for the practice must be consistent with the fair market value of the practice.
2. The remuneration must not be referral-sensitive.
3. The agreement would be commercially reasonable even without the possibility of referrals.
4. The agreement must meet other requirements that may be imposed by the Department of Health and Human Services.

The August 1995 final regulations issued on Stark I partially clarified this safe harbor. The new rule requires that there be no additional transactions between the parties for 6 months after the isolated transaction, except for transactions that are specifically excepted under other safe harbors. The new rule defined "transaction" to involve a single payment, and not long-term or installment payments such as a mortgage. Each installment payment would constitute a "transaction" for purposes of this rule and thus this safe harbor would not apply. If additional transactions fall under a safe harbor, then the initial transaction would still qualify as an isolated one.[19] The concern with extended payments is that the physician would be under a continuing obligation to refer patients to the purchasing entity in order to continue receiving payments.

Group Practice Arrangements with a Hospital.   Group practice arrangements with a hospital will fall under a safe harbor if several requirements are met:

1. The arrangement must be between a hospital and a group practice, as defined above.
2. The designated health services may be provided by the group practice but must be billed by the hospital.
3. For services provided to an inpatient of the hospital, the arrangement must meet the requirements in 42 U.S.C. § 1395x(b)(3) as to the provision of inpatient hospital services.
4. The arrangement must have begun before December 19, 1989, and must have continued without interruption.

5. Substantially all of the designated health services covered by the arrangement and furnished to patients of the hospital are furnished by the group practice.

6. The agreement must be in writing, and it must specify the services to be provided, along with the compensation to be paid.

7. The compensation paid over the term of the contract must be consistent with fair market value and not based upon referrals.

8. The compensation per unit of services must be fixed in advance and must be commercially reasonable even if no referrals are made.

9. The arrangement must meet other requirements as set forth by the Department of Health and Human Services.

Payments by Physicians for Items and Services.   The final safe harbor applicable to compensation arrangements relates to payments by physicians for items and services. This safe harbor has not been clearly defined in regulations to date, but the Department of Health and Human Services has promulgated two requirements:

1. The payments must be by a physician to a lab for clinical services.

2. The payments must be by a physician to an entity for other items or services and furnished at the fair market value price.

Discounts.   Discounts that a seller gives to a buyer on goods or services for which a claim may be submitted to Medicare or Medicaid are not defined as remuneration as long as several criteria are met:

Buyer's Duties
If the buyer reports costs on a cost report:

1. The discount must be earned based upon the purchases of that same good or service bought within a single fiscal year of the buyer.

2. The buyer must claim the benefit of the discount in the fiscal year in which the discount is earned, or the following year.

3. The buyer must fully and accurately report the discount on the cost report.

4. The buyer must provide the information given by the seller to DHHS upon request.

If the buyer is an HMO or Competitive Medical Plan with a risk contract under federal or state law, then it need not report the discount unless required by the risk contract.

If the buyer is neither of the above:

1. The discount must be made at the time of the original sale of the good or service.

2. If the item or service is separately claimed for payment with DHHS or the state, the buyer must fully and accurately report the discount.

3. The buyer must provide information supplied by the seller to DHHS or the state upon request.

A Competitive Medical Plan (CMP) is a state-licensed entity that provides healthcare on a prepaid, capitated basis through physicians employed by the CMP. The CMP assumes full financial risk and must have reserve protections similar to HMOs. It must also meet federal requirements for open enrollment, grievance, and quality assurance procedures.

Seller's Duties

If the buyer is an HMO or Competitive Medical Plan with a risk contract, the seller need not report the discount to the buyer.

If the buyer is any other individual or entity:

1. If the discount is required to be reported, the seller must fully and accurately report the discount on the invoice or statement submitted to the buyer and must inform the buyer of its duty to report the discount; or

2. If the discount is unknown at the time of the sale, the seller must fully and accurately report the existence of a discount program on the invoice or statement submitted to the buyer and must

tell the buyer of its duty to report and give the buyer documentation of the calculation of the discount when it becomes known. This information must include identification of the specific goods and services bought to which the discount applies.

The discounts safe harbor defines a "discount" to mean a reduction in the amount a seller charges a buyer for a good or service based on an arms'-length transaction. The buyer may buy either directly or though a wholesaler or group purchasing organization. A discount may be in the form of a rebate check, credit, or coupon directly redeemable from the seller only to the extent that such reductions in price are due to the original goods or services bought. A discount is defined not to include:

1. Cash payments.
2. Free or reduced charges in exchange for an agreement to buy a different good or service.
3. Reductions in price applicable to one payor but not to Medicare or Medicaid.
4. Reductions in price given to beneficiaries, such as routine reductions or waivers of coinsurance or deductibles owed by the beneficiary.
5. Warranties.
6. Services provided under personal services or management contracts.
7. Other remuneration in cash or in kind not explicitly described in the safe harbor.

Group Purchasing Organizations.   Payments by a vendor of goods or services to a group purchasing organization (GPO) as part of an agreement to furnish such goods or services to an individual or entity are defined as not comprising remuneration, if certain criteria are met. A group purchasing organization is defined as an entity authorized to act as a purchasing agent for a group of individuals or entities who are furnishing services payable by Medicare or Medicaid, and who are neither wholly owned by the GPO nor subsidiaries of a parent corporation that wholly owns the GPO, either directly or through another wholly owned entity. The criteria for this safe harbor are:

1. If the entity receiving the goods or services is a healthcare provider of services, then the GPO must disclose in writing to the entity at least annually, and to DHHS on request, the amount received from each vendor as to purchases made by or on behalf of the entity.
2. The GPO must have a written agreement with each individual or entity, for which items or services are furnished, that provides:
    a. That participating vendors, from which the individual or entity will purchase goods or services, will pay to the GPO only up to 3% of the purchase price of the goods or services provided by that vendor or
    b. If the fee paid to the GPO is not fixed at 3% or less, the contract must specify the maximum amount the GPO will be paid by each vendor, where the amount may be a fixed sum or percent of the value of the purchases made from the vendor by the group members under the contract between the vendor and the GPO.

Waiver of Beneficiary Co-Insurance and Deductible Amounts.   Under this safe harbor, remuneration is defined not to include a reduction or waiver of a Medicare or Medicaid program beneficiary's obligation to pay co-insurance or deductibles if the following criteria are met:

1. If the amount is owed to a hospital for inpatient hospital services payable through the prospective payment system:
    a. The hospital may not later claim the amount reduced or waived as a bad debt or otherwise shift the burden of the reduction or waiver onto Medicare or Medicaid, other payors, or individuals.
    b. The hospital must offer to reduce or waive the co-insurance or deductible without regard to the reason for admission, the length of stay, or the diagnosis-related group for which the claim is filed.

    c. The hospital's offer to reduce or waive the co-insurance or deductible amounts must not be made as part of a price reduction agreement between a hospital and a third-party payor, unless the agreement is part of a contract for the furnishing of items or services to a beneficiary of a Medicare supplemental policy issued under the terms of the Social Security Act, section 1882(t)(1).

2. If the amount is owed to a federally qualified healthcare center or facility under the Public Health Services Act and is owed by an individual who qualified for subsidized services under the Public Health Services Act or under titles V or XIX of the Social Security Act, then the healthcare center or facility may reduce or waive the co-insurance or deductible amounts for items or services payable under Part B of Medicare or Medicaid.

Increased Coverage, Reduced Cost-Sharing Amounts, or Reduced Premium Amounts Offered by Health Plans.   Another safe harbor defines remuneration not to include the additional coverage of any item or service offered by a health plan to an enrollee, or the reduction of some or all of the enrollee's obligation to pay the health plan or contract healthcare provider for cost-sharing amounts such as co-insurance, deductibles, or co-payment amounts, or for premium amounts attributable to items or services covered by the health plan, Medicare, or Medicaid, if certain criteria are met:

1. For risk-based HMOs, Competitive Medical Plans, Prepaid Health Plans, or demonstration projects, the plan must offer the same increased coverage or reduced cost-sharing or premium amounts to all enrollees unless otherwise approved by HCFA or the state.

2. For HMOs, Competitive Medical Plans, Healthcare prepayment plans, or prepaid health plans that have executed a contract with HCFA or a state to receive payment for enrollees on a reasonable cost or similar basis:

    a. The health plan must offer the same increased coverage or reduced cost-sharing or premium amounts to all enrollees unless otherwise approved by HCFA or a state.

b. The health plan must not claim the costs of the increased coverage or reduced cost-sharing or premium amounts against Medicare, Medicaid, or other payors or individuals.

Price Reductions Offered to Health Plans.   A reduction in price, which a contract healthcare provider offers to a health plan under the terms of a written agreement between the provider and the health plan for the sole purpose of furnishing to enrollees items or services covered by the health plan, by Medicare, or by Medicaid, is defined as not comprising remuneration, as long as the following criteria are met:

1. If the health plan is an HMO, Competitive Medical Plan, or prepaid health plan under contract with HCFA or a state under the Social Security Act, section 1876(g) or 1903(m), then the contract healthcare provider must not claim payment in any form from DHHS or a state for items or services furnished under the contract except as approved by HCFA or the state, and the provider may not otherwise shift the burden of such an agreement onto Medicare, Medicaid, other payors, or individuals.

2. If the health plan is an HMO, Competitive Medical Plan, healthcare prepayment plan, or prepaid health plan that has executed a contract with HCFA or a state to receive payments for enrollees on a reasonable cost or similar basis:

   a. The term of the agreement between the health plan and the contract healthcare provider must be for at least one year.

   b. The contract must specify in advance the covered items or services to be furnished to enrollees along with the methodology for computing the payment to the contract healthcare provider.

   c. The health plan must fully and accurately report, on the cost report or other claim form filed with DHHS or the state, the amount it has paid the contract provider under the agreement for the covered items or services furnished to enrollees.

    d. The contract provider must not claim payment in any form from DHHS or a state for items or services furnished under the agreement except as approved by HCFA or a state, and the provider may not otherwise shift the burden of such a contract onto Medicare, Medicaid, other payors, or individuals.

3. If the health plan is not described above, then both the health plan and provider must meet the following requirements:

    a. The term of the agreement between the plan and provider must be at least one year.

    b. The contract must specify in advance the covered items and services to be furnished to enrollees, which party is to file claims or requests for payment with Medicare or Medicaid for such items and services, and the schedule of fees the contract provider will charge for furnishing such items and services to enrollees.

    c. The fee schedule contained in the agreement must remain in effect throughout the term of the contract, unless a fee increase results directly from a payment update approved by Medicare or Medicaid.

    d. The party submitting claims or requests for payment from Medicare or Medicaid for items or services furnished under the contract must not claim or request payment for amounts in excess of the fee schedule.

    e. The contract provider and the plan must fully and accurately report on any cost report filed with Medicare or Medicaid the fee schedule amounts charged under the contract.

    f. The party who is not required to file claims under the contract must not claim or request payment in any form from DHHS or a state for items or services furnished under the contract, and it may not otherwise shift the burden of such a contract onto Medicare, Medicaid, other payors, or individuals.

ANTITRUST LAWS

Antitrust Statutes

The object of the antitrust laws is to protect and promote competition, but not competitors, as the method by which the nation allocates economic resources.[20] The antitrust laws seek to require firms to compete individually, "rather than by arranging treaties with [their] competitors."[21] Until 1975, when the Supreme Court held that the antitrust laws applied to the professions in Goldfarb v. Virginia State Bar,[22] the antitrust laws did not apply to the healthcare industry.[23]

There are four primary federal laws governing antitrust activities—the Sherman Act, the Federal Trade Commission Act, the Clayton Act, and the Robinson-Patman Act. All states, except Vermont and Pennsylvania, have antitrust statutes that are more or less comparable to the federal laws. These laws regulate healthcare activities in various forms, including credentialing of healthcare professionals, mergers and acquisitions, joint ventures, formation of integrated delivery systems, and exclusive contracting. Depending upon the specific circumstances, prohibited activities may include vertical price-fixing agreements, price discrimination, tying arrangements, exclusive dealing arrangements, vertical and horizontal mergers, group boycotts, and interlocking directorates between competitors.

Section 1 of the Sherman Act prohibits "every contract, combination . . . and conspiracy in restraint of trade or commerce . . . among the several states or with foreign nations."[24] Fundamentally, Section 1 prohibits concerted action by two or more parties to create an unreasonable restraint of trade. The actions of a single party, which includes a parent and subsidiary, or two subsidiaries of the same parent, cannot constitute a conspiracy and thus cannot violate Section 1 of the Sherman Act.

Section 2 of the Sherman Act prohibits monopolization, attempts to monopolize, and combinations or conspiracies to monopolize.[25] Unlike Section 1, unilateral activity as well as concerted activity can violate Section 2 of the Sherman Act. It is important to note that it is not illegal to have monopoly power, as long as it was not acquired through exclusionary or predatory activities. The antitrust laws recognize that successful organizations may become so through superior products, service, and efficiencies, without monopolization. The Department of Justice enforces the Sherman Act through civil and criminal actions. Private parties and state attorneys general are also authorized to bring suit under the Sherman Act.

The Federal Trade Commission Act[26] prohibits unfair methods of competition in interstate commerce, as well as unfair and deceptive acts or practices. The FTC Act does not apply to nonprofit entities, however.[27] This may protect some activities in the healthcare field, but it should be noted that the other antitrust statutes overlap the FTC Act to some extent and do apply to nonprofit entities. The Sherman Act, for example, would apply to mergers and acquisitions of nonprofit entities. The Federal Trade Commission is empowered to enforce the FTC Act as well as the Sherman Act; however, private parties are not authorized to bring causes of action under the FTC Act.

The Clayton Act[28] has two prohibitions. The first prohibits exclusive dealing arrangements involving the sale of commodities that have the effect of substantially lessening competition. The second prohibits mergers, joint ventures, consolidations, or acquisitions of stock or assets whose effect may be to substantially lessen competition or to create a monopoly. Both the Department of Justice and the Federal Trade Commission enforce the Clayton Act. Private parties and state attorneys general are also authorized to bring suit under this act.

The Robinson-Patman Act[29] prohibits price discrimination between different purchasers in the sale of commodities, although it permits quantity discounts and price differentials based upon different costs of manufacture, sale, or delivery. The Robinson-Patman Act does not apply to the provision of services. The Non-Profit Institutions Act[30] amended the Robinson-Patman Act and exempted nonprofit entities' purchase of drugs and supplies for their own use.

Other federal statutes related to antitrust include the Hart-Scott-Rodino Antitrust Improvements Act,[31] the McCarran-Ferguson Act,[32] the Health Care Quality Improvement Act,[33] the Local Government Antitrust Act,[34] and the Norris-LaGuardia Act.[35] The Hart-Scott-Rodino Act[36] is the primary means by which the federal government regulates mergers of larger entities. It requires premerger notification to the Federal Trade Commission and the Department of Justice where:

1. One of the merging entities has net sales or total assets exceeding $100 million, and the other merging entity has net sales or total assets exceeding $10 million.

2. The acquiring party will hold either at least 15% of the voting securities or assets of the acquired entity, or voting securities or assets of the acquired entity valued in excess of $15 million after the acquisition.

The McCarran-Ferguson Act[37] exempts the business of insurance from application of the federal antitrust laws if that business is regulated by the state and if the conduct does not constitute an illegal boycott, coercion, or intimidation. The Health Care Quality Improvement Act[38] exempts peer review activities from the application of the antitrust laws and consequent antitrust damages if the professional review action meets the requirements of the Act. The Local Government Antitrust Act[39] exempts the activities of local governments and their subsidiaries from damage awards, but not injunctions, in antitrust actions. Finally, the Norris-LaGuardia Act[40] exempts collective bargaining activities between employers and employees from application of the antitrust laws.

Other judicial doctrines provide defenses to antitrust claims in certain circumstances. The state action exception, first set forth in 1943 in Parker v. Brown,[41] exempts state-regulated activities from application of the antitrust laws if the activity meets two requirements: (1) the state has a clearly articulated state policy to replace competition with regulation in a certain area, and (2) the activities are subject to active governmental supervision. Private parties invoking this defense must meet both prongs of the test; however, governmental entities, such as municipal hospitals, need only meet the first requirement, since public entities are presumed to be acting in the public interest.

Another judicial doctrine that provides a defense to antitrust challenges is the Noerr-Pennington exception. This doctrine provides that private parties may petition the government in good faith to undertake anticompetitive activities on their behalf without violating the antitrust laws. The context in which this exception is typically used is in certificate of need activities.

Antitrust Analysis

Although all contracts and business arrangements have the effect of restraining trade, only those activities that *unreasonably* restrain trade are prohibited. Three modes of analysis are used to ascertain whether an arrangement violates the antitrust laws—the *per se* rule, the rule of reason, and the truncated rule of reason. The *per se* rule is a judicial determination that some forms of trade restraints have such a substantially detrimental effect on competition that they are unlawful of their face, without further inquiry. Some trade restraints "because of their pernicious effect on competition and lack of any redeeming virtue are conclusively presumed to be unreasonable and therefore illegal without elaborate inquiry as to the precise harm they have caused or the business excuse for their use."[42] Trade restraints that are deemed *per se* unlawful include price fixing, tying arrangements, and some group boycotts.

Courts use the rule of reason analysis for restraints on trade with less pernicious effects. This form of analysis involves the time-consuming and fact-intensive review of the various effects on competition from the challenged arrangement. Essentially, courts review and balance the procompetitive effects of the arrangement against its anticompetitive effects to determine whether the restraint gives the defendant market power. Anticompetitive effects include higher prices, restricted output, and lower quality and efficiency. Procompetitive effects include generating substantial efficiencies, increasing productive capacity, developing new products, and increasing quality. Market power exists when the arrangement gives the defendant the ability to raise prices or restrict output without challenge from competitors. Factors used in analyzing market power include the defendant's market share in the relevant geographic and product markets, a competitor's barriers to market entry, and the degree of seller concentration in the specific field.

The truncated rule of reason approach is used in some courts for restraints that have some redeeming effects on competition but which appear to be *per se* violations. Courts will briefly review the arrangement to determine if the procompetitive effects can outweigh the anticompetitive effects. If this result is unlikely, a court may hold the arrangement illegal without engaging in the fact-intensive analysis under the rule of reason approach. In Arizona v. Maricopa County Medical Society,[43] for example, the Supreme Court held that a fee schedule agreement involving 70% of the county's physicians was illegal *per se* despite claims that the fee schedule suppressed increases in insurance premiums.

Integration Activities in the Healthcare Field

Integration activities by definition involve joint undertakings and thus implicate the antitrust laws. Antitrust risks will primarily depend upon several factors:

1. The level of competition that existed between the participants prior to integration.
2. The extent of integration.
3. The market share of the integrated entity.
4. The type of joint action involved.

As for the first factor, the prior level of competition, there is little antitrust concern if the participants were not previously competitors, such that they did not provide the same types of services, or they did not operate in the same geographic market.[44] Under the second factor, the extent of integration is viewed as the level of joint risk sharing under the arrangement. The level of antitrust concern varies inversely with the level of risk sharing and integration involved in the arrangement. Unless there is some alteration of the status of the competitors as independent entities, then the antitrust risk will be high, particularly if it involves price fixing.[45] However, the precise level of integration required to justify price fixing is not completely clear. A 20% withhold of fees has been identified as "substantial risk sharing," for example, which also permits use of the rule of reason approach, as does the creation of a new product.[46] Minimizing antitrust concerns may include using a "messenger model" of integration, whereby an agent or third party negotiates the fees to be paid by payors and relates the fee information to each member on an individual basis only.

The third factor, market power, is also important in evaluating the antitrust risks of an integrated system. In general, the greater the market power of the integrated entities, the greater the concern that their specific activities have anticompetitive effects. The market power of an IDS is generally viewed from all angles and the market power of each participant in the venture is considered. In addition, the number of patients and physicians involved in the IDS is a factor.[47]

Finally, the antitrust risk of an integrated system is dependent upon the specific activities undertaken. Joint pricing is most risky, and should be undertaken through a messenger model if the withhold is less than 20%. Market or product allocation agreements are also suspect and should be ancillary to procompetitive benefits from the arrangement. In addition, initial discussions involved in forming the integrated system may implicate the antitrust laws.

To assist participants in the healthcare field in analyzing the antitrust risks of certain activities, the Department of Justice and the Federal Trade Commission jointly issued antitrust enforcement policy statements (Statements) as they relate to the healthcare field in September 1994 and again in August 1996.[48] These statements provide guidance, and safe harbors in some instances, on activities that are commonplace in the healthcare field. In addition, the agencies have established a business review procedure, whereby they will evaluate proposed conduct and provide a response within 90 days in most instances.

Mergers.   These agencies have indicated in the enforcement statements that, absent extraordinary circumstances, they will not challenge mergers of general acute care hospitals where one of the hospitals:

1. Has an average of fewer than 100 licensed beds over the last 3 years;

2. Has an average daily census of under 40 over the 3 most recent years; and

3. Is at least 5 years old. As with all safety zones, conduct falling outside of the zone is not necessarily prohibited.

For larger hospitals that cannot meet this safety zone, the agencies have indicated that they will follow the 1992 Horizontal Merger Guidelines in analyzing the proposed merger, such that they are not likely to challenge a hospital merger when:

1. After the merger the entity is not more likely to exercise market power because there are other strong hospitals remaining in the market, or because the merging hospitals provide sufficiently distinct services;

2. The merger would allow the hospitals to achieve economies of scale and efficiencies that could not otherwise be realized; and

3. The merger would eliminate a failing hospital whose assets would exit the market but for the merger.

Joint Ventures.   Joint ventures may involve arrangements in nearly any form between any of the participants in the healthcare field—physicians, physician groups, hospitals, managed care organizations, and payors. Antitrust risks emerge when these groups form ventures that involve cornering the market for specific products or services, joint pricing, or joint negotiations with payors or managed care organizations. The federal agencies have indicated in the joint enforcement statements that they will not challenge physician joint ventures if certain requirements are met:

1. If the network is exclusive, the network consists of 20% or less of the physicians in each specialty practicing in a specific geographic market.

2. If the network is nonexclusive, if the joint venture consists of 30% or less of the physicians in a nonexclusive network. If the market is small enough where there are only five physicians in a particular specialty (or four in the case of nonexclusive networks), the network may include one of those specialists on a nonexclusive basis.

3. The physicians in the network share substantial financial risk, such as capitated contracts or financial incentives for cost containment.

Ventures falling outside of this safety zone will still be analyzed under the rule of reason, and they will be upheld if they would generate procompetitive effects, such as the provision of a new service or efficiencies in patient care. However, exclusive ventures are subject to more scrutiny because their members may not compete with the venture, either by themselves or with another group.

The agencies have also set forth a safety zone that covers hospitals participating in joint ventures with other hospitals to share the costs of providing expensive, high-technology equipment, if certain requirements are met:

1. Only that number of hospitals whose participation is needed actually participate in the joint venture. Participation is sufficient when the costs of the equipment can be recovered over its useful life.

2. The safety zone applies to the purchase or operation of new or existing equipment but does not apply to the provision of specialized clinical services, which is analyzed under the rule of reason.

For high-technology joint ventures falling outside of this safety zone, the agencies will apply a rule of reason analysis to determine whether the joint venture substantially reduces competition, and whether it will produce procompetitive efficiencies that outweigh the potential anticompetitive effects.

Information Sharing among Providers. Providers may share and collectively provide non-fee-related information to purchasers of healthcare services without violating the antitrust laws as long as they do not attempt to coerce a purchaser's decision by engaging in boycotts if the purchaser does not accept the providers' joint recommendations. Examples of non-fee information sharing that would not be challenged include a medical society's collection of outcome data, and providers' development of suggested practice parameters.

On the other hand, an exchange of information regarding the price of medical services can violate the antitrust laws if it leads to price fixing or if it actually results in anticompetitive price increases. On the other hand, price information sharing can have procompetitive effects because it may generate competition to hold prices down. The agencies have set forth a safety zone whereby the collective provision of price information to purchasers by providers will not be challenged if the following requirements are met:

1. A third party manages the survey.

2. The information is more than 3 months old (although current price information may be provided to purchasers).

3. The data for each statistic comprises that of at least five providers, and the information is so aggregated that the prices or wages of an individual provider cannot be identified. No individual provider's data may represent more than 25% of a statistic.

This safety zone will not apply to the discussion of future prices, which would be illegal price-fixing, or to collective negotiations between unintegrated providers and purchasers who are contemplating an agreement among the providers on fees or other terms relating to reimbursement.

Joint Purchasing.   Agreements among providers to jointly purchase goods or services may implicate the antitrust laws if the volume purchased is so great that it would permit price fixing. This type of arrangement is highly unlikely to pose antitrust problems, since the barriers to entry for this type of arrangement are very low, and it would generate substantial procompetitive effects in the form of economies of scale and consequent reduced costs. The agencies have set forth a safety zone, however, which permits joint purchasing arrangements if certain requirements are met:

1. The purchases make up less than 35% of the total sales of the purchased product or service.
2. The cost of the products and services jointly purchased makes up less than 20% of the total revenues from all products or services sold by each participant in the joint arrangement.

Other factors that weigh in favor of upholding the arrangement include:

1. The agreement does not require the participants to purchase jointly all of their purchases of a specific product.
2. Independent employees or agents negotiate on behalf of the participants.
3. Communications between the participants and the purchasing group are not shared among the participants.

Physician Network Joint Ventures

The 1996 Statements of Enforcement Policy provide an expanded analysis of physician network joint ventures. The Statements define physician joint ventures as those that are physician controlled and in which the network's physician participants collectively agree on prices or price-related terms and jointly market their services. Whether the network falls within the safety zone depends upon whether it is in fact an exclusive or nonexclusive network. A network is exclusive if participants are restricted in their ability to individually contract or affiliate with other network joint ventures or health plans. If it is nonexclusive, then the network does not significantly restrict the participants' ability or willingness to participate in other networks, and the participants do in fact affiliate with other networks, as evidenced by their revenues from various sources.

Exclusive physician network joint ventures will fall under a safety zone if the physician participants share substantial financial risk, and if the participants constitute 20% or less of the physicians in each physician specialty with active hospital staff privileges who practice in the relevant geographic market. Where there are fewer than five physicians in a particular specialty in that market, then the network may include one physician on a nonexclusive basis. A nonexclusive venture will fall under a safety zone if its physician participants share substantial financial risk and if it constitutes 30% or less of the physicians in each physician specialty with active hospital privileges in that geographic market. Where there are less than four specialty physicians in that market, then the network may include one such specialist.

The agencies define the sharing of substantial risk as including agreements by the venture to provide services to a health plan at a capitated rate, or agreements to provide designated services or classes of services to a health plan for a predetermined percentage of premium or revenue from the plan. In addition, the sharing of financial risk is evidenced by the venture's use of significant financial incentives to the physician participants to achieve specified cost-containment goals, as shown by withholds distributed based on group performance, or bonuses and penalties based upon meeting cost and utilization targets. Risk sharing is also evidenced by agreements to provide complex or extended courses of treatment requiring the substantial coordination of care by physicians in different specialties for a fixed payment, where the costs of such treatment may vary greatly due to the patient's acuity and the choice of treatment.

As set forth in the 1996 Statements, a physician network that has entered into both risk-sharing and non-risk-sharing contracts does not fall under the safety zone. However, its activities would be analyzed under the rule of reason and would be permitted where the efficiencies from the capitated arrangements carry over to the fee-for-service business. A physician joint venture that includes more than the permitted number of specialists in the area would also not fall under the safety zone, but it would be analyzed under the rule of reason and permitted if its formation would not likely hamper the ability of health plans to contract individually with area physicians or with other physician network joint venturers, and if it would not enable the physicians to raise prices above competitive levels.

Where such ventures do not involve substantial risk sharing and thus do not fall under the safety zone, they may nonetheless be able to demonstrate sufficient integration to pass muster under the rule of reason. Integration may be sufficient where the venture is likely to produce substantial efficiencies, where it implements an active and ongoing program to evaluate and modify practice patterns by the physician participants, and creates a high degree of interdependence and cooperation among the physicians to control costs and ensure quality. This program may include: (1) establishing mechanisms to monitor and control utilization of healthcare services that are designed to control costs and assure quality of care; (2) selectively choosing network physicians who are likely to further these efficiency objectives; and (3) the significant investment of capital, monetary and human, in the necessary infrastructure and capability to realize the claimed efficiencies.

On the other hand, such networks may be substantially anticompetitive in nature and thus would not survive a challenge under the rule of reason. Indicators of an anticompetitive venture include: (1) statements evidencing an anti-competitive purpose; (2) a recent history of anticompetitive behavior or collusion in the market, including efforts to obstruct or undermine the development of managed care; (3) the obvious anticompetitive structure of the network, such as an exclusive network comprising a high percentage of the local area physicians; (4) the absence of any mechanisms with the potential for generating significant efficiencies or otherwise increasing competition through the network; (5) the presence of anticompetitive collateral agreements; and (6) the absence of mechanisms to prevent the network's operation from having anticompetitive spillover effects outside the network.

Decided before the 1996 Statements were issued, Blue Cross & Blue Shield United of Wisconsin v. Marshfield Clinic[49] was a seminal case involving a physician-owned HMO. On March 18, 1996, the United States Supreme Court denied review of the much-noted case. The Seventh Circuit had held that the HMO was not a separate market for physician services and thus did not have monopoly power over physician services when they employed less than 50% of the physicians in the relevant market. The Court found that Marshfield Clinic was not a monopolist but that it had illegally divided markets with another HMO. The Court ordered a retrial on the issue of damages, on the theory that this market-allocation arrangement had caused Blue Cross to pay excess fees.

Multiprovider Networks.   The 1996 Statements define multiprovider networks as ventures among providers that jointly market their healthcare services to health plans and other purchasers. They include networks involving otherwise competing providers, networks of providers offering complementary or unrelated services, networks of single-specialty providers, and PHOs.

The 1996 Statements specify that multiprovider networks will be analyzed under the rule of reason, and that they will not be viewed as *per se* illegal if the providers' integration is likely to produce significant efficiencies that benefit consumers, and any price agreements are reasonably necessary to realize those efficiencies. The same types of arrangements that demonstrate substantial financial risk sharing in physician networks is applicable to multiprovider networks, as outlined above. However, modes of integration may be different in multiprovider networks from physician networks and thus the agencies would review the specific facts of the arrangement. Price-setting and market allocation would be analyzed under the rule of reason and upheld if they were necessary to achieve the procompetitive effects of the arrangement.

For multiprovider networks, the relevant product markets used in the rule of reason analysis would include both the market for multiprovider networks as well as markets for the service components of the network that are or could be sold separately outside the network. In addition, since multiprovider networks involve companies that do not compete for the same types of customers, the agencies will review the network's ability to limit the ability of physicians to participate in other networks, and the ability of other networks or health plans to compete in the market. The exclusivity of the arrangement is also a factor, which will be reviewed as in physician networks, as outlined above.

Staff Privileges.   Credentialing decisions in hospitals are the most common source of antitrust suits in the healthcare arena. In 1986, Congress enacted the Health Care Quality Improvement Act,[50] which provides immunity from damages to participants in the peer review process as long as the participants comply with the Act's requirements. The Act requires that professional review actions be taken:

1. In the reasonable belief that the action furthers quality of care.
2. After a reasonable effort has been made to obtain the facts.
3. After adequate notice and hearing, or other fair procedures.
4. In the reasonable belief that the action was warranted.

Reviewing bodies are subject to liability if they are comprised of economic competitors of the excluded physician, and if they exclude a physician for anticompetitive purposes, as opposed to patient care reasons or objective credentialing and utilization criteria.

Exclusive Contracts.   Exclusive contracts most commonly permit a physician or group of physicians, typically hospital-based physicians, to be the exclusive providers of a specialty service within a hospital during the length of the exclusive contract. Such contracts also typically prohibit the hospital from granting medical staff privileges to noncontracting physicians in that specialty during the term of the exclusive contract. These arrangements benefit the contracting physicians by providing them with a relatively certain flow of patients; they benefit the hospital by enhancing efficiencies of operation within the department and assuring physician coverage. However, physicians who are excluded from practicing at the hospital by virtue of its exclusive agreement with another physician group have challenged such arrangements on antitrust grounds, alleging that they are unlawful tying arrangements or exclusive dealing contracts.

A key case upholding an exclusive contract was Jefferson Parish Hospital District No. 2 v. Hyde.[51] In Hyde, the Supreme Court held that the exclusive contract for anesthesiology services was in fact a tying arrangement; however, it held that it was not illegal because the hospital had legitimate business reasons for the arrangement, including increased operating efficiency in the department and the assurance of physician coverage. Although the hospital in Hyde had little market power, the Fourth Circuit upheld another exclusive contract in which the hospital did have substantial market power, in White v. Rockingham Radiologists, Ltd.[52] The Fourth Circuit so held because the hospital again justified the arrangement with legitimate business reasons.

Other exclusive contracting arrangements that may implicate the antitrust laws include health plans that contract with exclusive provider panels—either hospitals or physicians. Although there are fewer cases in this area, most courts have upheld the exclusive arrangements on various grounds. In St. Bernard General Hospital v. Hospital Service Association of New Orleans,[53] the court upheld the exclusive arrangement because it was the least restrictive means to achieving legitimate business objectives. Likewise in Northwest Medical Laboratories, Inc. v. Blue Cross Blue Shield,[54] the court held that the exclusive arrangement did not cause an adverse effect on competition because the HMO did not have market power in the relevant geographic area. In U.S. Healthcare, Inc. v. Healthsource, Inc.,[55] the court upheld an exclusive arrangement between an HMO and its employee physicians whereby the employees agreed not to contract with other HMOs. The court used the rule of reason approach and held that the arrangement did not foreclose a substantial part of the market in the state and thus was not a *per se* boycott. On the other hand, the court in Johnson v. Blue Cross Blue Shield[56] found that the exclusion of chiropractors from the health plan was due to a conspiracy and thus should be tested under the rule of reason.

TAX-EXEMPTION REQUIREMENTS UNDER SECTION 501(C)(3) OF THE INTERNAL REVENUE CODE

The rationale for tax exemption was stated succinctly in Geisinger Health Plan v. Commissioner,[57] where the court reasoned that "charitable exemptions from income taxation constitute a *quid pro quo:* the public is willing to relieve an organization from paying income taxes because the organization is providing a benefit to the public."

Unlike other statutory categories of tax exemption, section 501(c)(3) status gives its holders the ability to accept donations that are tax-deductible to their donors. Concurrent with this ability is an additional level of responsibility placed upon such organizations. To receive and maintain section 501(c)(3) classification, such organizations must meet several requirements:

1. The entity must be organized exclusively for charitable purposes—the "organizational test."
2. The entity must be operated exclusively for exempt purposes—the "operational test."
3. No substantial portion of the entity's activities can be for a private benefit. The entity must serve a public rather than a private interest.
4. No part of the entity's net earnings may inure to the benefit of an "insider."

These requirements are deceptively simple and may function as traps for the unwary in certain circumstances. As for the first requirement, the Internal Revenue Service held that the promotion of health is a charitable purpose under I.R.C. § 501(c)(3) in Revenue Ruling 69-545.[58] A hospital is engaged in the promotion of health if it meets the "community benefit" test, as follows:

1. The class of persons benefiting from the hospital's activities must be reasonably broad.
2. The hospital must operate an emergency room open to all persons without regard to their ability to pay.
3. The hospital must provide hospital care to everyone in the community who is able to pay directly or through private or public reimbursement.
4. The hospital must be governed by a board of trustees composed of independent civic leaders, as opposed to physicians or others with a private interest in the organization.
5. The hospital must maintain a medical staff open to all qualified physicians.

Other factors that the Internal Revenue Service has considered since the 1969 ruling include:

1. Whether the hospital provides specialized services if it does not operate an emergency room.
2. The hospital's provision of charity care, medical research, and educational activities.
3. The hospital's compliance with other laws, such as the Stark anti-referral laws and EMTALA—the Emergency Medical Treatment and Active Labor Act.

To meet the "organizational" test, a hospital's articles of incorporation must indicate that its purposes are limited to exempt purposes, such as charity. The hospital's organizational documents must also prohibit it from engaging in activities unrelated to its charitable purposes. Finally, the organizational documents must also indicate that the hospital's assets will be distributed to charitable organizations or for charitable purposes upon dissolution of the hospital.

The entity must also be operated exclusively for charitable purposes. No private benefit is permitted—no more than an insubstantial portion of its activities may further nonexempt purposes. No private inurement is permitted—no part of the entity's net earnings may inure to the benefit of an "insider." Any private benefit conferred by the organization must be qualitatively and quantitatively incidental to the charitable purpose of the activity or arrangement.[59] To be qualitatively incidental, the private benefit must occur only as a necessary concomitant of the activity that benefits the public—the benefit to the public cannot be achieved without necessarily benefiting private individuals. To be quantitatively incidental, the private benefit must be insubstantial when viewed in relation to the public benefit conferred by the activity. The analysis covers only the public benefit of that particular activity, not the overall good accomplished by the organization.[60]

Organizations that are tax-exempt under section 501(c)(3) may engage in profit-making activities that are unrelated to their exempt purposes only if such activities are an insubstantial portion of their activities, and such activities will be subject to the unrelated business income tax. An activity is subject to this tax if it is not substantially related to the entity's exempt purpose, and if it is regularly carried on. Examples of activities in the healthcare field that have been held to be subject to the unrelated business income tax include outpatient pharmacies and outpatient laboratory services sold to the general public, as opposed to hospital inpatients, parking lots serving physicians' private patients, laundry services, and hospital resale of supplies and medicines. Other activities have been held to be nontaxable, such as the operation of a gift shop for the convenience of patients, the rental of office space to physicians on staff, income from volunteer activities, and income from the cafeteria or parking lot if the activity primarily benefits patients or employees.

Although an insubstantial amount of private benefit transactions is permitted and subject to the unrelated business income tax, no private inurement is permitted, in any amount. Private inurement commonly involves the exempt entity's overpayment for property, goods, or services to an "insider." Conversely, private inurement may involve the entity's undercharging for services it provides to an insider. An insider is one who has the opportunity to control or influence the organization's activities because of his or her particular relationship with the organization. Medical staff members are generally presumed to be insiders.[61]

Private inurement commonly arises in the area of physician recruitment. Generally, recruitment incentives are permitted if certain requirements are met:[62]

1. The recruitment is necessary to further the hospital's exempt purposes.
2. The total compensation to the physician is reasonable and necessary to further the exempt purposes.
3. There is a demonstrable benefit to the hospital compared to the incidental benefits received by the physician.

Typically, violative arrangements involve excessive physician compensation, based on comparisons to similar positions demanding similar skills. Percentage compensation arrangements are generally scrutinized, and percent of net revenue arrangements are frequently viewed as *de facto* private inurement. However, percentage of gross arrangements are sometimes permitted. Private inurement may also involve the exempt organization's overpayment for the purchase of a physician practice, income guarantees, rent subsidies, provision of hospital support staff for a physician's private practice, or below-market loans or leases to an insider.

Following a dearth of guidance for nearly ten years in the area of physician recruitment, the Internal Revenue Service made public the contents of a closing agreement it entered with Hermann Hospital in Texas. Under the terms of the closing agreement, only new physicians or practitioners new to a hospital's service area could be permissible recruits. No incentives were permitted under the closing agreement to retain existing physicians. In addition, the IRS emphasized the requirement that the hospitals demonstrate a community need for the physician's services where they planned to use recruitment incentives.

In March 1995, the Internal Revenue Service issued a proposed revenue ruling[63] in the area of physician recruitment that permitted the recruitment of physicians already in the area to serve specific, identified community needs, such as for the indigent population, or for a distinct specialty. Once again, the IRS emphasized the need for hospitals to demonstrate the community need motivating the recruitment incentives.

Other activities implicating the private inurement prohibitions involve joint ventures between exempt entities and taxable entities. In 1991, the IRS held that a hospital would jeopardize its exempt status if it were to form a joint venture with members of its medical staff and sell to the joint venture a portion of its gross or net revenue stream from operations of a hospital department for a specified period of time.[64] The IRS's reasons for so holding were that the joint venture would cause the organization's net earnings to inure to private individuals; that it would benefit private interests more than incidentally; and that the joint venture may violate the anti-referral laws.[65] On the other hand, joint ventures are permitted if the venture expands existing resources for healthcare in the community; if it adds new healthcare providers to the community; if it improves treatment modalities; or if it reduces the costs of treatment.

Recently, the only express remedies available for violations of the tax-exemption requirements included revocation of the entity's tax-exempt status, and imposition of the unrelated business income tax on certain activities. On July 30, 1996, Congress enacted legislation to enhance these penalty provisions.[66] The legislation applies only to Section 501(c)(3) and 501(c)(4) organizations, and its primary focus is on the payment of excessive compensation, which of course must still be reported on relevant tax forms, such as Forms 990, 1040, W-2, and 1099. These modifications include imposition of intermediate sanctions and allow penalizing the recipients of excess benefits as well as any participating "organization manager."

The new legislation operates retroactively to September 13, 1995, to apply an excise tax of 25% of any excess benefit accruing to a disqualified person or insider after that date, subject to special transition rules for transactions before 1997.[67] Such penalties are in addition to possible revocation of an entity's exempt status. Organization managers who knowingly permitted the organization to engage in such a transaction are subject to a 10% penalty excise tax. Failure to correct an excess benefit transaction before notification by the IRS will result in an additional penalty of 200% of the excess benefit. However, if the violation was not due to willful neglect and has been corrected within the allotted time period, then the IRS must refund the penalty tax.

Another issue faces hospitals whose facilities were financed with tax-exempt bond proceeds. Nonprofit hospitals which are financed in part with tax-exempt bonds are restricted from using bond proceeds for private purposes. Generally, private use of tax-exempt bond proceeds is prohibited unless the arrangement meets the criteria set forth in IRS Revenue Procedure 93-19:[68]

1. Compensation for the use of the facilities must be based upon a reasonable, periodic, flat fee.
2. The maximum term of the contract must be up to 5 years.
3. Automatic increases in compensation must be determined by reference to an external index such as the Consumer Price Index.
4. The exempt organization must have the right to cancel the contract at the end of any 3-year period.

Private use would include the use of bond-financed facilities by persons unrelated to the exempt facility, such as independent contractor physicians. Generally, interest on the bonds will remain tax-exempt if the private use of bond proceeds is limited to 5% for tax-exempt organizations. Additionally, no more than 20% of the voting power on the private entity's board may be vested in the hospital or its employees or shareholders.[69] In a foundation model

PHO with a tax-exempt organization, "insider" physicians may not have majority control on the foundation board, nor may they set their own compensation through a board committee.

In December 1994, the IRS issued proposed regulations which, when final, will liberalize the provisions of Revenue Procedure 93-19. The proposed regulation expands the categories of qualified management contracts to include:

1. Contracts with terms not exceeding the lesser of 15 years or 50% of the useful life of the property if all the compensation is based on a periodic fixed fee.

2. Contracts with terms not exceeding the lesser of 10 years or 80% of the useful life of the property if at least 80% of the annual compensation is based on a periodic fixed fee.

3. Contracts with terms not exceeding 5 years if at least 50% of the compensation is based upon a periodic fixed fee.

4. Contracts with terms not exceeding 3 years if all the compensation is based on a per-unit fee.

The proposed regulations also provide clearer information on public use, and they also specify *de minimis* exceptions to the private business use test that are normally disregarded. For example, leases and other arrangements that are not renewable with terms of less than 1 year are usually disregarded. In addition, temporary use by developers of property to be sold to the public is also disregarded, as are incidental uses of a financed facility and qualified improvements to a facility.

INSURANCE LAWS

State insurance laws concern any entity that involves itself in "the business of insurance."[70] Accordingly, such laws typically regulate insurance companies, HMOs, and third-party administrators (TPAs). Some states are also beginning to regulate third-party utilization review companies as well. The difficulty with integrated delivery systems is ascertaining whether an entity has assumed an insurance-type risk, and if so, which of the entities in the integrated system has actually assumed that risk.

On the other hand, the federal Employee Retirement Income Security Act of 1974 (ERISA)[71] regulates the self-funded employee benefit plans structured by employers. ERISA pre-empts state insurance laws that relate to employee benefit plans, but not state laws regulating the business of insurance.[72] State laws cannot deem employee benefit plans to be the business of insurance under ERISA.

Insurance Risks

Insurance-type risks are not easily susceptible of a bright-line definition. However, it is generally recognized that insurance involves four elements: (1) the insured has an interest in his health that can be measured in dollar terms; (2) that interest is subject to a risk of loss through disease or accident; (3) an insurer can assume the risk as part of a program to share or distribute losses among a large group who bear similar risks in exchange for a premium; and (4) neither the insurer nor the insured have any substantial control over the risk.[73] State insurance codes are concerned with entities that indemnify or reimburse insureds for the expenses incurred in sustaining a loss.

Under the traditional fee-for-service reimbursement system, a state-licensed insurance company assumed the risk that losses would exceed its receipts; however, under managed care, new reimbursement methods have evolved that have shifted the risk onto different types of entities. Under a capitated payment system, an individual physician or hospital assumes the risk that excess care must be provided; however, such risk is not always pooled. Thus, some state insurance regulators view capitated payments as not an insurance-type risk. It is only when integrated organizations pool risk that some state insurance regulations apply. On the other hand, other state regulators view capitation as involving an insurance-type risk.[74] Withholds are typically viewed as a financial risk, not an insurance risk.

Hospitals reimbursed under the per diem or per case systems are not viewed as assuming an insurance-type risk, nor are physicians reimbursed under a global fee program, nor entities paid under a bundled fee arrangement. These reimbursement methodologies are more typically viewed as creative compensation arrangements and merely the financial-type risks of doing business. In Group Life & Health Ins. Co. v. Royal Drug Co.,[75] for example, the Supreme Court held that negotiated fee contracts with pharmacies participating in a network were not the business of insurance. Likewise in NGS American, Inc. v. Barnes,[76] the court held that claims processing and other administrative services were not the business of insurance because they were not part of the underlying contract with the insured. In Varol v. Blue Cross & Blue Shield,[77] the court held that a fee-for-service psychiatric program using Blue Cross's provider network, where the employer retained the risk for paying claims, was not an insurance product offered by Blue Cross but merely a cost management function.

Risk Bearers

Under the insurance laws of most states, insurance companies and HMOs are permitted to assume insurance risk if they comply with the respective state insurance laws. PPOs are not regulated under state insurance rules because they do not assume risk but broker services, and POS plans are regulated through the HMOs that sponsor them.

Integrated delivery systems, on the other hand, obtain cost savings by joining forces to pool resources and risk and thus may incur regulation under state insurance laws. A key issue is whether there is a regulated entity involved in the integrated system that is permitted under state law to assume or transfer insurance risk. Until state insurance regulations catch up with current movements in the healthcare industry, payment arrangements must be structured carefully to avoid the high reserve requirements and regulatory burdens imposed by the state insurance laws. Creative payment arrangements might include the use of bonuses for efficient service, which provide an upside risk but not a downside risk; charging losses to future management fees of the PHO; assumption of risk providers in an individual capacity; organizing the physician group as a professional corporation; and setting up joint ventures with insurance companies and HMOs. These payment arrangements may trigger application of other regulations and thus must be analyzed carefully.

Insurance Laws

If an entity is in the business of insurance, it will fall under a state's insurance laws governing insurance companies, HMOs, or health service organizations. Such laws typically require the entity to set aside financial reserves of a specific amount, and to submit insurance contracts to state regulators for approval.

Reimbursement and Payment Issues

Medicare is the largest third-party payor of health services in the country. As such, its rules for reimbursement percolate down to other payors in many instances. Since the reimbursement protocols for other payors are highly varied and subject to state insurance laws, only the Medicare program will be covered here.[78]

The Medicare program was enacted in 1965 as Title XVIII of the Social Security Act to provide a national health insurance program for the aged. Generally, Medicare covers medical services that are "reasonable or necessary" for the diagnosis or treatment of a disease or malformation; however, it does not cover experimental treatments. Although in recent years the Health Care Financing Administration has encouraged Medicare beneficiaries to enroll in managed care plans through risk contracts with HMOs,[79] Medicare is still primarily a fee-for-service reimbursement system.

"Part A" of the Medicare program covers care provided by or in institutional providers, such as inpatient hospital services, hospice care, skilled nursing facility care, and home healthcare, subject to an annual deductible. Medicare "Part B" pays for services provided by healthcare professionals and suppliers, as well as outpatient hospital services, home care, durable medical equipment, ambulance services, dialysis, and ambulatory surgery center services, subject to an annual deductible and a 20% co-insurance requirement.

Medicaid is a combination federal-state program that provides healthcare assistance to low income people who are aged, blind, or disabled, and to categorically needy persons.[80] States have the option to receive federal funding to help cover medically needy persons as well, who may have slightly higher incomes.[81] In the past, reimbursement under Medicaid was very similar to that under Medicare. As it relates to other third-party payors, Medicaid is intended to be the payor of last resort. However, since 1981, states have been permitted to develop their own reimbursement programs and methodologies within certain federal limits,[82] and thus their Medicaid reimbursement methodologies are becoming more widely varied.

Institutional Provider Participation in Medicare.   Hospitals electing to participate in Medicare must comply with the program's *Conditions of Participation*[83] and enter into a participation agreement with the HCFA agreeing to accept Medicare assignment. Assignment is mandatory for Part A services, which means that Medicare's payment is payment in full for all services rendered to all Medicare patients. Most hospitals are currently reimbursed under Medicare Part A for most services on a prospective payment system (PPS) basis, but other institutional providers must meet various conditions of participation and are generally reimbursed on a reasonable cost basis subject to cost or target rate limits. Certain specific services are also excluded from the PPS rate as well. HCFA sets the PPS reimbursement rates for hospitals, which it calculates to account for not only costs related to patient care, but also the overhead costs of the facility, necessary and proper interest costs related to patient care, and certain other specific categories of costs. By the year 2001, capital costs are scheduled to be fully included in the PPS rate as well. Certain patient care services are not reimbursable at all,[84] and certain other services are reimbursable on a non-PPS basis, typically calculated on a retrospective reasonable cost basis.

Fiscal intermediaries, under contract with HCFA, process claims and make PPS payments to hospitals based on the diagnosis-related group (DRG) in which a patient is categorized based upon the diagnosis at admission. The DRG reimbursement may vary for specific patients when their length of stay or costs exceed the norm by a certain factor—day outliers and cost outliers. In addition, one component of the DRG rate is adjusted for differences in area wages, thus payments for the same DRG will vary for hospitals in different areas. Finally, reimbursement rates vary for special categories of institutional providers, such as public hospitals, cancer hospitals, rural referral centers, hospitals in Alaska or Hawaii, disproportionate share hospitals, and sole community hospitals.[85]

Physician Participation in Medicare. Individual physicians may participate in Medicare and bill for their services under Part B in two different ways. First, the physician may elect to become a "participating provider," whereby he or she signs a yearly contract agreeing to accept Medicare assignment. Assignment means that Medicare's payment is payment in full for all services rendered to all Medicare patients. Physicians may charge patients only a 20% copayment amount and may not "balance bill" for excess charges. On the other hand, physicians may also participate in Medicare as "nonparticipating providers," whereby they accept assignment on a claim-by-claim basis. However, nonparticipating physicians are reimbursed 5% less than participating providers.

If the physician belongs to a group practice or is a member of a hospital medical staff, and that entity submits bills in its own name, then one participation agreement binds all physicians who work for that entity as to any services furnished for that entity.[86] However, if the physicians bill in their own names, they may decide individually whether to participate. In the case of university medical centers, individual departments can decide whether to participate.

Prior to 1992, Medicare carriers, under contract with HCFA, reimbursed physicians on a "reasonable charge" basis. A physician's "reasonable charge" was determined based on several factors: the physician's actual charge; the physician's customary charge; and the prevailing charges in the area for like services. Customary charges were based on the amount the physician charged in the majority of cases for a specific service to all third-party payors. If the physician was in a group practice, the group had a group customary charge if each physician in the group charged the same as the other physicians for the same services,[87] otherwise the physician had his or her own customary charge.

As of January 1, 1992, the Medicare program began to phase in the use of a fee schedule for reimbursement of physician services, to be completely in place by 1996. The Medicare program eliminated reimbursement based on customary charges and now reimburses physicians based on the lesser of the physician's actual charge for the service, or the amount determined under the Medicare fee schedule.[88] The fee schedule has three cost components: (1) the physician's time and the intensity of the work; (2) overhead costs;

and (3) malpractice insurance expenses. Each of these three components has its own relative value unit (RVU), each of which is adjusted for geographic differences. These adjusted RVUs are then multiplied by a conversion factor to ascertain the payment amount. There are three conversion factors based upon the type of services provided—surgical services, nonsurgical services, and primary care services. These conversion factors currently do not take into account any other specialty services.

Other services and items provided incident to a physician's services are also reimbursable under the Medicare program. Patient treatment supplies furnished incident to physician services are reimbursed as part of the fee schedule if they represent an actual expense to the physician, and the charges for supplies must be included in the physician's bills. Charges for drugs and biologicals that cannot be self-administered, that are provided incident to physician services, and that represent an expense to the physician are reimbursed as the lesser of the acquisition cost of the drug, or the national average wholesale price of the drug,[89] as long as the charges are included on the physician's bill.

The services of other medical paraprofessionals, such as physician assistants and nurse practitioners, are also reimbursable if commonly provided incident to a physician's services. However, such professionals must be employed by the physician or his or her clinic in order for the clinic to bill for their services. On the other hand, if these paraprofessionals perform tasks normally performed only by the physician, such as minor surgery or conducting physicals, then such services are not reimbursable because they are not provided "incident to" a physician's services, unless they are performed under the supervision of a physician in a hospital or nursing facility.[90]

As with the services of physician assistants and nurse practitioners, the services of physical, occupational, and speech therapy providers may also be reimbursable under Medicare under several different arrangements. First, they are reimbursable if they are furnished incident to a physician's services, the physician or clinic employs the therapist, the physician personally supervises the therapy, and the physician's bills include such charges. Second, physical therapy and speech pathology services may also be provided "under arrangement," by an outside service organization with a written contract. In such a case, they are reimbursable under Medicare if the clinic or physician bills for the services, if the clinic is qualified to provide such services under state law and assumes responsibility for their provision, and if receipt of payment by the clinic discharges the beneficiary's obligation to pay for the service.[91] Finally, physical and occupational therapists in independent practice may also be reimbursed under Medicare up to an annual limit per patient of $750 in billed charges, apart from therapy services furnished incident to a physician's services.[92]

Generally, diagnostic tests are reimbursable under the physician's fee schedule if furnished by a physician, by the physician's employees under the physician's supervision, or incident to a physician's services.[93] However, diagnostic services performed under arrangement with an outside supplier, regardless of where they are performed, are reimbursable only at the physician's cost of purchasing those outside services, and not at a marked-up cost.[94] All claims now must be submitted with documentation on purchased services or a statement to the effect that the claim includes no purchased services.

REIMBURSEMENT UNDER MANAGED CARE

In a nutshell, managed care is designed to permit greater controls on cost and quality in the delivery of healthcare by requiring healthcare providers to share the financial risk of providing that care. Health maintenance organizations (HMOs) are typically structured to provide all health services to enrollees on a prepaid basis, for a single capitated fee per enrollee per month, usually paid by the enrollees' employers. Enrollees must choose among the physicians on the HMO's panel, and a referral from a primary care "gatekeeper" physician is required for the enrollee to obtain care from specialists. HMOs are at financial risk to provide medical care required in excess of that paid for through premiums.

Variations on this model include the point of service (POS) plans, offered by HMOs, in which enrollees are permitted to decide at the point of service whether to use physicians outside the panel, for which they pay higher co-payments. Another variation is the preferred provider organization (PPO), which functions as a broker of discounted health services. Payors contract with a panel of providers, directly or through the PPO, who provide care at discounted rates. Enrollees must choose among the physicians on the panel, but they are not required to obtain referrals for specialty care services. Enrollees may be permitted to obtain care from providers outside the panel, but they must pay higher co-payments to do so.

Under managed care arrangements, physicians are compensated on a capitated basis, which may include withhold pools, or by global fee arrangements. A capitation payment is a fixed monthly fee per enrollee per month, which is designed to cover a comprehensive but specific set of health services. If enrollees require more care than is paid for through the monthly premiums, then the physician is at financial risk to provide that care. If the patient requires less care, then the physician can keep the excess. Withhold pools may be included, whereby a portion of the premium is withheld from the physician's salary and set aside to cover referrals to specialists and inpatient hospital care. Depending on the plan, physicians may or may not be at risk for amounts exceeding that covered by the withhold pool. If the withhold pool is not used up, the physicians share the excess. Under a global fee arrangement, physicians agree to cover the entire course of care for certain categories of patients, such as obstetrics patients, in exchange for a flat fee. The physician is again at risk to provide excess care and has an incentive to control costs.

Under managed care, hospitals may also be compensated on a capitated basis, perhaps including withhold pools. The reimbursement methodology under capitation is the same for hospitals as it is for physicians. Hospitals may also be reimbursed on a per diem basis or on a per case basis. Under a per diem system, the hospital is paid a pre-set rate for each day a patient receives in-patient care. If the hospital is able to control costs well, it can retain the difference between its costs and the per diem rate. On the other hand, the per case system functions much like the DRG system, in which hospitals are reimbursed for a patient's specific course of treatment.

Healthcare providers may also be reimbursed jointly where they are integrated into one provider system, such as a physician-hospital organization (PHO). In a PHO, providers may be compensated through global capitation, whereby providers are paid a global fee for rendering all hospital and physician care required by patients, and the PHO assumes the risk of excess care. To contain that risk, the PHO may purchase stop-loss insurance. On the other hand, under a bundled fee arrangement, the hospital may agree to accept a flat fee per case in a specific category, and it assumes the responsibility of compensating the physicians who provide the physician services in that category of case.

Distinctions for Integrated Delivery Systems under Medicare

Medicare reimbursement to providers may vary depending upon the structure of the integrated delivery system, and which entity is providing the reimbursable services. Examples of variances in reimbursement based on the structure of the IDS include:

1. Medicare considers new types of entities providing outpatient care, such as cancer centers and diagnostic imaging centers, as providing physicians' services. Thus, the facility cost is considered to be included in the physician's charges. However, if the entity is affiliated with a hospital it may obtain reimbursement under Part B as a hospital outpatient department.

2. Entities that are related by common ownership or control are limited in the manner in which they can account for transactions between themselves,[95] and related organizations must generally deal with each other at cost for reimbursement purposes under Part A.

3. When the ownership of a provider changes, the new owner's basis in the assets for Part A reimbursement purposes is limited to the lesser of the acquisition cost or the historical cost (the acquisition cost as of July 18, 1984). However, mergers between related parties, stock purchases, and affiliations are not considered to be a change in ownership.

4. The costs of administrative and supervisory services of hospital-based physicians are subject to special rules.[96]

5. The costs of services furnished under contracts with outside suppliers are subject to special rules.[97]

6. Start-up and organization costs, and the home-office costs of multi-entity providers are subject to special rules.[98]

7. Compensation paid to owners is subject to special rules.[99]

8. The prospective payment rate covers all services provided within 72 hours of hospital admission and which are admission-related if they are provided by a hospital-owned or -affiliated entity.[100]

9. In regard to reimbursement for skilled nursing facilities (SNF), routine service costs are reimbursed on a reasonable cost basis, subject to certain cost limits.[101] Ancillary services are also reimbursed on a reasonable cost basis, but they are not subject to cost limits. However, if services are contracted out, through an outside supplier, the SNF is reimbursed on a cost basis that is limited to the net amount actually paid to the supplier. If the SNF charges the outside supplier for billing or other administrative services, that amount must be treated as a discount to the provider and it may not be treated as income by the SNF.[102]

10. For home health services, Medicare reimburses the primary provider, even though services are provided by an outside supplier.[103]

11. Reimbursement rules governing hospice services restrict which types of services may be provided by outside suppliers. Generally, "core services" such as nursing services, medical social services, physician services, and counseling services must be provided by hospice employees.[104]

12. Outpatient surgical procedures are reimbursed depending upon where the service is performed. If done at an ambulatory surgical center, the service is reimbursed based on the lesser of the facility's reasonable costs or charges, or a blend of the reasonable cost and the ambulatory surgical center prospective payment rate. If done at a non-ASC site, the service is reimbursed on a reasonable cost basis.

13. Reimbursement to a hospital for durable medical equipment depends upon whether the hospital is a certified DME supplier. If it is so certified, the hospital is reimbursed based upon a fee schedule. If it is not certified, the hospital is paid on a reasonable cost basis.

14. Reimbursement for renal dialysis services likewise varies depending upon whether such services are provided within a hospital or at a free-standing provider. Under the Omnibus Budget Reconciliation Act of 1990, the Secretary of DHHS is required to develop a prospective payment system for more hospital outpatient services. In so doing, the Secretary will review the feasibility of varying payments based on whether the service is provided in a free-standing facility or in a hospital facility.[105]

In fact, in August 1996, HCFA issued a clarification of its reimbursement policy regarding which hospital-affiliated entities will qualify as provider-based or free-standing entities.[106] The concern is that facilities are classified as hospital-based when they should be classified as freestanding, and they are thus obtaining excess reimbursement. For example, hospitals are purchasing physician clinics located far from the hospital but are claiming them as outpatient departments of the hospital. HCFA's clarification listed eight criteria that must be met before an entity can be classified as provider-based:

1. The entity must be physically located close to where the provider is based, and both the entity and the provider must serve the same patient population.
2. The entity must be an integral and subordinate part of the provider where it is based, and it must be under common licensure.
3. The entity must be included under the accreditation of the provider where it is based.
4. The entity must be operated under common ownership and control.
5. The entity director must be under direct, daily supervision of the provider where it is located.
6. The clinical services of the entity and its parent must be integrated.
7. The entity must be held out to the public as part of the provider where it is based.
8. The provider and its parent must be financially integrated.

UNAUTHORIZED CORPORATE PRACTICE OF MEDICINE

Most states permit only natural persons to hold a license to practice medicine. Thus, general business corporations are prohibited from practicing medicine, and, in most states, are also prohibited from employing physicians to practice medicine on their behalf. This restriction can also apply to acquisitions of physician practices, prohibiting the transfer of assets such as patient medical records, and practice goodwill.

Violations of the corporate practice of medicine doctrine can result in fines and imprisonment in some states, or loss of licensure. On the other hand, most states permit professional corporations to "practice medicine" or to employ physicians if all shareholders of the professional corporation are licensed physicians. Some states permit hospitals to practice medicine under the hospital licensing statutes as well.

Although this doctrine has been in existence for some time, its persuasive hold on courts is diminishing in many states as pervasive changes affect the healthcare landscape. Originally, the rationales for the prohibition were to prohibit lay control over professional medical judgment, to avoid commercial exploitation of medical practice, and to avoid conflicts of interest between a physician's duty to the patient and to the physician's employer. Few states today strictly enforce the doctrine, or they statutorily decree that certain entities, such as hospitals and HMOs, are permitted to employ physicians. Where it is enforced, however, physicians typically enter into extensive contractual arrangements with corporations to work around the restriction. Primarily, the doctrine is seen as an obstacle to managed care initiatives, particularly in light of the fraud and abuse safe harbors protecting employment relationships.

SELECTED EMPLOYMENT ISSUES

The formation and operation of integrated delivery systems will implicate employment laws in several different ways. First, where workers who were classified as independent contractors are hired as employees, their employment will trigger the coverage of additional employment laws. The employer will also become liable for employee benefits and payroll withholding taxes.

Second, employment of physicians, typically highly compensated, will trigger protections under employee benefit laws, which prohibit discrimination in benefit plans in favor of highly compensated employees.

Third, although most employment laws cover most employers, some employment laws cover employers of a certain size or who have a certain number of employees. For example, an increase in the number of employees through aggregation of employers may trigger application of such laws as the Civil Rights Act of 1964 and the Family and Medical Leave Act. State laws may be similar. Examples of these federal size-sensitive laws include:

1. The National Labor Relations Act[107] applies to nearly all employers and governs the relationships between employees, employers, and labor unions, including union representation, unfair labor practices, and labor disputes.

2. The federal Fair Labor Standards Act[108] also applies to nearly all employers and most types of employees. It applies to enterprises having a gross annual volume of sales of at least $500,000, as well as all hospitals regardless of size. It governs minimum wage standards, overtime pay, and child labor restrictions.

3. The Civil Rights Act of 1964[109] contains 11 titles and bars discrimination in voting rights, accommodations, education, employment, and the use of federal funds. In particular, Title VII prohibits employment discrimination based upon race, color, religion, sex, and national origin. Title VII applies to employers having more than 15 employees. Compensatory and punitive damages awarded under Title VII are capped, but they depend upon the size of the defendant entity and range from $50,000 for entities with 14 to 101 employees, to $300,000 for entities with more than 500 employees.

4. Title VI of the Civil Rights Act of 1964[110] governs discrimination by any entity receiving federal financial assistance, which has been interpreted to include healthcare programs.[111] Patients are generally viewed as intended beneficiaries of this law,[112] but employees of healthcare institutions are not.[113] Depending upon the jurisdiction, physicians may be viewed as intended beneficiaries of this provision in regard to staff privileges claims.[114]

5. The Age Discrimination in Employment Act[115] prohibits discrimination in employment on the basis of age, for employees over 40 years of age. It applies to entities with at least 20 employees as well as to their agents, such as subsidiaries, that participate in the discriminatory practice.[116]

6. The Americans with Disabilities Act[117] prohibits discrimination in employment on the basis of disability. The Act covers employers having on average 15 or more employees during at least 20 calendar weeks of the current or previous year. The Rehabilitation Act of 1973[118] has similar provisions but it is slightly narrower in scope. It is limited to entities receiving federal funding, which includes hospitals and other healthcare institutions by virtue of their receipt of Medicare and Medicaid funds.[119]

7. The Family and Medical Leave Act of 1993[120] permits employees up to 12 weeks per year of unpaid leave for the arrival of a child or for a serious health condition of the employee or a family member. This Act applies to private employers who have 50 or more employees for at least 20 weeks of the current or prior year.

8. The Worker Adjustment and Retraining Notification Act of 1988[121] (WARN) requires employers to provide affected employees and the surrounding community with 60 days' notice of a plant closing or mass layoff. This Act applies to any business that employs 100 or more employees, not including part-time employees working less than 20 hours per week or who have worked for the employer less than 6 months. A "mass layoff" is defined as a reduction in force at a single site of employment of at least 33% of the employees (minimum of 50), or 500 employees for larger units.

SPECIAL LIABILITY ISSUES

Independent Contractors, Vicarious Liability, and Ostensible Agency

The general rule under common law is that an employer is not liable for the negligence of independent contractors.[122] An exception to this rule is the nondelegable duty doctrine, which holds that the employer cannot avoid liability by delegating certain functions to independent contractors.

Under the vicarious liability doctrine, an employer organization will be liable under the *respondeat superior* theory for the malpractice of its employed physicians. The physician's employment status is ascertained under common law, which typically focuses on the organization's legal right to control the ends and the means of the employee's work. The label given to the relationship in a contract is not controlling.[123] Most courts have held that the vicarious liability doctrine applies to staff model HMOs[124]; however, some courts have held that HMOs themselves do not render medical services and are thus not liable.[125] Other courts have also held that HMOs are liable for the negligent treatment of consulting physicians who are independent contractors.[126]

A substantial number of jurisdictions[127] follow the ostensible agency doctrine, which holds that hospitals or HMOs[128] are liable for the malpractice of their independent contractors if the hospital holds the contractor out to the public as its agent and a member of the public believes that the contractor is the hospital's agent. Cases relying upon this argument typically involve services provided in the hospital's emergency department, and perhaps other hospital-based services.

Corporate Negligence

The corporate negligence doctrine, effective in a substantial number of states, imposes a direct obligation upon hospitals to properly hire and credential physicians on its medical staff.[129] Depending upon the jurisdiction, this doctrine may also require hospitals and managed care organizations generally to ensure that patients receive quality care, to maintain safe and adequate facilities and equipment,[130] and to formulate and enforce policies to ensure quality care.[131] It also covers negligent utilization review, negligent benefit determinations, improper denials of coverage, and bad faith.

Financial Disincentives and Duty to Disclose

Most courts hold that managed care organizations are not liable for physician negligence by virtue of the financial disincentives to provide care in their compensation arrangements.[132] Although managed care organizations may not have a duty to disclose their compensation arrangements under common law,[133] many state legislatures are now requiring managed care organizations at least to disclose other forms of treatment that may be useful but that are not covered under the patient's benefit plan.

HOSPITAL AFFILIATIONS
Organizational Issues

Hospitals have been joining forces at a rapid pace across the country as managed care pressures mount, and they are doing so to control costs and provide higher quality and more comprehensive care.[134] This joining of forces typically takes the form of a merger, a joint venture, or an acquisition.

Organizational issues facing hospitals that are joining forces include how the new entity will be governed, and by whom. Consideration must be given to combining two separate corporate cultures as well. Religious-sponsored hospitals must comply with additional rules set forth by their religious sponsors, and nonprofit hospitals must comply with state laws governing the use and disposition of their assets.

Legal and Regulatory Issues

Antitrust is probably the most significant legal issue facing hospitals that join forces with other hospitals. Although the antitrust enforcement agencies have been steadfastly challenging hospital mergers, the agencies have not met with great success recently. In 1995, a federal district court in Dubuque, Iowa, approved the merger of the only two hospitals in the area, because the court viewed the relevant geographic area as including cities 70 miles away from the facilities.[135] The Department of Justice unsuccessfully challenged the proposed merger, arguing that it would not produce any efficiencies and would result in one facility controlling all inpatient services. Another merger involving hospitals in Grand Rapids, Michigan, also met with an unsuccessful challenge from the Department of Justice.

In a merger, the chief concern is the hospitals' postmerger market share, and whether that share gives the postmerger entity the capacity to raise prices or lower quality without restraint. However, antitrust risks are much lower for urban hospitals because each would typically have a smaller market share in a larger city. Since hospitals are generally of a large size, the Hart-Scott-Rodino premerger notification requirements would apply to hospitals planning to merge.

Hospitals that join forces but that do not purport to be merging run the greater risk of being challenged for "concerted activity." The chief concerns here are market allocation and price-fixing. Market allocation may take the form of allocating the clinical services that each hospital is to provide to the community. Price-fixing may take the form of jointly negotiating managed care discounts with payors. However, such alliances can generally produce significant cost savings by eliminating duplicative care and coordinating resources.

Joint ventures implicate the antitrust laws as well, since they involve less integration than do mergers. Since there is less integration, the hospitals are more likely to be viewed as separate entities and thus capable of conspiring under the antitrust laws.

In the early 1990s, nearly half the states enacted some form of statutory state-action exception to antitrust enforcement. However, few hospitals are seeking protection under these laws because they all must require ongoing supervision of the hospitals' activities. They instead opt to comply with federal antitrust requirements, which, once complied with, require no additional oversight from the federal agencies.[136]

Fraud and abuse restrictions are less of a concern with affiliating hospitals. Although inpatient and outpatient hospital care is a "designated health service" under the Stark laws, hospitals typically do not "refer" to each other as these laws define referrals.

Special Considerations for Tax-Exempt Organizations

Tax-exempt hospitals confront additional legal issues in the process of affiliation. Under the tax-exemption rules, exempt entities may not use their assets for substantial private benefit, nor may they permit private inurement of their resources. They must also operate primarily for a charitable purpose. Exempt entities which enter into joint ventures with nonexempt entities risk losing their exempt status if they engage in substantial activities that do not further their charitable purposes.[137]

Exempt entities may serve as general partners in a limited partnership with a taxable entity if they meet a two-pronged test:[138]

1. The partnership arrangement should be closely scrutinized to ensure that the exempt entity's duties under the Internal Revenue Code do not conflict with the objectives of the partnership. In essence, the exempt entity must be serving a charitable purpose through the partnership.

2. The partnership arrangement must permit the exempt entity to act exclusively in furtherance of its charitable purposes and only incidentally for the benefit of the taxable entity.

Since most exempt hospitals are also nonprofit entities under state law, additional concerns are raised when they are sold to for-profit entities. In addition, if they are sold, exempt entities must normally contribute their assets to a nonprofit foundation under state law. Particularly, the concern centers around whether community assets held by the hospital, which were obtained in the form of tax deductions, are being properly valued and distributed at the time of sale.

PHYSICIAN ORGANIZATIONS AND PHYSICIAN RELATIONSHIPS
Organizational Issues

Physicians collaborate in several different models of integrated systems.[139] Depending upon the form of the organization and the services offered, collaborating physicians may be able to contract directly with employers to provide care, since many employers are self-funded and prefer "one-stop shopping."

Traditionally, a physician participated in an integrated system by entering into a group practice with other physicians. Although there are typically few practice sites, the group practice is completely economically integrated into a single legal entity. It may have additional subsidiaries that provide specialized services, such as a real estate partnership or a management services company, which are separate for tax reasons.

A "group practice without walls" is made up of physicians at different sites who are shareholders and/or employees of a corporation in which they share overhead expenses but retain the individual assets of their own medical practices. Such groups typically permit physicians to remain independent practitioners while providing them with the stronger negotiating power of a group. On the other hand, such groups lack the legal protections that a single entity would have under the antitrust laws, which prohibit collusive activity between two or more parties, and under the fraud and abuse and anti-referral laws, which provide safe harbor protections to organizations legally organized as a single-entity "group practice." Multi-entity groups that merge their assets and employ physicians generally have such protections. Furthermore, where physician organizations share risk, they are under less scrutiny under the antitrust laws, since it is assumed that they do not have financial incentives to violate the antitrust laws or fraud and abuse laws.

An independent practice (or physician) association (IPA) is another integration model. In an IPA, physicians practice independently but partially integrate their practices to contract more effectively with third-party payors, including managed care contracting. IPAs are attractive to third-party payors because they provide one-stop shopping, for either a single- or multi-specialty group. An IPA can serve as the "messenger" of fee information to avoid antitrust risks, and it can assume economic risk by entering into capitation arrangements on behalf of the participating physicians. If the IPA does assume risk, it generally must comply with state insurance laws at some level.

IPAs can be formed as a business corporation, nonprofit corporation, professional corporation, or a limited liability form of corporation. If the IPA is formed as a business corporation, then it may sell shares of stock, but then it must also comply with securities laws unless an exemption applies. If it is formed as a professional corporation, then all of its shareholders must be physicians. If it is formed as a nonprofit corporation and obtains tax-exempt status, then it must comply with private inurement restrictions. Another model may involve minimal integration in the form of sharing overhead costs, such as leases, staffing, and equipment costs.

Physician Organizations (POs) are another form of physician integration. A PO provides the contract negotiation functions of an IPA combined with other functions. A PO may handle group purchasing and consolidate the billing functions of a group of physicians. A PO may be set up in the same corporate formats as an IPA, with the same advantages and disadvantages.

Governance of the integrated practice will depend in part on the corporate form of the practice. If it is a corporation, governance is vested in the board of directors, with approval on fundamental corporate changes reserved to shareholders. If it is a partnership, governance is typically handled by a managing partner. Ownership of shares in a corporation need not correspond to each shareholder's voting rights, however.

Legal and Regulatory Issues

Integration of physician practices raises several legal issues. First, the antitrust laws are implicated when the participants begin negotiations on the process of integration, since such discussions could be viewed as an attempt to monopolize, depending upon the size of the market. Antitrust laws are also implicated if such discussions involve market allocation or collective discussions on fees. Although most of the models discussed are not sufficiently integrated to avoid antitrust scrutiny, the group practice without walls may be sufficiently integrated to avoid scrutiny, such as when it contracts on a capitated basis, depending upon its actual structure.

Referrals of patients between affiliated entities may also raise fraud and abuse issues. Fraud and abuse concerns arise when the integrated practice provides "designated health services" but does not meet the requirements of a "group practice" under the safe harbors. Under the Stark anti-referral law, a group practice is defined as a group of two or more physicians legally organized as a partnership, professional corporation, foundation, nonprofit corporation, or similar association. Services provided must be provided through the joint use of shared office space, equipment, and staff, and substantially all of the services of the physician members must be provided through the group practice and billed under the group's billing number. Income must be treated as income to the group, not the individual physicians, although the physicians may be paid based upon the services they personally perform. The DHHS Office of the Inspector General has opined that a group practice without walls may be a sham structure, formed to avoid restrictions on joint ventures for ancillary services.

The form of the new entity will also determine where liability ultimately rests. If the integrated practice is a corporation, then liability will be limited to the corporation's assets in most cases. If the groups are integrated and formed as partnerships, then individual partners are personally liable for the partnership's debts. Securities laws are implicated if the integrated entity is formed as a corporation and seeks sources of outside capital, unless an exemption applies.

Physician integration may also implicate corporate practice of medicine restrictions. These restrictions limit the types of entities that may "practice medicine" and thus limit the forms of organization that can be used for physician integration. State law may require physicians to practice in and be employed only by professional corporations or HMOs, as opposed to general business corporations.

The formation of an integrated physician practice also raises tax implications, depending upon whether a separate entity is formed, or whether existing entities are merged.

Special Considerations for Tax-Exempt Organizations

Although physician groups are not typically formed as tax-exempt entities, they may be formed as such if they are organized and operated exclusively for charitable purposes and if they comply with the rules governing tax-exempt entities.

Additional issues arise if one merging entity is tax-exempt and the other is not, or even if a joint venture is formed between such entities. In a merger situation, the tax-exempt entity is prohibited from selling a portion of its gross or net revenue stream.[140] However, a tax-exempt entity may engage in insubstantial profit-making activities unrelated to its charitable purpose as long as it pays the unrelated business income tax on such activities.

HOSPITAL-PHYSICIAN ORGANIZATIONS

Organizational Issues

Physician-hospital affiliations are quickly becoming quite prevalent in the healthcare delivery system.[141] Generally, in these affiliations, physician and hospital services are integrated to provide more comprehensive services to patients and perhaps to provide capital to physicians. A physician-hospital affiliation may take several forms, including direct employment of physicians by hospitals, or a separate physician practice entity owned or controlled by the hospital, or a physician-hospital organization (PHO). Such affiliations provide the same advantages of IPAs in negotiating third-party payor arrangements, and since they include hospital services, they can provide more comprehensive services to payors.

Direct employment of physicians by hospitals is one form of affiliation between physicians and hospitals. Hospitals may seek direct employment of physicians to develop a more extensive primary care base or to penetrate new markets. However, direct employment may pose a problem under state corporate practice of medicine prohibitions in some states. In other states, hospitals are authorized to practice medicine under their licensing statutes and thus are exempt from this prohibition. Direct employment of physicians does have the benefit of avoiding referral problems under the Medicare fraud and abuse rules and related state statutes. It may also avoid private inurement problems if the hospital is tax-exempt.

Another form of affiliation may be a separate practice entity formed as a subsidiary of the hospital or as a subsidiary of a parent corporation over both the hospital and the practice entity. The physician practice entity may be formed as a nonprofit, tax-exempt subsidiary of the hospital, but it must meet certain criteria under IRS rules.

In a physician-hospital organization, a hospital integrates with its medical staff to negotiate and provide services under third-party payor contracts. The medical staff may be represented by a PO or an IPA, which would deal directly with the PHO. The PHO structure permits the hospital and medical staff to manage utilization review, peer review, and quality assurance functions, and it may handle management services functions as well. A PHO is appealing to payors because it provides one-stop shopping for comprehensive services. A PHO is often an intermediate step to more complete integration of medical services.

PHOs typically are legal entities separate from the hospital and physician group. They may be organized in several forms, including for-profit business corporations, nonprofit corporations, partnerships, or limited liability companies. A for-profit business corporation structure will require that the PHO comply with federal and state securities laws if stock is offered to numerous individuals, but it may be the most practical if the shareholders will hold their interests as an investment, to be sold at a later date perhaps. If the PHO is set up as a nonprofit entity, then the members obtain financial benefits through their contractual arrangements. If the PHO is structured as a corporation, it will incur double taxation, at the entity and individual shareholder levels, and thus compensation arrangements must be structured carefully. Most PHOs are not tax-exempt entities, even though they may be nonprofit corporations.

If the PHO is set up as a limited liability company, then it will have the advantages of taxation as a partnership and limited liability, although it may still need to comply with securities laws unless an exemption applies. As a partnership, the PHO would be taxed as a partnership but the partners would have joint and several liability.

One common form of the PHO is the "foundation model." Under this form, the hospital establishes a separate corporation, usually a tax-exempt organization, which builds or acquires all assets of a medical group clinic facility and then owns and operates the facility. If the foundation is tax-exempt, then the medical group cannot obtain an ownership interest in it. The PHO either employs or contracts with the medical group to provide the clinical services, depending upon the state's corporate practice of medicine prohibition. Unlike a management services organization (MSO), a foundation-model PHO is the provider of care and can bill for medical services rendered.

The Medicare billing rules applicable to MSO arrangements may also apply to the foundation model. Under these rules, a group medical practice may bill Medicare for services rendered by medical personnel only if those services are performed under the supervision of the physician. The group may reassign its right to payment only to an employer or to an organization in whose facilities the physician practices exclusively. To qualify under the supervision requirement, the services must be performed by the physician directly, by employees of the physician, or by ancillary personnel who have a common employer with the physician. Thus, if the physicians are independent contractors with the foundation, the medical group may not assign its payment rights to the foundation, and the foundation may not bill directly for the group's services. The foundation may provide billing services, but it must do so as a billing agent. As a billing agent, the foundation may not be compensated based upon collections or billable amounts. Although HCFA is currently reviewing this issue, there are some approaches to solving it. One is to treat the physicians as employees, in which case HCFA will approve the transfer of a provider number to the foundation. However, this approach implicates the corporate practice of medicine prohibition.

The "fully-integrated model" is a variant of the foundation model. In a fully integrated model, a corporate parent is created over the hospital and physician group subsidiaries. The parent may or may not be jointly governed by the hospital and physician group. This model may provide increased access to tax-exempt funding for all subsidiary organizations if the parent is tax-exempt. A fully integrated organization enjoys substantial power in the market-place through its ability to provide one-stop shopping and better control over costs. It also enjoys less scrutiny under the fraud and abuse laws if the entity employs the physicians, since there is only one entity, and it cannot refer to itself.[142] This single-entity status likewise applies to private inurement and antitrust concerns. But corporate practice, licensure, and CON issues may arise. If the physicians are employed, the entity may also need to employ auxiliary personnel and to lease physician space, in order to obtain reimbursement for auxiliary services provided "incident to" a physician's services without requiring the physician's direct supervision.

Legal and Regulatory Issues

There are several legal issues relating to who will own, control, and govern the joint organization. Antitrust is a chief concern with nearly all forms of integrated delivery systems where there is more than one legal entity involved in the system. If the system involves a parent-subsidiary relationship and the subsidiary is wholly owned, then generally no antitrust issues arise because there can be no conspiracy without two separate entities. An exception is where monopolization claims arise with a large system, since monopolization can be a unilateral activity.

The Justice Department has been particularly concerned with activities involving price fixing, boycotts, and monopolization. Price-fixing issues arise when two separate entities agree to set rates for specific services, or even discuss the rates they charge. Boycott issues arise when the ability of physicians to obtain medical staff membership at the hospital are limited because the medical staff is "closed" to new members. There are also significant antitrust issues if physicians are on the board of a PHO and the PHO is involved in managed care network activity, such as setting fee schedules.

Fraud and abuse issues are also a concern for most managed care activities involving hospitals, now that Stark II is in effect. One of the "designated health services" that triggers application of Stark II is "inpatient and outpatient hospital services." If the physicians are employees or independent contractors of the hospital or the PHO, then the arrangement generally will fall under a safe harbor if the compensation is reasonable and is not based upon the volume of referrals between the parties. However, an employment relationship may trigger the corporate practice of medicine prohibition in some states. If the integration process involves the merger or acquisition of physician practices, then the transaction must comply with the safe harbor requiring a single transaction not based upon the value of referrals. It should be noted, however, that the safe harbor for practice purchases does not cover hospitals at all, only physician-physician purchases from a retiring physician.

Insurance issues are also implicated in hospital-physician affiliations. If the PHO assumes risk, it must be regulated in some form by state insurance laws, either as a preferred provider or as an HMO. In addition, its utilization review functions may also be regulated under state laws.

Special Considerations for Tax-Exempt Organizations

The IRS set forth the tax-exemption requirements for hospital-affiliated medical practices in its rulings on the Friendly Hills Health Care Foundation and the Facey Medical Foundation in 1993 and 1994, which reiterate and expand the community benefit standard applicable to tax-exempt hospitals:

1. The hospital and the physician practice entity must provide an open emergency room to all persons regardless of their ability to pay.
2. The medical staff should be open to all qualified applicants.
3. The board of directors must represent a fair cross-section of the community, and no more than 20% of the board can be comprised of physicians with a financial interest in the organization.
4. Covenants not to compete must be limited, so as not to limit the community's access to medical care if the physicians leave.
5. Physicians must participate in Medicare and Medicaid programs in a nondiscriminatory manner.
6. The organization must comply with other tax-exempt requirements, such as operating for a charitable

purpose, and providing a community benefit, including a certain level of charity care.

7. Physician compensation must be reasonable and must not violate private inurement restrictions.

8. The acquisition of any medical practices must be done at fair market value according to approved IRS methodologies.[143]

There are also private inurement concerns if the hospital capitalizes the PHO in an amount that is disproportionate to the physician investors' share or if it engages in other activities that would expose the hospital's assets to a risk of loss that is greater than the physician investors' risk. Generally, the tax-exempt participant may not capitalize the PHO disproportionate to its profits, nor may it assume risks disproportionate to its interest in the PHO, and all services provided by or paid for by the exempt entity must be at fair market value. In addition, the exempt participant must be permitted to veto actions by the PHO, such as those implicating private inurement, which would jeopardize the exempt participant's tax-exempt status.

Physician recruitment is another area that implicates tax-exempt issues. Traditional recruitment incentives include loans, relocation assistance, income guarantees, malpractice insurance assistance, office and equipment leasing, and the provision of billing and support services. These recruitment incentives also create legal issues under the fraud and abuse rules, because such incentives can be viewed as inducements to refer.

In 1994 the IRS issued guidance in the area of physician recruitment with its publication of the Hermann Hospital closing agreement. This closing agreement specified the parameters within which recruiting would be permitted for tax-exempt hospitals:

1. The hospital must show a demonstrable community need for the physician's services. For example, the physician's specialty is deficient in the hospital's service area; there is a demand for service and long waiting periods; the area has been designated a health professional shortage area by DHHS; physicians are reluctant to relocate to the hospital due to its location; a physician is expected to retire; or there is a documented lack of physicians serving indigent or Medicaid patients in the service area.

2. Incentives used to retain existing physicians, who are nonemployee physicians with staff privileges, are prohibited.

3. Hospital subsidization of salary and benefit costs for support staff of nonemployee physicians in their private practices is prohibited.

4. Income guarantees cannot exceed 2 years.

Tax-exempt status is now more difficult to obtain for a foundation model PHO, and the IRS limits physician participation on the foundation board to 20%. Medicare is also concerned about granting provider numbers to the foundation entity, since physicians may assign their rights to payment only to an organization in whose facilities the physician practices—typically a hospital. Thus, the foundation may not be able to bill for physicians' services. Other IRS concerns include private use of tax-exempt bonds as well as acquisition of physician practices at fair market value.

PHYSICIAN PRACTICE ACQUISITIONS
Organizational Issues

Physician practice acquisitions generally take one of three forms: an asset acquisition, a stock acquisition, or a merger.[144] In an asset acquisition, the purchasing entity buys specific assets of the medical practice, and perhaps some specific liabilities. However, the purchaser can avoid buying contingent liabilities, such as for employment discrimination lawsuits, and the purchaser can also avoid being liable for questionable billing practices. Any employment or service contracts, or leases, typically will require that the other party to the contract consent to the assignment of the contract.

There are tax implications for using an asset acquisition, depending upon the corporate form of the practice. If it is an "S" corporation, a professional limited liability company, or a partnership, then the organization will be taxed at both the corporate and individual levels. The practice will be taxed at the corporate level on any gain recognized from the sale of its assets, and then the shareholders will be taxed on any cash they receive for the assets. However, tax planning can minimize this burden.

In a stock acquisition, the purchaser acquires the stock of the professional corporation from the physician shareholders, but the medical practice remains as a separate entity after the acquisition. The acquiring entity becomes the sole shareholder of the practice, and the practice becomes a subsidiary of the acquiring entity. Contracts and leases generally will not require consent for transfer in a stock acquisition, but some require consent when a controlling interest is transferred.

A stock acquisition is simpler to transfer ownership, but it is more risky because all assets and all liabilities of the practice are assumed. Thus, due diligence is more important in this form of acquisition, and the sellers are typically required to make comprehensive representations, warranties, and indemnities with regard to the practice. The transaction may involve setting aside a specific sum of money to handle contingent liabilities that may arise after the transfer.

A merger is similar to a stock transfer, except that after the merger only one entity exists. All of the assets and liabilities are transferred, but the medical practice is merged into the purchasing entity and ceases to exist.

Legal and Regulatory Issues

Historically, physician practice acquisitions have received little interest from the antitrust enforcement agencies because of their relatively small size.[145] The level of antitrust risk will depend upon which form of acquisition is used and the types of parties involved. If a hospital is acquiring a physician practice, then more market share is involved and thus more antitrust risk. In addition, the Hart-Scott-Rodino premerger notification requirements will apply if both entities are large enough. If two physician practices are merging, there is less risk because of the smaller market share. If a single entity remains after the acquisition, then Section 1 of the Sherman Act cannot apply to its future activities because concerted action is not possible. In addition, monopolization, while possible, is of little concern because of the relatively small market share of a physician's practice. In either case, the critical antitrust focus is whether the merged entity will be able to exercise market power such that it may raise prices or lower quality without constraint. The rule of thumb is that, after the merger, an entity with less than a 35% market share will not be able to exercise market power.

Physician practice acquisitions also raise legal concerns in the area of fraud and abuse. A key issue under the fraud and abuse laws is the acquisition price paid by a hospital for a solo practice or a group practice. The Inspector General's office recognizes that "what the hospital is really interested in is the future flow of business from the practice to the hospital."[146] The regulators are concerned that payments for future referral streams are disguised as goodwill payments or other payments for intangible items.[147] Specifically, the OIG views payments for goodwill, covenants not to compete, exclusive dealing arrangements, and patient lists as possible payments for referrals, although payments for tangible assets at fair market value do not raise legal concerns.

To comply with the fraud and abuse rules, the parties must obtain a complete and independent appraisal of the practice assets to ascertain fair market value. The transaction should also be structured without installment payments to avoid classification as an investment interest under the fraud and abuse rules.

In a fee-for-service system, another issue under the fraud and abuse laws involves payments to physicians after they have become employees or independent contractors with the purchasing hospital. In such a case, the safe harbors should be reviewed for compliance. This concern disappears, however, under a capitated payment system, which provides incentives for limiting services.

Finally, state certificate of need laws may be implicated if the acquisition cost for the practice exceeds a certain dollar limit or if it involves the acquisition of expensive medical equipment.

Special Considerations for Tax-Exempt Organizations

The key concern for tax-exempt entities is whether the physician practice is acquired at its fair market value. Excessive compensation for an acquisition jeopardizes the purchaser's exempt status because payments exceeding fair market value are private inurement. However, the IRS has recognized that practice acquisitions may be consistent with an exempt organization's charitable purpose, as long as the acquisition does not violate the fraud and abuse laws.[148] Since it is relatively easy to ascertain the fair market value of tangible items, these are not as great a concern to the IRS. However, payments for goodwill are an issue and must comply with relevant tax laws for valuing intangibles.

THE ACQUISITION PROCESS

The acquisition process normally begins with the parties discussing the desirability of the acquisition. The parties then sign a confidentiality agreement pertaining to the negotiations, and a letter of intent. Both parties then normally perform due diligence, and the practice is appraised. The parties then negotiate the specific terms of the acquisition and memorialize the agreement, which may include employment agreements for the selling physicians to work at the purchasing hospital. The sale is then closed according to the terms of the agreement.

MANAGEMENT SERVICES ORGANIZATIONS

Organizational Issues

Management services organizations (MSOs) can provide a broad range of management support and administrative services to physician practices.[149] Such support may include staffing and recruiting, billing, record keeping and information systems, equipment leasing, contract negotiation, consultation services, and the use of facilities. An MSO may have the capacity to provide all nonclinical services to medical practices. It may also purchase all of the assets of a physician practice and then contract with the physician practice to provide management services for a set fee. MSOs allow physician autonomy while providing centralized practice management and centralized managed care contract negotiations for physicians. MSOs are commonly used where enforcement of the corporate practice of medicine doctrine is strong and thus prohibits employment of physicians.

MSOs may be set up in various ways. Frequently, they are owned and governed by hospitals, less frequently by physicians, but they may also be jointly owned and governed in some instances. MSOs may function as a division or subsidiary of a hospital, or as a joint venture between the hospital and its medical staff, or as a separate entity. If a separate entity, its corporate form will depend upon whether any of its participants are tax-exempt entities, but it may be set up as a business corporation, a nonprofit corporation, or a partnership, or a limited liability version of those. The MSO itself generally does not qualify for tax-exempt status because it does not provide medical care services and thus does not have a charitable purpose. If it is a division of a tax-exempt hospital, then income from the MSO's operations is unrelated business income that is taxable to the hospital. In addition, the activities of the MSO division cannot be more than a "substantial" part of the hospital's operations, otherwise the hospital will jeopardize its tax-exempt status. On the other hand, the MSO may be set up as a separate limited liability company, in which case income can be passed through to the participants, including to a tax-exempt hospital. Private inurement restrictions will still apply in relation to physician contracts where a tax-exempt hospital is involved, however.

Hospitals can also be involved by contracting with a large group of physicians, although they remain separate entities, with the hospital providing many management services to the group, such as managed care contract negotiations, group purchasing, information systems, office management, provision of support staff, and leasing of space and equipment.

The MSO is typically a separate legal entity and perhaps is co-owned by the hospital and the physician group. The physician group may be a part-owner of the entity outright, or through another entity, such as a PHO. It may purchase the tangible assets of the group and lease them back to the group. Intangible assets such as patient records, managed care contracts, and the practice goodwill might not be acquirable because of state corporate practice restrictions, which may require these assets to be held by a professional corporation. In addition, asset appraisals are required if the MSO is affiliated with a tax-exempt entity, or generally for fraud and abuse concerns that excess payments are inducements to refer.

Medicare has special billing rules applicable to MSO arrangements. A group medical practice may bill Medicare for services rendered by medical personnel only if those services are performed under the supervision of the physician. To qualify under the supervision requirement, the services must be performed by the physician directly, by employees of the physician, or by ancillary personnel who have a common employer with the physician. Thus, even where the MSO provides comprehensive services, ancillary personnel normally are employed by the physician or his or her group practice, as opposed to being employed by the MSO. If the MSO provides billing services, it must do so as a billing agent and may not bill directly for the physician's services under Medicare reassignment rules.

Legal and Regulatory Issues

Antitrust considerations come into play with MSOs that are a separate legal entity. If the MSO employs the physicians, then it is a competitor with the hospital in the area of outpatient services. Antitrust risks will include price-fixing, concerted refusals to deal, and market allocation.

The corporate practice of medicine prohibition is implicated with MSOs in relation to both organizational and operational issues. In regard to organizational issues, this doctrine will determine whether the MSO can employ the physicians. In regard to operational issues, the physicians should retain the ability to exercise independent clinical judgment where the corporate practice prohibition is enforced.

Fraud and abuse issues also arise with MSOs. If an MSO is owned by a provider that might receive referrals from medical practices that the MSO services, then the arrangement must comply with fraud and abuse safe harbors. Although the MSO does not provide medical services, an indirect referral may exist when physicians own the MSO. Generally, the arrangement must comply with the safe harbors under the anti-kickback and anti-referral laws for employment and management services contracts. These safe harbors require that the contract be in writing and specify the services to be provided, and that it have a minimum term of 1 year. Compensation under the agreement must not be referral based, it must be set in advance, and it must be based upon the fair market value of the services. In addition, ancillary service personnel should remain employees of the medical practice in order to qualify as a group practice under the anti-referral laws.

Special Considerations for Tax-Exempt Organizations

Private inurement concerns arise when the MSO deals with a tax-exempt entity. In particular, private inurement is an issue if a tax-exempt hospital capitalizes the MSO in an amount that is disproportionate to its ownership interest or if the MSO under-charges the physicians for the services it renders. In addition, if a tax-exempt hospital receives services from the MSO, it must pay for them at fair market value.

NOTES

1. Letter from D. McCarty Thornton, Chief Counsel to the Inspector General, "Impact of the Anti-Kickback Statute and the Stark Amendment on Vertically Integrated Delivery Systems in the Health Care Industry," January 20, 1995.
2. Provisions in HR 3103 to Help Government Fight Federal, Private Fraud, in 5 Health L. Rep. (BNA) No. 32, at 1179 (August 8, 1996).
3. Ibid.
4. 42 U.S.C. § 1320a-7b(b).
5. Hanlester Network v. Shalala, 51 F.3d 1390 (9th Cir. 1995).
6. Ibid.
7. 760 F.2d 68 (3d Cir. 1985), cert. denied, 474 U. S. 988 (1985).
8. 871 F.2d 105 (9th Cir. 1989).
9. 42 U.S.C. § 1395nn.
10. Ibid.
11. 60 Fed. Reg. 41,914 (1995) (to be codified at 42 C.F.R. pt. 411).
12. "HCFA Aims to Curb Medicare Fraud with New Provider Application Form," in 5 Health L. Rep. (BNA) No. 33, at 1215 (August 15, 1996).
13. Ibid.
14. Ibid at 41,931. The final regulation for Stark I set forth a methodology for calculating this measurement. "Patient care services" are defined as any task performed by a group practice member that addresses the medical needs of specific patients, regardless of whether they involve direct patient encounters. Patient care services are measured by the total patient care time each member spends on the services. If 8 members of a 10-member group practice devote 100% of their patient care time to the group practice, 1 devotes 80% of his time to the group practice, and the other physician devotes only 10% of his time to the group practice, then the 10 participants devote a total of 890% of their total time to the group. That percentage is then divided

by the number of physicians in the group, or 890/10, for a quotient reflecting that 89% of the patient care services are provided through the group. This requirement applies unless the group practice is located in a health professional shortage area. If members of an urban practice devote a portion of their medical services to a shortage area, then that amount of time is not calculated in determining whether the group meets the "substantially all" test.

15. 60 Fed. Reg. 41,914 (1995) (to be codified at 42 C.F.R. pt. 411).
16. 42 U.S.C. § 1395ww(d)(2)(D).
17. 60 Fed. Reg. 41,914, 41,981 (1995) (to be codified at 42 C.F.R. pt. 411). The final regulation clarifies that the physician being recruited must not be precluded from establishing staff privileges at another hospital or referring business to another entity.
18. 800 F. Supp. 1451 (E.D. Tex. 1992).
19. 60 Fed. Reg. 41,914, 41,960 (1995) (to be codified at 42 C.F.R. pt. 411).
20. City of Lafayette v. Louisiana Power & Light Co., 43 U. S. 389 (1978).
21. United States v. Citizens & Southern Nat. Bank, 422 U. S. 86 (1975).
22. 421 U. S. 773 (1975), reh. denied, 423 U. S. 886 (1975).
23. See, generally, John J. Miles, *Health Care and Antitrust Law.* Deerfield, IL: Clark Boardman Callahan, (1995).
24. 15 U.S.C. §§ 1–7.
25. 15 U.S.C. §§ 1–7.
26. 15 U.S.C. §§ 41–58.
27. 15 U.S.C. § 44.
28. 15 U.S.C. §§ 12–27.
29. 15 U.S.C. § 13.
30. 15 U.S.C. § 13c.
31. 15 U.S.C. § 18a.
32. 15 U.S.C. §§ 1011–15.
33. 42 U.S.C. §§ 11101–52.
34. 15 U.S.C. §§ 34–36.
35. 29 U.S.C. §§ 101–10; 113–15.
36. 15 U.S.C. § 18a.
37. 15 U.S.C. §§ 1011–15.

38. 42 U.S.C. §§ 11101–52.

39. 15 U.S.C. §§ 34–36.

40. 29 U.S.C. §§ 101–10; 113–15.

41. 317 U. S. 341 (1943).

42. Northern Pacific Ry. Co. v. U. S., 356 U.S. 1, 5 (1958).

43. 457 U. S. 332 (1982).

44. See FTC Staff Advisory Opinion to Maryland Medical Eye Associates, May 15, 1987.

45. See, e.g., Michigan State Medical Society, 101 F.T.C. 191 (1983); Southbank IPA, Inc., 114 F.T.C. 783 (1991); FTC v. Indiana Federation of Dentists, 476 U. S. 447 (1986).

46. See U.S. Dept. of Justice & Fed. Trade Commission, Statements of Enforcement Policy and Analytical Principles Relating to Health Care and Antitrust (September 27, 1994); Hassan v. Independent Practice Assoc., P.C., 698 F.Supp. 679 (E.D. Mich. 1988) (capitation payments and risk withhold of 15% or 12% sufficient).

47. See, e.g., U.S. Healthcare, Inc. v. Healthsource, Inc., 986 F.2d 589, 591 (1st Cir. 1993) (5% of patients controlled, and 25% of physicians).

48. U.S. Dept. of Justice & Fed. Trade Commission, Statements of Enforcement Policy and Analytical Principles Relating to Health Care and Antitrust (September 27, 1994); U. S. Dept. of Justice & Fed. Trade Commission, Statements of Antitrust Enforcement Policy in Health Care (August 28, 1996).

49. Blue Cross & Blue Shield United of Wisconsin v. Marshfield Clinic, 65 F.3d 1406 (7th Cir. 1995), cert. denied, U. S. Sup. Ct. No. 95-1118 (Mar. 18, 1996), as reported in "U.S. Supreme Court Declines to Consider Marshfield Clinic Antitrust Case Issues," 5 Health L. Rep. (BNA) No. 12, at 441 (March 21, 1996).

50. 42 U.S.C. §§ 11101–52.

51. 466 U. S. 2 (1984).

52. 820 F.2d 98 (4th Cir. 1987).

53. 712 F.2d 978 (5th Cir. 1983), cert. denied, 466 U. S. 970 (1984).

54. 775 P.2d 863 (Or. Ct. App. 1989), aff'd, 794 P.2d 428 (Or. 1990).

55. 986 F.2d 589 (1st. 1993).

56. 677 F. Supp. 1112 (D.N.M. 1987).

57. 985 F.2d 1210, 1215 (3d Cir. 1993), aff'd, 30 F.3d 494 (3d Cir. 1994).

58. Rev. Rul. 69-545, 1969-2 C.B. 117.

59. Gen. Couns. Mem. 37,789 (Dec. 18, 1978).

60. Gen. Couns. Mem. 39,862 (Nov. 21, 1991).

61. Gen. Couns. Mem. 39,498 (Apr. 24, 1986).

62. Ibid.

63. IRS Ann. 95-25, 1995-14 I.R.B. (Apr. 3, 1995).

64. Gen. Couns. Mem. 39,862 (Nov. 21, 1991).

65. Ibid.

66. P.L. 104-68.

67. Ibid.

68. See Rev. Proc. 93-19, 1993-1 C.B. 526; Rev. Proc. 82-15, 1982-1 C.B. 460.

69. Ibid.

70. See, generally, Douglas A. Hastings et al., *Fundamentals of Health Law* (1995); Phyllis Brasher, "Evolving Managed Care and IDS Regulatory Initiatives under State Insurance, HMO and Related Laws: Can NAIC and State Regulators Keep Pace?" in Twenty-Ninth Annual Meeting of the American Academy of Healthcare Attorneys 113 (1996).

71. 29 U.S.C. § 1001 et seq.

72. 29 U.S.C. § 1144.

73. See Couch on Insurance 3d § 1 (1995).

74. See Memorandum from National Association of Insurance Commissioners, Health Plan Accountability Working Group, to State Insurance Commissioners (August 10, 1995).

75. 440 U. S. 205 (1979), reh. denied, 441 U. S. 917 (1979).

76. 805 F.Supp. 462 (W.D. Tex. 1992), aff'd, 998 F.2d 296 (5th Cir. 1993); see also Insurance Bd. of Bethlehem Steel Corp. v. Muir, 819 F.2d 408 (3d Cir. 1987).

77. 708 F.Supp. 826 (E.D. Mich. 1989).

78. See, generally, Douglas A. Hastings et al., *Fundamentals of Health Law* (1995).

79. As of July 1996, approximately 3.8 million Medicare beneficiaries, or 10% were enrolled in managed care plans. 2 Managed Care Reporter (BNA) No. 34, at 814, (August 21, 1996).

80. See Social Security Act § 1902(a)(10)(A).

81. See Social Security Act § 1902(a)(10)(C).

82. See, e.g., Social Security Act § 1915 (permitting a gatekeeper arrangement).

83. See 42 C.F.R. pt. 42.

84. See Social Security Act § 1862; 42 C.F.R. § 411.

85. See Social Security Act § 1886(d)(5) and 42 C.F.R. § 412.106.

86. *Medicare Carriers' Manual* § 17001(E)(1).

87. *Medicare Carriers' Manual* § 5207.

88. Social Security Act § 1848(a)(1).

89. See 42 C.F.R. § 405.517.

90. *Medicare Carriers' Manual* § 5259.

91. See 42 C.F.R. § 405.1701 et seq.

92. Social Security Act §§ 1861(g) and (p); 1833(g).

93. Social Security Act § 1861(s)(3).

94. See Social Security Act § 1842(n).

95. See *Provider Reimbursement Manual* § 1004.1 et seq.

96. *Provider Reimbursement Manual* § 2108.

97. *Provider Reimbursement Manual* § 2118.

98. *Provider Reimbursement Manual* § 2150.

99. 42 C.F.R. § 405.426.

100. See 42 C.F.R. 412.2; *Medicare Intermediary Manual* § 3610.3.B.

101. See 42 C.F.R. § 413 et seq.; *Provider Reimbursement Manual* § 2300 et seq.

102. *Provider Reimbursement Manual* §§ 2118, 2118.1.

103. See 42 C.F.R. §§ 484.14(f) and (h).

104. See 42 C.F.R. § 418 Subparts D and E.

105. 42 U.S.C.A. § 1320b-5 note (West supp. 1996).

106. Transmittal No. A-96-7, August 1996, as reported in "HCFA Clarifies, Tightens Rules Regarding Provider-Based Entities," in 5 Health L. Rep. (BNA) No. 33, at 1223 (August 15, 1996).

107. 29 U.S.C. §§ 151–69.

108. See 29 U.S.C. § 201 et seq.

109. See 42 U.S.C. § 2000 et seq.

110. 42 U.S.C. § 2000d.

111. Bryan v. Koch, 492 F.Supp. 212 (S.D.N.Y. 1980), aff'd, 627 F.2d 612 (2d Cir. 1980).

112. Marable v. Alabama Mental Health Bd., 297 F.Supp. 291 (M.D. Ala 1969); but see Griggs v. Lexington Police Dept., 672 F.Supp. 36 (D. Mass 1987), aff'd, 867 F.2d 605 (1st Cir. 1988) (patient failed to allege status as intended beneficiary).

113. Mosley v. Clarksville Memorial Hosp., 574 F.Supp. 224 (M.D. Tenn. 1983); Flora v. Moore, 461 F.Supp. 1104 (N.D. Miss. 1978), aff'd, 631 F.2d 730 (5th Cir. 1980), reh'g denied, 636 F.2d 314 (5th Cir. 1981).

114. United States v. Harris Methodist Fort Worth, 970 F.2d 94 (5th Cir. 1992); but see Vuciecevic v. MacNeal Memorial Hosp., 572 F.Supp. 1424 (N.D. Ill. 1983); Vakharia v. Swedish Covenant Hosp., 824 F.Supp. 769 (N.D. Ill. 1993).

115. 29 U.S.C. § 621.

116. Crawford v. West Jersey Health Systems, 847 F.Supp. 1232 (D.N.J. 1994).

117. 42 U.S.C. §§ 12111–13.

118. 29 U.S.C. § 704 et seq.

119. United States v. Baylor Univ. Medical Center, 736 F.2d 1039 (5th Cir. 1984), cert. denied, 469 U. S. 1189 (1985).

120. 29 U.S.C. § 2611 et seq.

121. 29 U.S.C. § 2101 et seq.

122. See, generally, H. Lee Barfield, "Liability of Managed Care Organizations," in American Academy of Healthcare Attorneys Fundamentals of Healthcare Law 9th Annual Institute 319 (1995).

123. Keller v. Missouri Baptist Hosp., 800 S.W.2d 35 (Mo. Ct. App. 1990).

124. See, e.g., Sloan v. The Metropolitan Health Council of Indianapolis, Inc., 516 N.E.2d 1104 (Ind. Ct. App. 1987).

125. See, e.g., Mitts v. H.I.P. of Greater New York, 104 A.D.2d 318 (N.Y. App. Div. 1984); Williams v. Good Health Plus, 743 S.W.2d 373 (Tex. Ct. App. 1987).

126. Schleier v. Kaiser Foundation Health Plan, 876 F.2d 174 (D.C. Cir. 1989).

127. See Uhr v. Lutheran General Hosp., 589 N.E.2d 723 (Ill. App. Ct. 1992).

128. Boyd v. Albert Einstein Medical Center, 547 A.2d 1229 (Pa. Super. 1988); but see Raglin v. HMO Illinois, Inc., 595 N.E.2d 153 (Ill. App. Ct. 1992).

129. See, e.g., Darling v. Charleston Community Memorial Hosp., 211 N.E.2d 253 (Ill. 1965), cert. denied, 383 U. S. 946 (1966); Elam v. College Park Hosp., 132 Cal. App. 3d 332 (1982); Rule v. Lutheran Hospitals & Home Society of America, 835 F.2d 1250 (8th Cir. 1987); Johnson v. Misericordia Community Hosp., 301 N.W.2d 156 (Wis. 1981).

130. Candler General Hosp., Inc. v. Purvis, 181 S.E.2d 77 (Ga. Ct. App. 1971).

131. Wood v. Samaritan Institution, 161 P.2d 556 (Cal. Ct. App. 1945).

132. See, e.g., Sweede v. Cigna HealthPlan of Delaware, Inc., 1989 WL 12608 (Del. Super. 1989); Pulvers v. Kaiser Foundation HealthPlan, 99 Cal. App. 3d 560 (1979). But see Bush v. Dake, No. 86-25767 (Saginaw County, Mich., 1989) (unpublished opinion).

133. Teti v. U. S. Healthcare, 1989WL 143274 (E.D. Pa. 1989), reh'g denied, 904 F.2d 696 (3d Cir. 1990).

134. See "How Close Is Too Close in Hospital Partnerships?" *Modern Healthcare* (Apr. 17, 1995) 2.

135. United States v. Mercy Health Services, No. 94-1023 (N.D. Iowa 1995).

136. See "Little Activity Seen under State Laws Granting Antitrust Immunity," 4 Health L. Rep. (BNA) No. 9, at 303 (Mar. 2, 1995).

137. See, e.g., R. Todd Greenwalt and Ronald G. Tefteller, "Joint Ventures, Conversions, and Other Transactions Involving Tax-Exempt and Proprietary Organizations," in Twenty-Ninth Annual Meeting of the American Academy of Healthcare Attorneys, 585 (1996).

138. Gen. Couns. Mem. 39,005 (Jun. 28, 1983); see also Priv. Ltr. Rul. 95-17-029 (Jan. 27, 1995) (regarding use of the limited liability company form).

139. See, generally, Peter N. Grant, "Forming Integrated Delivery Systems: Legal Issues Related to the Formation and Restructuring of Integrated Medical Groups and New Models in Hospital-Medical Group Affiliation," in 2 American Academy of Hospital Attorneys 26th Annual Meeting, § 10 (1993); Thomas S. Stukes, "Overview of Integrated Delivery Systems and Selected Regulatory Issues in North Carolina," in 1995 Health Law Primer, Dec. 15, 1995 (North Carolina Bar Foundation).

140. Gen. Couns. Mem. 39,862 (Nov. 21, 1991).

141. See, generally, Peter N. Grant, "Forming Integrated Delivery Systems: Legal Issues Related to the Formation and Restructuring of Integrated Medical Groups and New Models in Hospital-Medical Group Affiliation," in 2 American Academy of Hospital Attorneys 26th Annual Meeting, § 10 (1993); Thomas S. Stukes, "Overview of Integrated Delivery Systems and Selected Regulatory Issues in North Carolina," in 1995 Health Law Primer, Dec. 15, 1995 (North Carolina Bar Foundation).

142. See Medicare Compliance Alert, Sept. 27, 1993 (safe harbor may not be needed where a parent-subsidiary relationship is involved, since there is not a referral to be protected).

143. See *IRS Continuing Professional Education Technical Instruction Manual for Exempt Organizations,* 1995 and 1996.

144. See, generally, Thomas S. Stukes, "Overview of Integrated Delivery Systems and Selected Regulatory Issues in North Carolina," in *1995 Health Law Primer,* Dec. 15, 1995 (North Carolina Bar Foundation).

145. See, generally, John J. Miles, "Antitrust Concerns and Operational Issues Arising from Physician Network Formation and Acquisition of Physician Practices," in 1 Twenty-Ninth Annual Meeting of the American Academy of Healthcare Attorneys 398 (1996).

146. Letter from D. McCarty Thornton, Chief Counsel to the Inspector General, "Impact of the Anti-kickback Statute and the Stark Amendment on Vertically Integrated Delivery Systems in the Health Care Industry," January 20, 1995.

147. See letter from D. McCarty Thornton to T.J. Sullivan, reported in Tax L. Rep. (BNA), Feb. 24, 1993; Letter from D. McCarty Thornton, Chief Counsel to the Inspector General, "Impact of the Anti-kickback Statute and the Stark Amendment on Vertically Integrated Delivery Systems in the Health Care Industry," Jan. 20, 1995.

148. See Gen. Couns. Mem. 39,862 (Nov. 22, 1991).

149. See, generally, Peter N. Grant, "Forming Integrated Delivery Systems: Legal Issues Related to the Formation and Restructuring of Integrated Medical Groups and New Models in Hospital-Medical Group Affiliation," in 2 American Academy of Hospital Attorneys 26th Annual Meeting, § 10 (1993).

PART

IV

THE FUTURE OF
INTEGRATED SYSTEMS

7

THE NEW FRONTIER

The continuing process of physician, hospital, and community integration should be sought not as the end result, but as the beginning of the latest, most effective means to finance and deliver healthcare services. This final chapter is a postscript on integrated systems thinking, a culmination of what systems should consider, the why and how of it. Many pressures drive changes in local geographic subsystems of healthcare delivery: economic, political, clinical, social, and cultural. Integrated community healthcare results from the successful partnering and appreciation of system assets and community needs to achieve its designed goals. The previous chapters discussed the background and many of the specific issues in developing provider networks and integrated systems. This final section highlights special interests to more fully frame concerns of increasing importance to the successful economic and clinical delivery of healthcare.

EMPHASIS AND DEDICATION TO PRIMARY HEALTHCARE AND DEVELOPING PHYSICIAN LEADERSHIP

Integrated provider networks must dedicate themselves to supporting care given at the appropriate level of the continuum of care. For obvious reasons, care delivered in the primary care setting is less expensive than healthcare of a highly technical, advanced, and invasive nature. Primary care physicians are attaining the pinnacle of career desirability: they are valued at a premium, an indispensable commodity for delivery systems. These physicians make the judgment on the ongoing referral of services at greater and greater intensities, delivering care at the least expensive level before progressing as medically indicated. Recall Stephen Shortell's organized delivery systems approach: a total rededication to outpatient primary care is the cornerstone of the system of the future.[1] This type of commitment does not come easily, as Shortell points out; making the commitment to primary care has been a difficult one for many developing IDS organizations, and a dangerous career decision for healthcare executives.

Physician leadership and participation is vital. Without substantial (50%) physician direction, providers won't buy into the massive changes required to complete the development of an effective IDS. The direction that an organization takes is a function of leadership and values more than of elegant protocols.[2] One example is the development of a physician-hospital organization in the mid-Atlantic region of the U. S. with a 20% managed care penetration: despite a 50–50 ownership by a physician group and hospital, 50% physician board membership, an active physician advisory committee, and additional strong physician involvement, specialist participation and acceptance has grown very slowly. At this level of managed care penetration, physicians are concerned but not ready to commit to new, untested ventures and risk assumption, despite reasonable assurances that their market dependence (in the given market) on managed care will not change overnight. Maintaining physician involvement and leadership is a sign not only of giving voice to a large, key constituency, but of recognizing the need for clinical perspectives at both the organization and operation levels. Competent clinical leadership is what assures the checks and

Recognizing Partner Contributions

Hospitals' Contributions	Physicians' Contributions
Existing Market Presence	Patients
Capital for Network Development	Care Management Expertise
Inpatient Hospital Network	Existing Market Presence
Ancillary Services	Organized Network of Physicians
Outpatient Clinics	Extenders and Outpatient Services
Emergency Services	Primary Care Gatekeepers
Hi-Tech Tertiary Care Programs	Physician Leadership
Management Information Systems	Direct Patient Care Expertise
Nursing Support Staff	QA Practice Protocols
Preventive/Community Education	Utilization Management
In-Home Services	Education/Research
UR/QA Services	Specialist Contracting

Integrated Delivery System

Coordinates Entire Continuum of Care	Provides Capital for Development
Eliminates Redundant Systems	Manages Comprehensive Medical Record
Eliminates Fragmentation	Provides Single Management Structure

balances that lead to proper cost-effective care delivery. Without a complete com-mitment to involving physicians in leadership and operational activities, it is difficult at best, and perhaps impossible to create sus-tainable delivery systems (see Exhibit 7–1).

CONTINUED SUPPORT OF SPECIALTY HEALTH SERVICES

We will lose much if we do not continue to support the development of technology (hardware, software, systems approaches, and technological thinking) as well as placing the important role specialists play in high esteem. If we accept that the U. S. healthcare system is (the most) technologically advanced and technologically focused in the world, the strides made in medicine and related scientific fields are the product of that environment. Our system has much room for improvement, and our public policy definitions have much to grow before we can make the advances in primary care, maternal, fetal and child health that characterize other nations' developed healthcare systems. One may well argue that a measure of the health status of a community is based more on the preventive and primary healthcare available than the highest level of technology available to a select few individuals. Irrespective of the public policy, the further development of healthcare systems must support a baseline scope of service at least to the level that U. S. consumers have become accustomed. Clinical pathway or protocol development may lead to significant reductions in unnecessary testing (fewer MRIs, chest films, full spectrum lab panels) but only after these approaches are proven clinically and scientifically.

The continued support of specialty health services recognizes the vast knowledge base that exists among clinicians. Tapping into this knowledge base, keeping the physicians as active partners in the system development and reform, is an important component in effective partnership and maintaining collegial growth among system stakeholders.[3] These issues touch both the dumbing down of medicine and the maintenance of quality through volume of activity. Systems in this country cannot and should not become a mirror image of the systems in England or Canada. Not only would the public not support this change (by employers and payors not contracting), but it would ultimately affect the development of the field of knowledge of medicine adversely. We have a social and ethical responsibility to maintain the growing body of knowledge in the field. We cannot fulfill this mission without sufficient commitment of resources and adequate volumes of patients to support either our physical plants or our clinical expertise.

DEVELOPING INTEGRATED PHYSICIAN RELATIONSHIPS

Whether it is a developing, midstage, or nearly mature IDS, creating pluralistic physician relationships (a.k.a. physician integration) will remain arguably an important area for most systems. The strategies differ vastly by stage of the system, managed care penetration, market readiness, and other factors, but the relationships must continue to be developed, nurtured, formalized, and solidified. Much of this text has discussed the need to partner with physicians and other community care providers in order to create a healthcare system with sufficient infrastructure to manage the clinical and administrative components demanded in the delivery systems of today. Developing integrated physician relationships means not only bringing together the clinicians to render care, but means true partnership, win-win relationships, and equal and proportional risk sharing for common and individual benefit. Few communities will develop successful, sustaining delivery systems without true partnering behavior. It is true that some markets are created by strong-arming the physicians into some structure but these strategies are not likely enduring. Primary care physicians can relocate so many places that they may be bound only by contracts. Specialists may have to make tough personal decisions about their practice locations in order to find the right mix of professional and personal contentment.

HEALTH PLANS MUST SERVE THE PHYSICIAN

In an integrated environment all system components share the success or failure of the system. Health plans (the insurance/risk component) must serve to facilitate the provision of care by the physician. HMOs, in concept, are not in the business of restricting or blocking access to care or of earning profits. They are in the business of establishing a continuity of care. Health plan surveys, internally and externally conducted, serve as one measure of satisfaction with the plan, both from the clinical and patient care perspectives. Part of the dilemma surfaces: is the investor-owned community going to remain satisfied with the return on healthcare stocks, and is this really appropriate? Does this create a perverse incentive? Although the issue is not the tax structure of the entity, it is the underlying nature of the entity and how they use their profits to enhance and enlarge the ability to produce high-quality, cost-effective healthcare. There is nothing wrong with profit as a byproduct of service delivery, providing that the focus remains on care. The concern is that as the level of arbitrage in the system is reduced by greater and greater competition and lower per-member, per-month fees, at what level does reimbursement fall below that which is acceptable to provide care? In California, some plans are in the low $90s pmpm rate; some might question whether we have arrived at that level. With medical loss ratios as low as 69% in some systems (most are between 75% and 85%), premium and capitation amounts continue to drop due to premium impaction, competition, the merger of major HMOs, risk spreading, and aggressive direct contracting. The battle is for a finite amount of money as the system arbitrage increases. Some regional or national systems are willing to sustain certain markets as losses to maintain presence and market power. At some point, does the return on investment become so low that investors will seek other opportunities and leave the healthcare system in shambles? Does this mean that the for-profit HMO is a short-term phenomenon? Perhaps for systems whose main purpose is investor return.

Coordination of healthcare—organized medicine—has been the most obvious benefit of managed care. The byproduct of this has been physician organization and integration, which has created the opportunity to direct the outcomes of care processes, and to identify what is appropriate care under any given set of circumstances and what yields the best results. This approach is new because of the influence of, or the driving of managed care, as a positive outcome. Managed care should enhance the relationship between the patient or enrollee and his or her family physician, and through that partnership, the result should be the best health outcome for the individual. While patients under the old fee-for-service system may have been satisfied with the relationship they had with their physician, the realities of the marketplace are changing the conditions by which virtually all patients interact with their care providers.

It has been said that managed care provides physicians with feedback on the quality of care they provide so they can recognize what they do well and identify opportunities for improvement. Under an enrolled population, the access to meaningful data is considerable; how these data are used is the issue. Physicians must be given not only the data but the tools they need to analyze and derive accurate responses that will positively affect their ability to provide care in a managed or coordinated fashion. Data should not be used as a hammer or negative incentive to order physician behavior. Information is the goal; it should be used as an obligation owned by the health plan to improve care delivery and financing with the goals of profit and reduction in cost. Plans and physicians must learn together what works within the construct of medicine and economics and each must respect the other. Managed care education must be provided to physicians to help them identify the impact of their clinical decisions, why and how care is financed, and how small changes in practice patterns can make significant changes in operations. Physicians need to understand the impact of their decisions in order for them to guide the clinical redesign. Through core groups of clinicians, the concept is then spread to other physicians and throughout the system. As with the data, the tools to effect this redesign and education are the responsibility of the health plan or integrated system.

Hospital-based physicians present another level of challenge. The PEAR physicians (pathology, emergency medicine, anesthesiology, radiology, and radiation therapy) have lived in a utilization- and request-driven world. Many of the activities of these physicians are directed by, or are the result of care processes ordered by referring or admitting physicians. Their practices are vastly different from other practicing physicians and their orientation to practice or care costs has likewise been foreign in respect to managed care. Bringing these PEAR physicians into the managed care arena, the cost-consciousness fold, is challenging for a number of reasons: (1) these physicians often do not worry about technology or supply overhead; (2) they are primarily concerned with income from professional services only (they derive little or no ancillary income); (3) they have not been forced to bargain with payors to the same extent that non-hospital-based physicians do; and (4) they have little incentive to make any changes in the way they practice. Looking at each of these PEAR physician groups, health plans can begin to identify means to contract with them and create positive incentives for the plan, or system, while bringing them into the cost-consciousness fold and finally, incentivizing them toward cost-effective care.

The degree to which these physicians could share in risk, both in upside risk (surplus allocation) and downside risk (deficit coverage) may be limited to their opportunity to effect meaningful change in the system. For example, among the hospital-based physicians, anesthesiology and pathology may be considered to have low discretionary utilization because of their nature to respond to the needs of other physicians and the limited choices they can make in providing many of their services. Radiology and radiation therapy may be considered to have a medium discretionary utilization, recognizing that even while radiation therapy has small system costs overall, the potential for real cost savings at the patient level is realizable. Emergency medicine physicians have high discretionary utilization and may well be appropriate for inclusion in risk-sharing payment models. Looking at discretionary utilization in other subspecialties, infectious disease and geriatrics are low, developmental pediatrics is medium, neonatology is medium to high, and oncology and physiatry are high. Plans should delve into researching local treatment and market issues in structuring effective incentive plans for these physicians.

Plans should not have as a goal, a contract relationship with physicians. Physicians must be involved with the health plan that allows them the autonomy to practice clinical medicine while respecting the economic impact of their clinical decisions, within the scope of appropriate care of the patient. As we know, care is delivered between one patient and one doctor at a time. Plans must recognize that they serve in a supportive role to the delivery of care to the patient. If a relationship is built in which physicians are actively involved in the design of the system of delivery and the way in which utilization management is conducted and implemented, and if they reap some of the reward, you have a true partnership. The danger is that the provider-sponsored organization begins to see how it can function without the expertise of the health plan. The approach should be more like a modified direct contracting model, a number of functional elements that health plans bring must be included or replicated to be effective. If the goal was simply price discounting, then providers would make up the differences in volume without appropriate concern to quality. Health plan investors or partners should therefore take out only the amount of money relative to what it brings, or puts in for the skills and risks involved.

Lastly, some general thought on pursuing health plan partnerships for emerging integrated environments. The following represents some points for guiding the thought process in partnering with free-standing health plans. Note that for any given criterion, the issue may be of greater or lesser importance as plans, relationships, and markets evolve.

Product Type of Plan.   The type of product a particular plan brings to the network may be more or less valuable than other types depending on the nature and existence of established plans in the marketplace. For example, HMO plans, gatekeeper, and point of service (POS) models may well be more attractive than PPO-POS or straight PPO plans. The network should establish relative guidelines on what they intend to establish, in what time frame, and by what means in order to assess which plans they should seek contracts with and which they should avoid, or delay until the major players are already contracted.

Provider Relationship. The type of provider relationship, be it with a plan that is fully insured or self-insured may play a role in deciding which to pursue first. Typically, fully insured plans offer greater short-term financial stability, market depth (current and potential/projected), and staying power. In some markets, most notably Florida, Medicare plans are of considerable importance. In other markets, the potential for Medicare and Medicaid relationships will not only become important, but may serve as a significant source of revenue as these plans develop and refine their private contracting arrangements. As one example, the North Carolina Medicaid population was approximately 1.2 million lives in October 1996, with direct healthcare expenditures of $3.5 billion. Add another 7% for administrative costs and you can see why these populations can become very valuable to the network that can efficiently manage this population.

Network Relationship. Contracting with a given plan that offers many different products in your market area is generally more desirable than plans that offer fewer choices. Although each market offers its own unique set of contracting opportunities (number of employers, existence and penetration of competing plans, proximity and volume of large numbers of workers covered by one plan, e.g., state or federal employee groups), the specific types of products offered, the existing enrollment, and the competitive nature of these products may make contracting or partnering with a plan not only attractive, but in some cases imperative.

Risk Sharing Potential. What are the opportunities and conditions for risk sharing on behalf of the contracting network in working with health plans? The ability to manage risk is the goal of most provider networks, unless the market has been so defined as to make the opportunity a last-ditch effort for the physician network to remain in existence (a niche player, a bottom-dweller who is the low-cost leader). Networks should evaluate the need and time frame to accept risk for their system, whether it is limited to a physician professional component (primary care and specialty care) or includes hospital services. The scenarios vary considerably from global capitation to specific capitation to percent of premium, and other methods; the iterations are almost limitless. Caution should be extended to gaining competent legal and actuarial guidance in evaluating risk assumption, particularly related to contracting issues and variations for negotiating acceptable terms that are favorable to, and reward the efforts of the physician/hospital network.

Plan Growth and Market Leadership Potential.   Related to the network relationship above, pursuing a plan relationship with major players may be an imperative in some cases, but the majority of cases involve choosing which plan(s) to pursue first, and why they should be considered. For obvious reasons, large plans with significant penetration in the market area should be evaluated initially. Plans with known expansion plans or new products should also be considered, perhaps as a second-tier effort. The goal for maturing networks will be to increase the number of covered lives within its defined area of interest, whether that is through relationships with only the major plans, modified or individual direct contracting, or through a shotgun approach, contracting with many different payor sources.

Exclusivity.   A network's ability to negotiate exclusive provider status is often a difficult task, frequently agreed to only for defined periods of time by plans. The specific type of exclusivity depends on the contracting nature between the plan and the provider network. Being the only provider network involved in risk contracting may well be of greater value than being able to negotiate a complete exclusive provider arrangement. Considering the fact that many nationally operating health plans are beginning to contract with the MedPartners and PhyCors of the world, the likelihood of excluding a competing physician group in your community may be impossible. Depending on the size, however, negotiating the only at-risk contract in your area may be possible. And the reality is, that is where you want to be anyway. Plan relationships that are something less than exclusive may be of importance to developing provider networks. The concept of a positive, mutually beneficial relationship implies that the parties respect each other and that the goals of each, at least the internal, incremental goals, continue to be serviced to the satisfaction of each party. Defining what one's relationship ought to be is as much an issue internal to each potential partner as it is to the partners envisioning what it might be together.

CREATING A SHARED SENSE OF PURPOSE
WITHIN THE SYSTEM

Aligning incentives within the IDS infrastructure is much easier in a single economic entity (e.g., a mature system) than in a developing or midstage IDS. As capitation has its own way of aligning physician incentives, albeit with some real problems in the absence of quality indicators, a shared sense of purpose must be developed by all components of the IDS to effect substantive, sustaining change. Physicians must begin to understand one another and share responsibility and risk proportionate to their individual, group, and system goals within the scope of good clinical medicine. In the academic environment, many autonomous faculty believe they have no immediate superior; they function and make decisions on their own and without responsibility to any person, department, or institution. They are simply treating patients. Helping the cardiovascular surgeon understand that they are truly economic partners with the cardiologist, internist, and family physician often takes more than sharing the same incentive risk pools. The location of care (turf) is secondary to the delivery of appropriate care, at the appropriate time, in the appropriate setting. Unless physicians are given the opportunity and resources to look past their own wallets, incentives are not aligned among them.

Bringing together the elements of the system, hospital services, physician services, health plan or risk-bearing capacity, and all other supplemental (carved out) services requires each entity to be incentivized so that the whole succeeds. How is that effected? On the macro level, focusing on the inflow of premium dollars identifies the first part of the equation. Administrative details such as payment periods, claims periods, and interest payments are negotiated to full advantage. System elements, as discussed under health plans above, must create incentives for distinct populations of physicians based on their ability to control costs and make substantive changes in the system, but these physicians must also believe that the total system orientation is one of cooperation and support of common goals. For obvious reasons, the incentive mechanisms for a primary care physician are likely to be very different from those of a cardiologist or pathologist. The issue is to examine what the environment is dictating and what can reasonably be accomplished in your given system. As an example, in any given system the contracting mechanisms may vary from discounted fee for service to capitation to patient premium or a percent of premium for specified services. The approach to creating a shared sense of purpose addresses the impact of each constituent group on their ability to effect meaningful change. In most health plans, the majority of expense falls into the hospital services pool, followed by the specialist physician pool, followed by the primary care pool and carveouts. Allowing the hospital to manage its expenses based on certain elements of cost and utilization (over which it has no control) is one beginning. Specialists can accept risk through capitation, although only when developed quality standards are in place to prevent the natural ill consequences of delivering care under capitation. Recognizing that most physicians will do the right thing for the patient regardless of the mechanism for payment, IDS organizations, physician networks, and health plans should make the development of a quality standard a top priority in order to assist the fringe physicians and ensure continuous improvement in the whole system. Unfortunately for many developing systems, it may be several years before enough covered lives are in the system to effectively capitate the specialist component. Specialists can also accept risk through other mechanisms such as payment drafts against risk pools. Obviously, the more narrow the risk pools the more comfortable the physicians will feel that they are able to manage care, because they are more likely to see the result of their efforts. Grouping small numbers of physicians of similar specialties together, provided with appropriate data, is one means of assisting these self-managed teams to higher levels of managed care operations. Primary care physicians lend themselves well to either of the techniques outlined for specialists, although because the volume of lives needed for a primary care physician is considerably less than for specialists, capitation works well, again, only after appropriate quality standards are in place.

Administrative functions must also be aligned to a common purpose within the system. Senior management must feel empowered to make decisions by a supportive board and understand that the environment is flat, fluid, and fast. Physicians are only going to go along with making major cultural changes on their behalf it they perceive the same type of pressure is on administration. Administration must bend over backwards and recognize that physicians are in the driver's seat. Successful integration will only occur when hospital and system leadership recognizes this imperative. As healthcare delivery moves toward assumption of the health status of a community (a defined geographical area such as a county), the shared sense of purpose is facilitated by total system economic alignment and systems of rewards shared by all.

PHYSICIAN COMPENSATION

Physician compensation for employed physicians must be driven by a number of factors including the specialty of physician, predominant payment mechanisms for the practice, payor mix, and group/system status. Physician payment mechanisms should include components of a base salary (or salary draw on an established amount) and an incentive, which can be variable based on specific, objective targets established for the physician, group, and system. A difficult issue to overcome is the concept of equal compensation for unequal physicians. Two internists may have similar practices and years of experience, but drastically different work habits reflecting unequal workload. Manuel Valasquez, professor of management at Santa Clara University and business ethicist, notes: "The fundamental principle of distributive justice is that equals should be treated equally and unequals, unequally."[4]

Although no one algorithm can be said to work in all circumstances, the following guidelines should be considered:

Essential and Value-Added Physician Functions

Essential Physician Functions
- Maintain office hours for 4½ days per week.
- Provide call coverage for practice/hospital with other medical staff members.

- Conduct patient rounds as time beyond office hours.
- Complete medical records within time frame established by employer.
- Attainment of budgeted number of patient encounters and/or revenue targets as established in operating budget/*pro forma* for the practice.
- Provide service outside office setting, through community health provider entities that the hospital and physicians deem as a significant contribution to the community.
- Achieve positive scores (number is negotiable) on patient and employee satisfaction surveys.

Value-Added Physician Functions

- Serve as Medical Director (e.g., Rural Health, Community Outreach Clinic).
- Serve as Medical Student/Residency Preceptor.
- Provide contract services to Department of Public Health.
- Provide contract services to read EKGs, Holter monitors, Stress tests, etc.
- Attain outstanding scores on patient and employee satisfaction surveys.
- Proactively manage utilization of healthcare services and operating expenses of inpatient and outpatient services.
- Enhance administrative-clinical interface in providing higher-quality, cost-effective care.

Compensation Formula Review.   The compensation formula should be based on specific physician production targets in the form of revenue for physician professional services. Historical practice performance can be the baseline for establishing revenue targets that may be monitored against national comparative physician production data, e.g., Medical Group Management Association physician productivity or RVU models. Input can be derived from practice physicians and management to assess realistic levels of revenue from which to base the compensation plan. Monthly reports keep physicians and management appraised of performance.

The practice physicians and management participate in performance reviews biannually in conjunction with payment of "Incentive Pool Dollars." The formula should be reviewed annually by the hospital and practice governing board.

Two-Tiered Incentive. The incentive should be based upon an assessment of progress in achieving annual performance (based on the annual operating budget/*pro forma*) and by measuring progress toward value-added physician functions and 3- to 5-year strategic objectives.

Incentive Pool. The incentive pool should be based on attainment of revenue targets and variable indicators of performance.

Incentive Pool Dollars. As the incentive plan is based initially on the attainment of revenue targets, the first part of the incentive pool can be dollars that are paid to physicians based on performance at the prescribed intervals each year for attaining identified revenue targets. These amounts are carried in the operating budget/*pro forma* as line item expenses with the assumption that they will be attained. The second part of the incentive pool, paid after the close of the fiscal year, are those dollars remaining after meeting practice operating expenses (as defined by the budget or actual incurred expenses) and net of payback of the annual contribution for any purchase price for the practice or other negotiated overhead expenses. Any dollars remaining will constitute the second-tier incentive pool dollars for distribution to the hospital and physicians. These dollars will consist of a maximum amount to the physician of X% of their base salary draw and be paid according to specified goals in practice performance, quality of care indicators, patient and staff satisfaction, resource utilization, and medical records maintenance.

Division of Incentive Pool. Division of incentive pool dollars among physicians can be based on each physician's net contribution to margin consisting of gross revenue minus physician resource consumption (resource consumption items defined in individual income statements showing total revenue, compensation, benefits, allocation of office overhead, etc.). Gross revenue is defined as the net total of revenue received from all activities per physician as of the close of the fiscal year.

Incentive Funds Distribution. Incentive funds are typically distributed approximately 45 days after the close of the mid- and end-of-fiscal-year periods. Each physician has a period to review individual and group financial reports, request clarifications, and approve the reports. If a physician cannot accept the baseline reports before the close of the review period, payment will automatically defer, with no financial penalty to the practice, until agreement is reached. Those physicians voluntarily leaving the practice will have their subsequent incentive calculated based upon the standard formula but with revenue defined as *in-hand* as of the date of termination plus an estimate of collected accounts receivable as of the normal cutoff dates, whichever date occurs first.

Treat capitated income differently from noncapitated income and pay it out differently. For example, one may treat the distribution of the capitated income stream by a share formula or by a performance-based formula.

Share-Based Distribution. Income may be divided based on equal shares or pro rata shares in the event of a significantly disparate number of assigned patients or workload distribution.

Performance-Based Distribution. Income may be distributed by absolute or relative performance of each physician. For example, the ratio of actual to expected member costs, or the total $ member costs of care rendered compared to the expected cost of care (by age and sex). Other means might profile actual costs compared to some benchmarked amount or comparing actual costs (or encounters) with an established treatment corridor based on encounters. As an example of the corridor model, a range of expected treatments (encounters, referrals, etc.) can be established based on utilization assumptions for a given patient population and specialty of practice, e.g., a general surgery estimate may be 17 to 23 procedures per 1,000 population. The amounts distributed to the physician may be a function of actual to expected encounters derived from this range. Indeed this model, and derivations, have been used by Kaiser Health

Plans and others to establish capitated payment amounts and reconciliation formulas.

THE PERILS FACING ACADEMIC MEDICAL CENTERS AND THE EDUCATION OF HEALTH PROFESSIONALS

Academic centers must be supported in order to prevent a total collapse of the healthcare system as we know it. Economic incentives presently existing in managed care will not support the academic center environment, and without subsidy the face of healthcare must change. Academic centers are scrambling to develop financially integrated clinical entities in attempts to survive the changing landscape of managed care and reimbursement. Their responsibility for a triple mission of patient care, research, and education divides their resources such that greater and greater amounts of their operating funds are derived from clinical care, but may not necessarily be returned as investment: they are often returned as specialist income without the opportunity for capital growth. Support may come in the form of government intervention of some means to support these pillars or face a continual dumbing down of medicine.

Academic centers have not been terribly successful in negotiating better managed care contracts due to their comprehensive nature or the image of quality at the teaching institution. In contracting, the issue of cost still leads the pack in deciding which institutional provider wins the contract. In network participation, having an academic center may be desirable but only because the package includes the tertiary and quaternary care. Plans can pay a small premium for the highest level of care because it makes little impact on the health plan in total, depending on the population enrolled. When the dollar value impact differs significantly, the history to date has been to exclude the academic environment in favor of a significantly lower cost. According to Richard Janeway, MD, academic centers have been competing successfully, particularly in areas of high managed care penetration, on the basis of value added as long as the price differential is not greater than 3% to 5%.[5] Whether this strategy is sustainable is uncertain.

Teaching hospitals and their medical faculties must begin to address areas of business in the care of patients, with the core of acknowledging that support of the academic mission of education and research are of considerable importance. Janeway indicates that the key to bringing the mission elements together is that it is incumbent on the education and research functions of the medical school that they apply productivity and efficiency measures to the educational and research environment to prove themselves worthy of support. Sustaining these efforts may come about through several means including the development of, as Janeway calls it, a single clinical enterprise, or through the merger of major institutions, for instance, merging Mt. Sinai and New York University Medical Center, Columbia-Presbyterian Hospital and Cornell Medical Center with the possibility of bringing in Memorial Sloan Kettering.

Academic centers cannot remain in the tertiary and quaternary business only. Replicating primary care may be beyond the means of most academic centers who have significant investment in higher-level, inpatient resources and specialists. The answer generally is in the alignment with primary care and feeder networks to provide the base for continued operations; an IDS that has value for each participant member and which creates the effective continuum of care. Academic centers often lead the initiative and cause the alignment of all the other service providers, but they should not really appear to be the hub of the system. The hub is the understanding that the total physician driven care delivery process is supported by the economic asset infrastructure to make it work. Purchasing or developing networks of employed physicians may serve the feeder role for specialists and hospital services, but only as an incremental source; the bulk of income still feeds the physicians, both primary care and specialists.

Academic centers must embrace the challenge that the previous systems approaches were hospital-hospital driven, which was not destined for success. The formula for success relies on physician leadership and participation, for instance, organized physician approaches. The physician organization, with attached hospitals, is likely to be among the most successful arrangements. Hospitals typically become the capital partner of the system, only because physicians were not organized to create capital resources to mount such a venture. In some states, corporate practice of medicine laws prevent hospitals effectively from becoming the center of such a system.

The federal government holds some responsibility and cannot be let off the hook, for preserving and maintaining the important functions of medical education and research at academic medical centers, which are largely responsible for making American medicine the standard of the world. Quoting Dr. Janeway, "If there is not some recognition of the special nature of the academic medical center, the intellectual backbone of modern American medicine will get a very bad case of osteoporosis."[6] If the academic medical center is forced to compete in the clinical arena solely on economic terms, a dumbing down of medicine will occur, with the longer-term result of national importance. The Association of American Medical Colleges, the Association of Academic Health Centers, and the American Medical Association are working diligently to spread this message. The reality is that the public has no awareness of the academic medical center or of its importance to the healthcare infrastructure of the United States. Given the many of issues facing the U.S. Congress related to healthcare, the message of the academic environment sometimes falls quiet.

CLINICAL AND MANAGEMENT INFORMATION SYSTEMS AND PROCESSES: MANAGING QUALITY OF CARE WITHIN CLINICAL VARIATION

Information systems are the heart of administrative operations for developing IDS organizations. As mentioned above, health plans must provide the tools, data, and support for integrated provider networks to achieve optimum functioning in the clinical, administrative, and financial realms. Investment in this technology is not an issue to be taken lightly. Many regional and national systems are making investments in the range of $10M to $50M or more to effect immediate information transfer in satellite locations and along a continuum of care. Electronic paperless clinical records are beginning to become more commonplace with numerous products on the market. Integrating the clinical record with the administrative record across locations, and adding the ability to extract information and automate claims processing completes the picture. Regional communications systems allow real-time access to patient records, in an appropriate manner, to identify episodes of care in the patient's home via home care providers, in the physician office, the hospital or clinic, the pharmacy, or the nursing home. Regional communications eliminate or significantly reduce redundant tests and, in some cases, patient procedures, as patients move from one setting to another. Integrating clinical, administrative, and financial information brings all elements of the system closer together while sharing expenses in system development. Telemedicine links play a strong role in the transfer of information as well.

Medical management systems must be physician driven. Medical management systems must also satisfy the demands of managed care organizations while maintaining high-quality care. These systems are primarily people-oriented groups and frequently include an information systems component. These committees, therefore, seek to maximize the proliferation of high-quality care across their plan or system. A PHO or IPA, for example, may have a quality committee (or utilization management system) comprised of physicians with support by case managers and hospital quality assessment staff. The physicians give clinical direction while staff ensure that committee guidelines are disseminated. The goal must be to create a stream of communication that does not question clinical judgment or create an administrative burden on practicing physicians, thereby reducing their time delivering patient care. In fact, much of a physician's pattern of practice may well be a developed behavior external to the optimum level of clinical decision making. How else can an advanced organization such as Med-Partners/Mullikin achieve 150 inpatient days or less per thousand commercial patient population when the national average for HMOs is about 350? Including staff from the hospital business office and systemwide information systems may also be desirable. Attaining the optimum utilization targets is neither an easy task, nor does it occur overnight. One method to move the process in the right direction is to establish interim utilization goals, perhaps one-half of the way from where current utilization exists and the identified optimum. Essentially, payment accounts for each specialist are based on treatment or encounter volume against which actual billed charges are profiled. Withhold and gainsharing incentives can then be paid based on the ratio of actual to target utilization, remembering that year one is an interim year. Individualizing withhold return and incentive requires more sophisticated data management but is likely to foster a better and fairer working relationship with partnering physicians. Medical management systems or committees also implement health risk assessments to patients to begin to identify areas where preventive intervention may reap rewards in patient care management.

These systems begin to establish data on the local treatment patterns of their participating physicians, often assisted from outside sources such as Iameter or Milliman and Robertson, from which clinical guidelines and treatment protocols may be developed. Again, effective patient management under capitation requires that quality indicators exist. Development of clinical guidelines may be the easier part of the task; implementing guidelines across physicians is likely to be the more difficult issue, especially dealing with the potential for malpractice suits. The focus for most systems beginning to develop guidelines are with common illnesses and procedures of high system volume; high cost, high impact areas are the rule. Some examples include urinary tract infection, hypertension diagnosis, breast cancer detection, and low back pain. Teams on the quality committee can begin to assemble interested clinicians by subspecialty, beginning with primary care (OB/GYN, Pediatrics, and Adult Medicine) and motivated specialty care physicians.

Outcomes measurement along a journey of Continuous Quality Improvement (CQI) should be one of the primary goals of any medical management/quality assessment program. It is one thing for a system to understand its deficiencies and opportunities for improvement but it is another to be able to objectively quantify one's accomplishments and indicate plans of action for continuous improvement. Benchmarking the best practices of other integrated systems is also an excellent method to expand the knowledge base and identify local issues relevant to these benchmarked practices. Nationally a number of comparative data sets exist including the Health Plan Employer Data and Information Set (HEDIS) created by the National Committee for Quality Assurance (NCQA). One word of caution: HEDIS and NCQA data report cards include a variety of administrative and systems measurements that may or may not be beneficial (i.e., meaningful) based on the stage of system development and the goals identified by your physician leaders for your community. Arguably, the development and adherence to administrative and procedural standards is laudable; however, clear clinical and administrative conditions should be set based on local market and medical staff concerns. Outcomes measurements derived from processes that are objective are among the most powerful data for integrated systems. These data allow management and implementation teams to focus efforts in narrow ranges identified by the monitors in order to continually improve in care delivery. Clean outcomes data can be very powerful in managed care and direct contracting as well. As the key to successful risk bearing is accurate estimation of cost and utilization, outcomes data allow plans to narrowly define their risk profile and compete successfully for contracts.

Care management systems begin to make inroads when creative clinical and administrative minds seek patient-centered alternatives to traditional care processes. Gone are the days of double-digit hospital stays, even after traumatic events. In are the intensive, highly-skilled, follow-up procedures provided under the direction of surgeons and medical physicians through specialized, though lower-cost delivery centers. Consider the trauma victim who is now stabilized through inpatient care and discharged to a rehabilitation setting with home care follow-up. The cost savings begin to add up (in healthcare, saving $30,000 here and $50,000 there begins to look like real money). Adding physician assistants and nurse practitioners to certain points of entry and follow-up are also making significant inroads in most areas of the country. Adding a nurse triage or call system has become one of the most beneficial additions to care networks through the establishment of toll-free phone numbers, specific triage protocols, and high-touch patient contact.

Information exchange between the system, plan, or other entity becomes crucial to allow physicians to understand how their actions affect the system. By understanding your medical staff and the local market, you can determine the lowest-cost setting and procedures to deliver quality healthcare services. These activities bring exceptional value to integrated systems at considerably less cost than any historical alternative. This is the type of thinking that systems must embrace in order to survive in the next generation.

BUILDING RELATIONSHIPS IN THE FACE OF CHANGE

The mistake many organizations are making, not only in healthcare but across all industries, is expecting change, i.e., the future, to remain linear. One of the most referenced phrases regarding the healthcare industry describes it as going through a paradigm shift. From traditional business and economic principles, we refer to this as *second order change*. It is a clear time of chaos when the immediate future is the only reality we can cling to; anything beyond the immediate year is unknown. From the global perspective, change is not occurring in a linear manner; it is growing exponentially. Partnerships appear among competitors to create unions of great strength nationally and in some cases, globally. Forty percent of the 1980 Fortune 500 have disappeared through acquisition, breakup, or bankruptcy.[7] The rate of change creates levels of uncertainty that drive reactions from staid organizations never before considered. Industry examples of sustaining revenue declines of 30% or more within a 6-month period send heretofore stable entities to the auction block. Organizations limited by traditional thinking will be lost to those who dream and do. Nothing stops an organization faster than people who believe that the way they worked yesterday is the best way to work tomorrow.[8]

Nicholas Imparato and Oren Harari describe the environment: "The combination of turbulence we are experiencing today—in values, in commerce, economic order, technology, politics, and social structures—requires business to rethink its core assumptions—its missions and procedures."[9] Imparato and Harari also share an excellent example of how the business world changes demands on its workers (imagine managed care demands on physicians):

> It is as if they were hired to play baseball in the major leagues, and with supreme effort, they all developed into fantastic players with batting averages around .300. One day the manager shows up dribbling a basketball, announcing that the era of baseball is ending. To the players, his behavior may appear shocking and unfair. But if the manager reflects the real world, is it reasonable to assume that the players will succeed in the new era by putting in additional hours honing their batting and fielding skills, or by denying the realities of basketball hoops and man-to-man defense, or by hoping that the speed on the base paths and a strong throwing arm will help them camouflage their deficiencies until retirement?[10]

Looking to other industries, over the next decade, a considerable amount of new revenue in healthcare may well come from services that do not presently exist. Does one need to ponder at length why HBO & Company is moving into the information services market, in healthcare, and in home care? How soon will they joint venture with the Baxters and Searles? With concomitant developments in telemedicine, just how soon will cable-based interactive home care be available, reimbursable, and become an acceptable standard of care, for physician extenders? The healthcare delivery system is changing as rapidly as technology and imagination allow. The rage of Baby on Board placards of the 1980s will become HBO's established ancillary services line in the year 2000 with health education channels and in-home patient/provider video consultations.

Provider networks will begin to grow into dominant forces once the major regional physician management companies and savvy local networks bring the physician delivery component to a refined science. As most businesspeople recognize, overcoming resistance to change is where we get productivity leaps in the hearts and minds of people.[11] How organizations begin to understand the role and responsibilities of their personnel in the face of the new business environment will make all the difference in the world when it comes to them living the reality of the marketplace.[12] Imparato, Harari, and others report that middle management in many organizations has only partial or no understanding of corporate objectives, and that the situation worsens lower down the corporate ladder.[13,14] Imagine the housekeeping staff recognizing that their job directly and materially affects the ability to gain contracts or satisfy patient perceptions about treatment at their facility. One can go so far as to explain and distribute the strategic plan to clerks, receptionists, telephone operators, and housekeepers in efforts to help to understand the environment. It is the ability to internalize all facets of the operating environment into our employees, because they see it as important to them, that will differentiate successful organizations.

A parting thought was shared by historian and psychologist Arnold Toynbee: success arises from inward articulation or self-determination more than from conquering external obstacles.[15] With this blessing, your journey to continually improving the health and well-being of your community will prosper, and you along with it.

NOTES

1. Stephen M. Shortell, "Creating Organized Delivery Systems: The Barriers and Facilitators," *Hospital & Health Services Administration,* Winter 1993, pp. 447–66.
2. Nicholas Imparato and Oren Harari, *Jumping the Curve* (San Francisco: Jossey-Bass, 1996) p. 182.
3. Systems cannot be perfected overnight and they cannot be perfected without clinical input. This doesn't mean that physicians will command the same level of respect as in the past 20 to 30 years (as surgeons joke, you can teach a monkey to do surgery), but they must be acknowledged and made complete partners in the reform, i.e., the system of the future.
4. Manuel Velasquez, *Business Ethics: Concepts and Cases* (Englewood Cliffs, NJ: Prentice-Hall, 1992), p. 91.
5. Richard Janeway, MD, from an interview in Winston-Salem, NC, August 26, 1996.
6. Ibid.
7. Oren Harari, "Don't Let It Go to Your Head," *Small Business Reports* (18, no. 10 (1993), pp. 59–61.
8. Unknown quote; some have attributed it to Jon Madonna, CEO of KPMG Peat Marwick.
9. Imparato and Harari, *Jumping the Curve,* p. 4.
10. Ibid., p. 56.
11. Attributed to James Baughman, as quoted by Frank Rose in "A New Message for Business?" *Fortune,* October 8, 1990, p. 162.
12. Paul Lawrence and Jay Lorsch, "Differentiation and Integration in Complex Organizations," *Administrative Science Quarterly,* 12, 1967, pp. 1–47.
13. Imparato and Harari, *Jumping the Curve,* p. 202.
14. Steven J. Heyer and Reginald Van Lee, "Rewriting the Corporation," *Business Horizons* 35, no. 3 (1992), pp. 13–22.
15. Arnold J. Toynbee, *A Study of History: Abridgment of Volumes I–IV, Part I of II,* edited by D. C. Somervell (New York: Oxford University Press, 1957), p. 199.

APPENDIX

APPENDIX

A

SELECTED READINGS

Bledsoe, D. et al. "Tying Physician Incentive Pay to Performance." *Healthcare Financial Management,* December 1995.

Bohlmann, R.G. "New Group Formation and Mergers." *Medical Group Management Journal,* May/June 1993.

Bonds, R.G. "Structuring Competitive Physician Compensation Programs." *Healthcare Financial Management,* December 1995.

Bordens, T.C. and Halpern, J. "Reclassifying Physicians as Employees for Federal Tax Purposes." *Healthcare Financial Management,* February 1994.

Collins, H. and Lee, V. "Operational Assessment: A Must for Gauging Practice Efficiency." *Healthcare Financial Management,* March 1996.

"Docs Get Their Way." *Modern Healthcare,* January 8, 1996.

Friend, P.M. "PHO Growing Pains." *Healthcare Executive,* May/June 1996.

Gapenski, L.C. and Langland-Orban, B. "Predicting Financial Risk under Capitation." *Healthcare Financial Management,* November 1995.

Gold, M. et al. "A National Survey of the Arrangements Managed-Care Plans Make with Physicians." *New England Journal of Medicine,* December 21, 1995.

Goldberg, M.A. "New Tax Traps in Buy-Sell Agreements." *Medical Economics,* October 10, 1994.

Griffith, G.M. "IRS View on Physician Control of Integrated Networks." *Healthcare Financial Management,* November 1995.

Guzzetta, D. "Developing an Incentive System for PHO Physicians." *Healthcare Financial Management,* February 1996.

Harris, C., Hicks, L.L., and Kelly, B.J. "Physician-Hospital Networking: Avoiding a Shotgun Wedding." *Health Care Management Review,* Fall 1992.

HFMA Principles and Practices Board. "Practice Acquisition: A Due Diligence Checklist." *Healthcare Financial Management,* December 1995.

Hill, J. and Mullen, P. "Exploring Practice Management Options." *Healthcare Financial Management,* January 1996.

Hudson, T. "The Great Debate." *Hospitals and Health Networks,* January 20, 1996.

Hudson, T. "There's No Place Like Home." *Hospitals and Health Networks,* February 5, 1996.

Hunt, D.E. "How Mergers Go Wrong." *Medical Economics,* December 26, 1994.

King, J.P. "Legal Issues Affecting IPA Formation." *Healthcare Financial Management,* November 1995.

Louiselle, P. "Conducting Financial Due Diligence of Medical Practices." *Healthcare Financial Management,* December 1995.

Lutz, S. "How Much?" *Modern Healthcare,* February 12, 1996.

McGarry, L.J. "Practice Valuation: The Impact of Large Medical Groups and Managed Care on Goodwill Determination." *College Review,* Fall 1994.

Manecke, S.R. and Davis A. "Managing the Transition after Acquisition." *Healthcare Financial Management,* January 1996.

Mangan, D. "A Surefire Way to Lure a Young Doctor." *Medical Economics,* February 1994.

Peregrine, M.W. and Glaser, L. "Legal Issues in Medical Practice Acquisitions." *Healthcare Financial Management,* February 1995.

Peters, G.R. and Schantz, T.S. "Tax and Other Issues Affecting Physician Integration Activities." *Group Practice Journal,* May/June 1994.

"Promises, Promises." *Modern Healthcare,* February 19, 1996.

Rimmer, T.B. "Physician Practice Acquisitions: Valuation Issues and Concerns." *Hospital and Health Services Administration,* Fall 1995. **Note.** Also read response letter in Winter 1995.

Robinson, J.C. and Casalino, L.P. "The Growth of Medical Groups Paid through Capitation in California." *New England Journal of Medicine,* December 21, 1995.

Sandrick, K. "How to Succeed with Doctors by Really Trying." *Hospitals and Health Networks,* February 5, 1996.

Sauve, M. "Reassessing the Number and Mix of System Physician Needs." *Healthcare Financial Management,* February 1996.

Schiller, D.J. "What You Should Bargain for in a Restrictive Covenant." *Medical Economics,* July 11, 1994.

Slomski, A.J. "Got the Urge to Merge? You're Not Alone." *Medical Economics,* April 11, 1994.

Slomski, A.J. "How Hospitals Are Luring Doctors onto Their Payrolls." *Medical Economics,* November 1994.

TABLE 1

Present Value of One Dollar Due at the End of *n* Periods

$$PV = \frac{\$1}{(1 + r)^n}$$

PV = present value; *r* = discount rate; *n* = number of periods until payment

n	1%	2%	3%	4%	5%	6%	7%	8%	9%	10%
1	.99010	.98039	.97007	.96154	.95238	.94340	.93458	.92593	.91743	.90909
2	.98030	.96117	.94260	.92456	.90703	.89000	.87344	.85734	.84168	.82645
3	.97059	.94232	.91514	.88900	.86384	.83962	.81630	.79383	.77218	.75131
4	.96098	.92385	.88849	.85480	.82270	.79209	.76290	.73503	.70843	.68301
5	.95147	.90573	.86261	.82193	.78353	.74726	.71299	.68058	.64993	.62092
6	.94204	.88797	.83748	.79031	.74622	.70496	.66634	.63017	.59627	.56447
7	.93272	.87056	.81309	.75992	.71068	.66506	.62275	.58349	.54703	.51316
8	.92348	.85349	.78941	.73069	.67684	.62741	.58201	.54027	.50187	.46651
9	.91434	.83675	.76642	.70259	.64461	.59190	.54393	.50025	.46043	.42410
10	.90529	.82035	.74409	.67556	.61391	.55839	.50835	.46319	.42241	.38554
11	.89632	.80426	.72242	.64958	.58468	.52679	.47509	.42888	.38753	.35049
12	.88745	.78849	.70138	.62460	.55684	.49697	.44401	.39711	.35553	.31863
13	.87866	.77303	.68095	.60057	.53032	.46884	.41496	.36770	.32618	.28966
14	.86996	.75787	.66112	.57747	.50507	.44930	.38782	.34046	.29925	.26333
15	.86135	.74301	.64186	.55526	.48102	.41726	.36245	.31524	.27454	.23939
16	.85282	.72845	.62317	.53391	.45811	.39365	.33873	.29189	.25187	.21763
17	.84438	.71416	.60502	.51337	.43630	.37136	.31657	.27027	.23107	.19784
18	.83602	.70016	.58739	.49363	.41552	.35034	.29586	.25025	.21199	.17986
19	.82774	.68643	.57029	.47464	.39573	.33051	.27651	.23171	.19449	.16351
20	.81954	.67297	.55367	.45639	.37689	.31180	.25842	.21455	.17843	.14864
21	.81143	.65978	.53755	.43883	.35894	.29415	.24151	.19866	.16370	.13513
22	.80340	.64684	.52189	.42195	.34185	.27750	.22571	.18394	.15018	.12285
23	.79544	.63414	.50669	.40573	.32557	.26180	.21095	.17031	.13778	.11168
24	.78757	.62172	.49193	.39012	.31007	.24698	.19715	.15770	.12640	.10153
25	.77977	.60953	.47760	.37512	.29530	.23300	.18425	.14602	.11597	.09230

(Continued)

TABLE 1

Present Value of One Dollar Due at the End of *n* Periods
(Continued)

n	11%	12%	13%	14%	15%	16%	17%	18%	19%	20%
1	.90090	.89286	.88496	.87719	.86957	.86207	.85470	.84746	.84034	.83333
2	.81162	.79719	.78315	.76947	.75614	.74316	.73051	.71818	.70616	.69444
3	.73119	.71178	.69305	.67497	.65752	.64066	.62437	.60863	.59342	.57870
4	.65873	.63552	.61332	.59208	.57175	.55229	.53365	.51579	.49867	.48225
5	.59345	.56743	.54276	.51937	.49718	.47611	.45611	.43711	.41905	.40188
6	.53464	.50663	.48032	.45559	.43233	.41044	.38984	.37043	.35214	.33490
7	.48166	.45235	.42506	.39964	.37594	.35383	.33320	.31392	.29592	.27908
8	.43393	.40388	.37616	.35056	.32690	.30503	.28478	.26604	.24867	.23257
9	.39092	.36061	.33288	.30751	.28426	.26295	.24340	.22546	.20897	.19381
10	.35218	.32197	.29459	.26974	.24718	.22668	.20804	.19106	.17560	.16151
11	.31728	.28748	.26070	.23662	.21494	.19542	.17781	.16192	.14756	.13459
12	.28584	.25667	.23071	.20756	.18691	.16846	.15197	.13722	.12400	.11216
13	.25751	.22917	.20416	.18207	.16253	.14523	.12989	.11629	.10420	.09346
14	.23199	.20462	.18068	.15971	.14133	.12520	.11102	.09855	.08757	.07789
15	.20900	.18270	.15989	.14010	.12289	.10793	.09489	.08352	.07359	.06491
16	.18829	.16312	.14150	.12289	.10686	.09304	.08110	.07078	.06184	.05409
17	.16963	.14564	.12522	.10780	.09293	.08021	.06932	.05998	.05196	.04507
18	.15282	.13004	.11081	.09456	.08080	.06914	.05925	.05063	.04367	.03756
19	.13768	.11611	.09806	.08295	.07026	.05961	.05064	.04308	.03669	.03130
20	.12403	.10367	.08678	.07276	.06110	.05139	.04328	.03651	.03084	.02608
21	.11174	.09256	.07680	.06383	.05313	.04430	.03699	.03094	.02591	.02174
22	.10067	.08264	.06796	.05599	.04620	.03819	.03162	.02622	.02178	.01811
23	.09069	.07379	.06014	.04911	.04017	.03292	.02702	.02222	.01830	.01509
24	.08170	.06588	.05322	.04308	.03493	.02838	.02310	.01883	.01538	.01258
25	.07361	.05882	.04710	.03779	.03038	.02447	.01974	.01596	.01292	.01048

(Continued)

TABLE 1

Present Value of One Dollar Due at the End of *n* Periods
(Concluded)

n	21%	22%	23%	24%	25%	26%	27%	28%	29%	30%
1	.82645	.81967	.81301	.80645	.80000	.79365	.78740	.78125	.77519	.76923
2	.68301	.67186	.66098	.65036	.64000	.62988	.62000	.61035	.60093	.59172
3	.56447	.55071	.53738	.52449	.51200	.49991	.48819	.47684	.46583	.45517
4	.46651	.45140	.43690	.42297	.40960	.39675	.38440	.37253	.36111	.35013
5	.38554	.37000	.35520	.34111	.32768	.31488	.30268	.29104	.27993	.26933
6	.31863	.30328	.26878	.27509	.26214	.24991	.23833	.22737	.21700	.20718
7	.26333	.24859	.23478	.22184	.20972	.19834	.18766	.17764	.16822	.15937
8	.21763	.20376	.19088	.17891	.16777	.15741	.14776	.13878	.13040	.12259
9	.17986	.16702	.15519	.14428	.13422	.12493	.11635	.10842	.10109	.09430
10	.14864	.13690	.12617	.11635	.10737	.09915	.09161	.08470	.07836	.07254
11	.12285	.11221	.10258	.09383	.08590	.07869	.07214	.06617	.06075	.05580
12	.10153	.09198	.08339	.07567	.06872	.06245	.05680	.05170	.04709	.04292
13	.08391	.07539	.06780	.06103	.05498	.04957	.04472	.04039	.03650	.03302
14	.06934	.06180	.05512	.04921	.04398	.03934	.03522	.03155	.02830	.02540
15	.05731	.05065	.04481	.03969	.03518	.03122	.02773	.02465	.02194	.01954
16	.04736	.04152	.03643	.03201	.02815	.02478	.02183	.01926	.01700	.01503
17	.03914	.03403	.02962	.02581	.02252	.01967	.01719	.01505	.01318	.01156
18	.03235	.02789	.02408	.02082	.01801	.01561	.01354	.01175	.01022	.00889
19	.02673	.02286	.01958	.01679	.01441	.01239	.01066	.00918	.00792	.00684
20	.02209	.01874	.01592	.01354	.01153	.00983	.00839	.00717	.00614	.00526
21	.01826	.01536	.01294	.01092	.00922	.00780	.00661	.00561	.00476	.00405
22	.01509	.01259	.01052	.00880	.00738	.00619	.00520	.00438	.00369	.00311
23	.01247	.01032	.00855	.00710	.00590	.00491	.00410	.00342	.00286	.00239
24	.01031	.00846	.00695	.00573	.00472	.00390	.00323	.00267	.00222	.00184
25	.00852	.00693	.00565	.00462	.00378	.00310	.00254	.00209	.00172	.00142

C

MEDICAL PRACTICE ACQUISITION DUE DILIGENCE CHECKLIST

Buyer: _____   Buyer's Counsel: _____

Seller: _____   Seller's Counsel: _____

Practice Name: _____

Date Due Diligence Started: _____

Date Due Diligence Filed and Delivered to: _____

Coordination of Documents:	**Team Member Responsible Name/Phone Number**
Settlement Statement	_____
Asset Purchase Agreement	_____
Assets	_____
Excluded Assets	_____
Assumed Liabilities	_____
Contracts	_____
Bill of Sale	_____
Opinion of Seller's Counsel	_____
Employment Agreement	_____
Permits, Authorizations, Certificates, and Licenses	_____
Opinion of Buyer's Counsel _____	_____
Review of licenses, permits, accreditation or franchises relating to the use or running in favor of the practice	_____
Certificate of Existence (Seller)	_____
Certificate of Existence (Buyer)	_____

	Team Member Responsible Name/Phone Number
Coordinator of Due Diligence File:	_____
A. Financial Review:	_____
B. Reimbursement/Medical Billing Issues:	_____
C. Professional Credentials/Clinical Review Patient Demographics Review:	_____
D. Personnel Review:	_____
E. Practice Efficiency/Physical Layout:	_____
F. Legal and Regulatory:	_____

A. FINANCIAL REVIEW

Procedure: **Assigned To/Due Date:**

1. Perform analytical review of financial statement from the past 3 to 5 years and query any major changes _____

2. Assess profitability, growth, and productivity trends and compare them to those of other practices and to industry averages _____

3. Test tracing of trial balance detail into financial statements _____

4. Trace/reconcile financial statements to tax returns _____

5. Review cash disbursement ledger (A/P postings) _____

6. Review cash receipts journal (A/R postings) and trace to daily deposits _____

7. Test tracing of patient charges from bills to A/R for a selected sample _____

8. Review office bad debt/account adjustment policies and history of bad debt write-offs _____

9. Review payroll tax returns and examine tax payment canceled checks _____

Procedure: **Assigned To/Due Date:**

10. Review bank reconciliations
    for selected months   _____

11. Verify purchase documents for major
    items on fixed-asset listing   _____

12. Inventory physical presence and
    condition of fixed assets (used as the
    basis for asset allocation during
    valuation process)   _____

13. Confirm major receivables from
    Medicare, Medicaid, HMOs, PPOs,
    and other third parties. Review
    appropriateness based on contract   _____

14. Confirm loan balances (in excess of
    $10,000 each) and terms of debts to
    be assumed   _____

15. Review equipment and real estate
    leases, obtain market comparability
    information, and assess transferability   _____

16. Perform search for unrecorded
    liabilities   _____

17. Review adequacy of financial and
    patient accounting system and any
    related computer systems   _____

18. Interview medical office manager to
    determine if computer data are
    transferable to applicable software   _____

19. List and investigate other special issues   _____

B. REIMBURSEMENT, MEDICAL BILLING REVIEW

Procedure: **Assigned To/Due Date:**

1. Review appropriateness of charge
   master and billing forms (superbill)   _____

2. Pull sample of three months'
   explanation of medical benefits
   (EOMBs) from third-party payers   _____

Procedure: **Assigned To/Due Date:**

3. Select appropriate sample of patient
   encounters from EOMBs and from
   self-pay patients   _____

4. For selected encounters:

   a. Review appropriateness of
      diagnosis based on medical record
      documentation   _____

   b. Review for proper application of
      charge schedule   _____

   c. Review reasonableness of laboratory
      and ancillary service orders   _____

   d. Review referrals made,
      appropriateness thereof   _____

   e. Review payments received,
      appropriateness thereof   _____

   f. Document adequacy of medical
      records   _____

5. Document known and proposed
   changes in reimbursement that will
   influence future practice revenues   _____

6. Calculate accounts receivable collection
   ratios and days outstanding and
   compare to other practices and
   industry averages   _____

7. Review laboratory and ancillary service
   facility certifications, as applicable   _____

8. Prepare file memo on work performed
   and conclusions drawn therefrom   _____

C. PHYSICIAN CREDENTIALS, MEDICAL RECORDS, PATIENT DEMOGRAPHICS REVIEW

Procedure: **Assigned To/Due Date:**

1. Review continuing medical education
   status for each physician   _____

Procedure: **Assigned To/Due Date:**

2. Confirm current specialty board status
   of each physician   _____

3. Review physician records with respect
   to patient complaints to practice and to
   governmental agencies or professional
   societies   _____

4. Select sample of patient records and
   form opinion on overall compliance
   with medical records standard   _____

5. Gather patient demographic information
   including payment source, age, sex,
   and geographic dispersion   _____

6. Examination of life insurance policies   _____

7. Review any suits filed or pending   _____

8. Prepare file memo on work performed
   and conclusions drawn therefrom   _____

D. PERSONNEL REVIEW

Procedure: **Assigned To/Due Date:**

1. Review personnel listing, compare
   salaries to those of other local facilities
   and buyer's criteria   _____

2. Gather history of physician salaries and
   compare to local and regional market
   and specialty standards   _____

3. Interview selected personnel and
   determine compatibility of functions
   with buyer's other organizations   _____

4. Review all employment contracts
   or "special deals"   _____

5. Review compatibility of employee
   benefits with those of other local
   facilities and buyer's criteria   _____

Procedure: **Assigned To/Due Date:**

6. Review retirement plan for adequacy
   of funding, outstanding accruals, and
   for reasonableness of continued benefits
   under the plan   _____

7. Review vacation policy and accrued
   vacation days   _____

8. List other areas not covered   _____

9. Prepare file memo on work performed
   and conclusions therefrom   _____

E. PRACTICE EFFICIENCY, PHYSICAL LAYOUT REVIEW

Procedure: **Assigned To/Due Date:**

1. Visit practice site(s) and assess overall
   condition and physical appearance of
   office(s) and equipment   _____

2. Review adequacy and timeliness of
   office filing systems for both financial
   and patient records   _____

3. Review and assess efficiency
   of office layout   _____

4. Assess space for practice expansion
   modification within current facility   _____

5. Estimate capital improvements and
   additions needed for next 2 years   _____

6. Prepare file memo on work performed,
   conclusions drawn, and note statement
   of how this practice fits into purchaser's
   strategic plan   _____

F. LEGAL AND REGULATORY REVIEW

Procedure: **Assigned To/Due Date:**

1. Review corporate status   _____

2. Run UCC search on practice,
   shareholders, spouses, etc.   _____

3. Review lease obligations to be assumed   _____

4. Review all loan documents for liabilities
   to be assumed   _____

5. Review all managed care contracts
   for limitations and exclusivity clauses   _____

6. Interview medical office manager
   to determine if practice has been
   rejected by any payors   _____

7. Review malpractice insurance to
   determine basis of coverage
   (occurrence vs. claims made), history
   of malpractice claims, and outstanding
   claims   _____

8. Obtain and review all requested legal
   opinions from seller's attorney   _____

9. Do title search if real property
   is involved   _____

10. Review regulatory issues applicable
    to the practice   _____

11. List other legal/regulatory issues
    (as specified in advance)   _____

12. Resolve questions regarding practice
    name, logo, and use of existing
    telephone numbers   _____

13. Prepare file memo on work performed
    and conclusions drawn therefrom   _____

D

THE INSTITUTE OF BUSINESS APPRAISERS BUSINESS APPRAISAL STANDARDS

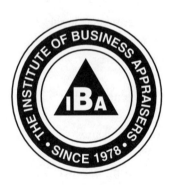

CODE OF ETHICS

1. The Appraiser shall achieve and maintain a high level of competence, shall stay informed as to all matters involving or affecting business values, and shall accept only those assignments for which he/she has the necessary background and qualifications.

2. An appraisal assignment is a confidential undertaking between the Appraiser and the client. No information regarding the appraisal assignment shall be disclosed to any third party without the express consent of the client.

3. Although an Appraiser may express an informal or preliminary opinion as to the value of a business, he/she shall not do so until after he/she has obtained all of the pertinent facts and given them due consideration.

4. All formal appraisal reports shall be in writing, shall be signed by the Appraiser, and shall include the following as a minimum:

   a. A statement of the purpose for which the appraisal was made and a definition of the value estimated.

   b. A description of the business or business interest being appraised.

   c. A summary of the facts upon which the appraisal is based.

   d. A description of the appraisal method(s) employed.

   e. A statement of the conclusions reached, together with any applicable qualifications or limitations on the conclusions.

   f. A statement of the assumptions and conditions applicable to the appraisal and to the conclusions reached.

   g. A statement that the Appraiser has no present or contemplated future interest in the business being appraised, or a full and complete description of any such interest that may exist.

5. The engagement to perform an appraisal and the fee charged shall be independent of the value reported.

6. In the conduct of his/her business, the Appraiser will at all times observe both the letter and the spirit of applicable laws, regulations, and good business practices.

THE INSTITUTE OF BUSINESS APPRAISERS
STANDARD ONE

1.0   **Professional Conduct & Ethics**

1.1   Competence. The achievement of certification as a business appraiser (CBA) is a result of specialized training, study, practice, the successful completion of a proctored examination, and a favorable review of the candidate's actual appraisal reports by The Institute of Business Appraisers' Qualifications Review Committee. To maintain certification, a CBA will adhere to continuing education requirements and periodic recertification as required by IBA.

Prior to accepting an engagement to perform a business appraisal, the appraiser must judge his competence to complete the assignment. Should the appraiser have a meaningful lack of knowledge and experience, the appraiser <u>must</u> immediately disclose that fact to the client. If the client desires the appraiser to continue with the assignment, the appraiser shall take those steps necessary to perform the appraisal in a competent manner, or take those steps necessary to complete the assignment under the supervision of an appraiser who has the requisite skill, or with the permission of the client, refer the engagement to a qualified business appraiser.

It is essential that a business appraiser communicate the research and thought processes which led to his opinions and conclusions in a manner that is clear, meaningful and not mis- leading. Said communication, whether oral or written, shall not be rendered in a careless or negligent manner.

The appraiser as an individual must be competent. Software valuation programs and/or excessive reliance on rules of thumb are not surrogates for individual competence.

The professional business appraiser recognizes and understands that compliance with these standards and ethics is an essential part of competence.

1.2   Confidentiality. The very fact an appraiser has been retained to value all or a portion of a business enterprise, or its securities, is in itself confidential. Consequently, it is considered unethical for a business appraiser to disclose either the assignment itself or any of the reasonably identifiable contents of an appraisal report without the client's express permission.

1.3   Disinterestedness. It is unethical for a business appraiser to accept any assignment when the appraiser has a present or contemplated interest in the property being appraised, or a bias for or against any person associated therewith, either directly or indirectly. Such interests include, but are not limited to, present, contemplated or prospective activity with the business enterprise, its officers, directors, or owners, including possible acquirers or investors.

However, if a prospective client, after full disclosure by the appraiser of said interest or bias, still elects to engage the appraiser, the appraiser may accept the assignment. When accepting such an assignment, the business appraiser <u>shall</u> include a Statement of Departure as required by Standard 1.21(b). The Statement of Departure <u>shall</u> include a complete disclosure of the interest or bias.

1.4   Nonadvocacy v. Advocacy. Nonadvocacy is considered to be a mandatory standard of appraisal.

The appraiser's obligation to serve the public interest assures that the integrity of valuations will be preserved. Hence, the appraiser may only be an advocate for his unbiased process and conclusions. The appraiser <u>must</u> be guided by nothing other than his informed judgment, the dictates of the client (as permitted under these standards), applicable administrative rulings, and the law.

In the event the appraiser is engaged to function not as an appraiser but as an advisor or consultant, he may serve as an advocate. In such instances the appraiser <u>shall</u> include a statement of departure which states, that any positions taken were taken as an advocate for the client.

1.5   Engagement. Prior to performing an appraisal assignment, a business appraiser <u>should</u> obtain a written agreement signed by the client or his agent. At the very least, the engagement agreement <u>should</u> specify what the appraiser is being engaged to appraise, the function (use) of the appraisal, the purpose (standard of value) including the definition thereof, the effective date of the appraisal, the scope of the appraisal, that the appraisal will be performed on a nonadvocacy basis (see Standard 1.4), the amount of or method for calculating the appraiser's fee, together with the method for payment of same, and an indication of when the client may expect the report.

1.6   Coherence and Production. Appraisal reports must have logical organization. Readers's questions that can reasonably be anticipated should be answered. Data in one part of the report should not contradict other portions without reconciliation.

The appraiser should develop contributing conclusions from the various components of the appraisal process drawing them together in a cross-supporting manner that logically brings the reader to the appraiser's conclusion.

The report should be produced in a manner and style which brings credit to the appraiser and the profession. Typographical errors and the like <u>shall</u> be eliminated. In formal reports, page and exhibit numbers <u>should</u> be used together with a table of contents or index to enhance readability.

1.7   Supportable Opinion. The essence of business appraisal is a supportable opinion.

While it is intuitively logical that on a case-by-case basis certain opinions will be based on the informed, but subjective, judgment of the appraiser to a greater degree than others, the appraiser's goal is to have a supportable opinion. The reader should not be expected to accept critical elements such as adjustments to financial statements, the selected capitalization or discount rates or weightings, without support—even in those instances where the vicissitudes of the assignment dictate that support be primarily based on the informed judgment of the appraiser.

1.8   Replicability. The appraiser's procedures and conclusions in the formal report <u>must</u> be presented in sufficient detail to permit the reader to replicate the appraisal process.

1.9   Appropriateness. The standard of value, the type of report and the valuation approaches/methods utilized should be appropriate to the assignment. The material included in the report should be relevant, clear and cogent.

1.10   Jurisdictional Exception. If any part of these standards is contrary to the law or public policy of any jurisdiction, only that part shall be void and of no force and effect in that jurisdiction.

1.11   Fiduciary Duty to Clients, and Other Duties.

<u>Client</u>   The one employing the business appraiser.

<u>Third Parties</u>   Others who could be expected to review the report, e.g., attorneys, accountants, lenders, buyers, investors, regulatory agencies, courts, etc.

<u>Public</u>   Society at large.

(a)   <u>Specialized Character of Business Appraisal</u>. Seldom are others intimately familiar with the process of business appraisal. Therefore, it is anticipated the business appraiser will use his professional abilities properly, as more fully described throughout these standards.

(b)   <u>Loyalty, Obedience and Reasonable Skill and Care</u>. Agents have such duties to clients. While no fiduciary or other affirmative duty is owed to others, services provided in accordance with these standards should be clear as to meaning and not be misleading to others.

1.12   Duty to Profession.

(a)   <u>Professional Cooperation and Courtesy</u>. It is unethical to damage or attempt to damage the professional reputations or interfere with the performance of other business appraisers practicing within the scope of these standards through false or malicious statement or innuendo.

(b)   <u>Conduct</u>. Every member is reminded that his demeanor and general conduct represents his profession and fellow practitioners, and unprofessional conduct damages more than his individual reputation.

(c)   <u>Cooperation</u>. Each member <u>shall</u> cooperate fully with the efforts of the Institute and/or its Ethics and Discipline Committee when investigating possible activities which are contrary to these standards.

1.13   Substance v. Form. The form of an appraisal report can be oral or written with variations of each. However, it is only the form of the report that varies. The appraiser's responsibilities to gather data, analyze the data, and draw supportable conclusions as applicable to the type of assignment undertaken does not change. Regardless of whether the final valuation is reported orally, in a summarizing letter report or a formal report, the appraiser <u>must</u> have first completed an appropriate valuation determination process.

A preliminary report is an exception to the above requirement for a thorough, complete work process. By its nature, a preliminary report results from a more cursory evaluation. (See Standard Six, Preliminary Reports.)

1.14   Professional Fees. The fees charged for the services of an appraiser are a product of the marketplace, however, a business appraiser is ethically denied the selection of a fee that could in itself call to question the objectivity of the appraiser.

(a)   <u>Finder's Fee</u>. No appraiser will pay fees, or offer gain in any form, to others to promote the appraiser's work in such a way, or under any circumstances, that will diminish the dignity of, or reflect discredit or disrepute upon, the appraisal profession.

(b)   Referral Fees. It is the right of an appraiser and, therefore, not unethical to pay a referral fee to another professional for the referral of appraisal assignments.

(c)   Percentage Fees. To accept any engagement for which the compensation is based on a percentage of the valuation conclusion impairs independence and is thus unethical.

1.15   Access to Requisite Data. The business appraiser, must decide what documents and/or information are requisite to a competent appraisal.

(a)   Reliability of Data. An appraiser may rely upon documents and/or information provided by the client and/or his agents without further corroboration; provided, the report clearly states he has done so. This right, however, does not abrogate the appraiser's duty to ask or otherwise inquire regarding information which on its surface clearly appears to be incomplete or otherwise inaccurate.

(b)   Pertinent Data. In situations where access to "pertinent" data is denied to the appraiser, the appraiser may, at his option, withdraw from completing the assignment. However, should the appraiser elect to compete the assignment, the report must include a Statement of Departure as required under Standard 1.21(b). Such Statement of Departure must describe the limitation and/or restriction and its potential effect on the appraiser's conclusion.

(c)   Essential Data. When the business appraiser is denied access to data considered essential to a proper appraisal, the business appraiser should not proceed with the assignment.

1.16   Valuation Approaches/Methods. The approaches/methods used within a given assignment are a matter that must be determined by the business appraiser's professional judgment. The task is generally decided through consideration of the approaches/methods that are conceptually most appropriate and those for which the most reliable data is available.

1.17   Definitions.

(a)   <u>Terms</u>. The appraiser should be careful in the use of ambiguous or esoteric terms. Such terms require definition to prevent the reader from applying a different definition.

(b)   <u>Computations</u>. All computations, particularly those used to compute ratios and weightings should be clearly defined.

1.18   Principal Sources and References.

(a)   <u>Formal Report</u>. A formal report <u>must</u> include a list of the principal sources of nonconfidential information and references whenever their inclusion will materially contribute to the clarity and understanding of the report.

(b)   <u>Oral and Informal Reports</u>. The appraiser's workpapers <u>must</u> include a general description of the principal sources of information and references.

1.19   Site Tours and Interviews.

(a)   <u>Tour</u>. Familiarity with an appraisal subject is a compelling necessity to a credible valuation. For this reason, it is desirable that a business appraiser make personal inspections or tours of appraisal subject sites whenever possible. When such activities are not performed, the appraiser's report <u>shall</u> disclose that the appraisal process did not include a site tour.

(b)   <u>Interview</u>. An appraiser <u>should</u> not perform an appraisal without interviewing the management and other parties considered appropriate in the circumstances.

1.20   Eligibility of Data. An appraisal shall be based upon what a reasonably informed person would have knowledge of as of a certain date. This shall be known as the appraisal's "date of valuation" or "effective date" and accordingly reflect the appraiser's supportable conclusion as of that date. Information unavailable or unknown on the date of valuation <u>must</u> not influence the appraiser or contribute to the concluding opinion of value.

(a)   <u>Imminent Change</u>. The appraiser is sometimes faced with the knowledge of a material imminent change in the business; a change not known of on the "date of valuation," but known as of the appraisal's "report" date. In such an event, the imminent change (positive or negative) <u>should</u> not affect the valuation conclusion, unless a reasonably informed person could have anticipated the imminent change. However, it is not uncommon for an appraiser to disclose such a change within the narrative portion of the report.

(b)   <u>Data on Guideline Companies</u>. When an appraiser selects guideline companies, the data on the companies judged sufficiently similar <u>should</u> be information knowable, although perhaps not yet compiled, on or before the appraisal's date of valuation. Additionally, the data on the guideline companies should be for the same accounting period; however, if it is as of a different period, said different period <u>must</u> be on or before the appraisal's date of valuation.

This restriction should apply whether the guideline companies are specific companies or aggregate industry statistics or ratios.

1.21   Departure. A business appraiser may be engaged to perform an appraisal assignment that calls for something different from the work that would routinely result from the appraiser's compliance with all <u>must</u> standards; provided, that prior to entering into an agreement to perform such an assignment.

(a)   The appraiser is of the opinion that the assignment is not so limited in scope that the resulting report would tend to mislead or confuse the client or other anticipated readers; and

(b)   The appraiser has advised the client that the assignment calls for something different than that which would normally result from compliance with applicable standards and, therefore, the report <u>shall</u> include a statement of departure.

1.22   Hypothetical Reports. An analysis or appraisal may be prepared under a hypothetical assumption, or series thereof, even though they may appear improbable. However, such a report must clearly state (i) the hypothetical assumption and (ii) the purpose of the analysis or appraisal, and any opinion of value must clearly be identified as resulting from a hypothetical assumption.

1.23   Dissenting Opinion.

(a)   <u>Dissenting Opinion With Other Appraisers</u>. Collaborating appraisers, and review appraisers must sign the report. When a signing appraiser disagrees in whole or in part with any or all of the findings of other appraisers, said dissenting opinion must be included in the report, signed by the dissenting appraiser.

(b)   <u>Dissenting Opinion With Case Law and/or Administrative Regulation</u>. As any other member of society, appraisers are required to comply with statutory law and statutory definitions as they may exist from time to time and from jurisdiction to jurisdiction. However, case law and/or administrative regulations do not have the same force as statutory law. Therefore, the business appraiser may, when he believes it is warranted, express within the appraisal report a dissenting opinion to case law and/or an administrative regulation.

1.24   Membership Designations. It is considered unethical conduct for any individual to explicitly or implicitly indicate he is a Certified Business Appraiser (CBA) when he has not been awarded the designation.

(a)   <u>Certified Business Appraisal Reports</u>. An appraisal report may be considered a "Certified Report" when it is signed by a Certified Business Appraiser who is taking technical responsibility for its content.

(b)   <u>Misuse of Certification</u>. Each Certified Business Appraiser is honor-bound to refrain from any use of his professional designation in connection with any form of activity that may reflect discredit upon his designation, or the organization that conferred it, or deceive his client, or the public. As with actual appraisal conclusions, this has been left as a matter of individual judgment and conscience, those who abuse this privilege could be subject to disciplinary action by IBA's Ethics and Discipline Committee.

1.25   Certification. Each written report <u>must</u> contain a certification signed by the appraiser. Additional appraisers signing the report <u>must</u> accept responsibility for the full contents of the report. [In the event of a dissenting opinion, see Standard 1.23(a).] The certificate must be similar in content to the following:

(a)   That to the best of the appraiser's knowledge, the statements of fact contained in the report are true and correct.

(b)   That the reported analyses, opinions, and conclusions are limited only by the reported assumptions and limiting conditions, and are the appraiser's personal, unbiased professional analyses, opinions and conclusions.

(c)   That the appraisal was performed on a basis of nonadvocacy, including a statement that the appraiser has no present or contemplated interest in the property appraised and has no personal bias with respect to the parties involved, or a complete disclosure of any such interest or bias.

(d)   That the appraiser's compensation is not contingent on an action or event resulting from the analyses, opinions, or conclusions in, or the use of, the report.

(e)   That the appraiser's analyses, opinions, and conclusions were developed and that the report has been prepared in conformity with the Business Appraisal Standards of The Institute of Business Appraiser's.

(f)   That no one provided significant professional assistance to the person signing the report. However, if there are exceptions to this, then the name of each individual providing significant professional assistance must be disclosed.

1.26   Qualifications of the Appraiser. The reader cannot fully judge the quality of the appraisal report without being given the opportunity to judge the appraiser's qualifications. Therefore, each appraisal report <u>must</u> include the appraiser's qualifications in a manner the appraiser believes accurately presents his appraisal experience, certification, professional activities, and other qualifications.

1.27   Force and Effect. These standards shall be in full force and effect on the date of their issuance. (Earlier compliance is encouraged.) Any and all prior standards regarding business appraisal practices, reports, conduct, or ethics are superseded. Future amendments, to be effective, <u>shall</u> be initiated and passed in accordance with Standard 1.29.

1.28   Enforcement. The enforcement of these standards, including amendments or modifications as may occur in accordance with Standard 1.29, <u>shall</u> be the responsibility and duty of all members as to their own performance, and otherwise by the standing Ethics and Discipline Committee of The Institute of Business Appraisers and/or such other individuals or committees as are designated from time to time by the governing body of The Institute of Business Appraisers.

1.29   Amendments to Standards. The Standards Committee of The Institute of Business Appraisers is a standing committee. Certified members desiring to propose amendments, additions, or deletions to these standards should submit a clear expression of the proposed change to The Institute of Business Appraisers, Attention: Chairperson, Standards Committee. The chairperson reserves the right to return any submitted change for further clarification as to the precise change proposed. The chairperson shall distribute copies of the proposed change to the members of the Standards Committee for their opinions on the proposed change. Should two-thirds or more of the Committee support the change, it shall be endorsed by the Committee and an exposure draft will be provided to all CBAs. The exposure draft shall provide for a thirty-day period for the vote of all CBAs. In the event that those certified members who vote "No" exceeds 50%

of all CBAs (those voting plus those not voting), the Committee's vote will be overruled and the proposed change will die for lack of support. Otherwise, the change will be adopted as of the first day of the month following the date copies of the amendments are provided to all members.

(a)   Automatic Amendment. It is the intent of the Business Appraisal Standards Committee (BASC) of The Institute of Business Appraisers (IBA) that these standards not conflict with standards nine and ten of the Uniform Standards of Professional Appraisal Practice as promulgated by The Appraisal Foundation. In the event of such a conflict, these standards will be amended as necessary. Pending said amendment, the conflicting portion of these standards will be temporarily suspended. However, nothing contained herein is intended to imply that these Business Appraisal Standards, promulgated by the IBA cannot restrict or require standards in excess of the restrictions or requirements of The Appraisal Foundation.

1.30   Signing Reports. Each written report <u>must</u> be signed by the appraiser and any other appraisers, including those signing as a "Review Appraiser" or "Collaborating Appraiser," <u>shall</u> accept responsibility for the full content of the report. [In the event of a dissenting opinion, see Standard 1.23(a).]

(a)   Exception. Should the policy of a given firm be that all reports are to be signed by a person authorized to sign reports on behalf of the firm, an exception to Standards 1.30 and 1.25 is permitted. However, in this event:

(i)   The designated signer <u>shall</u> take technical responsibility for the full content of the report; and

(ii)   The report may not be considered a "Certified Appraisal Report" unless a Certified Business Appraiser taking technical responsibility signs the report.

(iii)   The fact that a given appraisal report is signed under 1.30(a) is not intended in any way to justify or excuse deviation from any standard that would otherwise apply.

STANDARD TWO

2.0   **Oral Appraisal Reports**

   2.1   Usage. In general written reports are preferred; however, oral appraisal reports are permitted when ordered by the client.

   2.2   Mandatory Content. When presenting an oral report, the business appraiser <u>shall</u> in a manner that is clear and not misleading communicate the following:

      (a)   <u>Introduction</u>. Identify the client, and set forth the property being appraised, the purpose and function of the appraisal, the definition of the standard of value, and the effective date of the appraisal.

      (b)   <u>Assumptions and Limiting Conditions</u>. Disclose any extraordinary assumptions or limiting conditions that in the appraiser's judgment affected the value.

      (c)   <u>Disinterestedness</u>. That the appraisal was performed on a basis of nonadvocacy, including a statement that the appraiser has no present or contemplated interest in the property appraised and has no personal bias with respect to the parties involved, or a complete disclosure of any such interest or bias [See Standard 1.3]

      (d)   <u>Valuation Conclusion</u>. Represents a concluding opinion of value expressed as:

         (i)   a statement of a specific opinion of value; or

         (ii)   a range of values; or

         (iii)   a preliminary estimate which <u>must</u> include a statement that an opinion of value resulting from a formal report might be different and that difference might be material. (See also Standard Six, Preliminary Reports)

   2.3   Conformity. Oral appraisal reports should comply with all applicable sections of Standard One, Professional Conduct and Ethics.

2.4   Written Follow-up. By its nature, the oral report is less detailed than the written report. Therefore, whenever feasible, it is suggested that oral reports be followed by a written presentation of the salient features of the oral report. In general, the written follow-up should include:

(a)   Assumptions and Limiting Conditions. All applicable assumptions and limiting conditions.

(b)   Support. In general, a brief presentation of the information considered, the appraisal approaches used and the research and thought processes that support the appraiser's analyses, opinions and conclusions.

(c)   Appraiser's Certification as specified in Section 1.25.

2.5   Recordkeeping. An appraiser should retain written records of appraisal reports for a period of at least five (5) years after preparation or at least two (2) years after final disposition of any judicial proceeding in which the appraiser gave testimony, whichever period expires last.

STANDARD THREE

3.0   **Expert Testimony**

3.1   Definition. Expert testimony is an oral report given in the form of testimony in a deposition and/or on the witness stand before a court of proper jurisdiction or other trier of fact.

3.2   Mandatory Content. The appraiser shall answer all questions put to him in a manner that is clear and not misleading. When giving testimony, the appraiser shall not advocate any position that is incompatible with the appraiser's obligation of nonadvocacy, i.e., it is unethical for the appraiser to suppress any facts, data, or opinions which are adverse to the case his client is trying to establish, or to over-emphasize any facts, data, or opinions which are favorable to his client's case, or in any other particulars become an advocate. The expert witness must at least comply in a manner that is clear and not misleading with the following:

(a) <u>Introduction</u>. Identify the client, and set forth the property being appraised, the purpose and function of the appraisal, the definition of the standard of value, and the effective date of the appraisal.

(b) <u>Assumptions and Limiting Conditions</u>. Disclose any extraordinary assumptions or limiting conditions that in the appraiser's judgment affected the value.

(c) <u>Disinterestedness</u>. That the appraisal was performed on a basis of nonadvocacy, including a statement that the appraiser has no present or contemplated interest in the property appraised and has no personal bias with respect to the parties involved, or a complete disclosure of any such interest or bias. (See Standard 1.3)

(d) <u>Valuation Conclusion</u>. Any concluding opinion of value may be expressed as:

(i)   a statement of a specific opinion of value; or

(ii) a range of values; or

(iii) a preliminary estimate which <u>must</u> include a statement that an opinion of value resulting from a formal report may be different and that difference may be material. (See also Standard Six, Preliminary Reports.)

3.3   Conformity. Expert testimony reports <u>should</u> comply with all applicable sections of Standard One, Professional Conduct and Ethics.

3.4   Recordkeeping. An appraiser <u>should</u> retain written records of appraisal reports for a period of at least five (5) years after preparation or at least two (2) years after final disposition of any judicial proceeding in which the appraiser gave testimony, whichever period expires last.

STANDARD FOUR

4.0   **Letter Form Written Appraisal Reports**

4.1   Definition. An appraiser's written report can be in the form of a letter report or a formal report. The letter report, which is shorter than the formal report, presents conclusions together with brief generalized comments. This type of report is often referred to as a short-form report, letter opinion, or an informal report.

By its nature, the letter form report is an instrument of brevity. It should contain at least a summary of the material factors that led to its conclusions, but it is usually intended by the parties to reduce the normal appraisal burden of writing a comprehensive report, and thereby allow the client to realize some economic benefit. However, the appraiser is still required to perform materially the same investigation and analysis as would be required for a comprehensive formal report and maintain in his file the workpapers necessary to support the conclusions stated in the letter report.

4.2   Conformity. The letter form written report <u>must</u> comply with all applicable provisions of Business Appraisal Standards, Standard One, Professional Conduct and Ethics.

4.3   Mandatory Content. All letter form written appraisal reports <u>shall</u> minimally set forth in a manner that is clear and not misleading.

(a)   Identify the client, and set forth a description of the business enterprise, security or other tangible and/or intangible property being appraised.

(b)   Form of the organization and if incorporated, the state of incorporation, together with a description, adequate to the assignment, of all classes of securities outstanding and a list of shareholders whose interest should, in the appraiser's judgment be specified. If a partnership, the type and the state of filing, together with a list of those partners, whether general or limited, whose interest should, in the appraiser's judgment, be specified.

(c)   The purpose (standard of value) of the appraisal.

(d)   The function (use) of the appraisal.

(e)   The definition of the standard of value that is the purpose of the appraisal.

(f)   The effective ("as of") date of the appraisal.

(g)   The date the appraisal report was prepared.

(h)   The report's assumptions and limiting conditions.

(i)   Any special factors that affected the opinion of value. Such factors include, but are not limited to, buy-sell agreements, restrictive stock agreements, corporate articles, bylaws and resolutions, partnership agreements, litigation, regulatory compliance, or environmental hazards.

(j)   Applicable discounts and premiums such as minority interest, control, marketability or lack thereof.

(k)   A certification consistent with the intent of section 1.25.

4.4   Distribution of Report. The letter report <u>should</u> include a clear statement of the expected distribution of the report.

4.5   Valuation Conclusion. The letter report <u>must</u> include a clear statement of the appraiser's concluding opinion of value expressed as appropriate to the assignment:

(a)   a statement of specific opinion of value; or

(b)   a range of values; or

(c)   a preliminary estimate which <u>must</u> include a statement that an opinion of value resulting from a formal report might be different and that difference might be material. (See also Standard Six, Preliminary Reports.)

4.6   Transmittal Letter. If a transmittal letter is used, it <u>should</u> include a summary of the engagement. It may be structured in the form of a letter, an executive summary, or a similar rendering. However, regardless of the structure used, if a transmittal is used, it <u>shall</u> refer to the report in a manner sufficient to discourage any attempt to remove and use the transmittal without the report.

4.7   Recordkeeping. An appraiser <u>should</u> retain written records of appraisal reports for a period of at least five (5) years after preparation or at least two (2) years after final disposition of any judicial proceeding in which the appraiser gave testimony, whichever period expires last.

STANDARD FIVE

5.0   **Formal Written Appraisal Reports**

5.1   Definition. The formal appraisal report is a comprehensive business appraisal report prepared to contain at a minimum, the requirements described within this standard. It is sometimes called the long form, narrative or comprehensive report.

5.2   Conformity. The formal written report <u>must</u> comply with all applicable provisions of Business Appraisal Standards, Standard One, Professional Conduct and Ethics.

5.3   Mandatory Content. All formal appraisal reports <u>shall</u> minimally set forth the following items in a manner that is clear and not misleading, including detail sufficient to permit the reader to reasonably replicate the appraiser's procedures:

(a)   Identify the client, and set forth a description of the business enterprise, security, or other tangible and/or intangible property being appraised.

(b)   Form of the organization and if incorporated, the state of incorporation, together with a description, adequate to the assignment, of all classes of securities outstanding and a list of shareholders whose interest should, in the appraiser's judgment be specified. If a partnership, the type and the state of filing, together with a list of those partners, whether general or limited, whose interest should, in the appraiser's judgment, be specified.

(c)   The purpose (standard of value) of the appraisal.

(d)   The function (use) of the appraisal.

(e)   The definition of the standard of value that is the purpose of the appraisal.

(f)   The effective ("as of") date of the appraisal.

(g)   The date the appraisal report was prepared.

(h)   The report's assumptions and limiting conditions.

(i)   The principal sources and references used by the appraiser.

(j)   The consideration of relevant data regarding:

(i)   The nature and history of the business.

(ii)   The present economic conditions and the outlook affecting the business, its industry, and the general economy.

(iii)   Past results, current operations, and future prospects of the business.

(iv)   Past sales of interests in the business enterprise being appraised.

(v)   Sales of similar businesses or interests therein, whether closely-held or publicly-held.

(vi)   The valuation approaches/methods considered and rejected, the approaches/methods utilized, and the research, sources, computations, and reasoning that supports the appraiser's analyses, opinions and conclusions.

(vii)   Any special factors that affected the opinion of value. Such factors include, but are not limited to, buy-sell agreements, restrictive stock agreements, corporate articles, bylaws and resolutions, partnership agreements, litigation, regulatory compliance, or environmental hazards.

(viii)   Applicable discounts and premiums such as minority interest, control, marketability or lack thereof.

(ix)   When valuing a majority interest in a business on a "going concern" basis, consider whether the business' highest value may be achieved on a liquidation basis.

(k)   A Certification consistent with the interest of section 1.25.

5.4   Distribution of Report. The formal report <u>should</u> include a clear statement of the expected distribution of the report.

5.5   Valuation Conclusion. The formal report <u>must</u> include a clear statement of the appraiser's concluding opinion of value expressed as appropriate to the assignment:

(a) a statement of a specific opinion of value; or

(b) a range of values.

5.6   Transmittal Letter. If a transmittal letter is used, it <u>should</u> include a summary of the engagement. It may be structured in the form of a letter, an executive summary, or a similar rendering. However, regardless of the structure, if used, the transmittal <u>shall</u> refer to the report in a manner sufficient to discourage any attempt to remove and use the transmittal without the report.

5.7   Recordkeeping. An appraiser <u>should</u> retain written records of appraisal reports for a period of at least five (5) years after preparation or at least two (2) years after final disposition of any judicial proceeding in which the appraiser gave testimony, whichever period expires last.

STANDARD SIX

6.0   **Preliminary Reports**

6.1   Definition. A brief oral or written report reflecting the appraiser's limited opinion.

A preliminary report <u>must</u> clearly identify any valuation as a "limited" opinion of value as the appraiser has not performed the detailed investigation and analysis essential to a cogent appraisal. [See Standard 6.5]

6.2   Conformity. The preliminary report <u>must</u> comply
with all applicable provisions of Business Appraisal Standards,
Standard One, Professional Conduct and Ethics.

6.3   Usage. The preliminary report has use when a client
desires the appraiser's limited opinion.

6.4   Disclosure. The presentation of a preliminary opinion
without disclosing its limitations is unethical.

6.5   Departure. If an appraiser makes a preliminary report
without including a clear statement that it is preliminary, there is
the possibility a user of the report could accord the report and its
limited opinion of value a greater degree of accuracy and reliability than is inherent in the preliminary report process. Therefore,
all preliminary reports <u>shall</u> include a Statement of Departure in
accordance with Standard 1.21(b). The Statement of Departure
<u>shall</u> include a statement that the report is preliminary and the
conclusion subject to change following a proper appraisal and
that said change could be material.

6.6   Oral v. Written. All preliminary reports whether oral
or written are subject to Standard Six.

6.7   Recordkeeping. An appraiser <u>should</u> retain written
records of appraisal reports for a period of at least five (5) years
after preparation or at least two (2) years after final disposition of
any judicial proceeding in which the appraiser gave testimony,
whichever period expires last.

INDEX